Topical Reviews in
Radiotherapy and Oncology

Topical Reviews in

Radiotherapy and Oncology

Volume 1

EDITED BY

Thomas J. Deeley FRCR

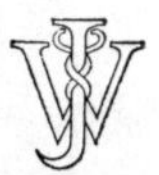

Bristol
John Wright & Sons Ltd,
1980

Published by John Wright & Sons Ltd., 42–44 Triangle West, Bristol BS8 1EX.

British Library Cataloguing in Publication Data

Topical reviews in radiotherapy and oncology.
– (John Wright 'topical reviews' series).
Vol. 1
1. Cancer – Radiotherapy
2. Oncology
I. Deeley, Thomas James II. Radiotherapy and oncology
616.9'94'0642 RC271.R3

ISBN 0 7236 0538 6

Printed by John Wright & Sons Ltd.,
at The Stonebridge Press, Bristol BS4 5NU.

Preface

This is the first volume in a new series designed to look at a few chosen aspects of oncology in depth. The literature available is enormous, conflicting and dispersed through many journals, magazines and books. The busy worker finds some difficulty in his search through the literature in locating pertinent articles, in determining a balance between conflicting points of view, in assessing the value of the articles written, in making a forecast of possible lines of future developments, in obtaining details from the foreign literature and in sorting out a mass of information all having a bearing on the same subject. He is helped by the expert in a particular field, who devotes his whole work to a relatively small piece of the oncology jigsaw. Limiting the work to a few chosen subjects has enabled the authors to write in some detail so that each chapter stands on its own.

It is the duty of the Editor to show why he has selected these subjects from the whole field of oncology. It is, of course, very difficult to select pertinent subjects for the first edition; the desire to make an impression or to pick the spectacular is difficult to repress. Ideally it should include subjects that will have an impact when the book is published; it will, of necessity, cover aspects which are growing in importance or which offer scope for further work or discussion. It must also include topics that have become somewhat neglected and need impetus to provoke new ideas. Some developments that held promise may have proved to be misleading or lack the value that was expected, but this may need to be said and such a review volume would be a suitable forum for the changed ideas to be made known. The literature often contains conflicting evidence and it is difficult for the reader to obtain a clear view; such a review offers an excellent opportunity for an expert to summarize and to make a survey, admittedly biased. Some subjects have suffered from familiarity, there has been little or no progress over a period for many years, these will benefit from an objective appraisal. Finally, the student in oncology should be catered for by providing an up-to-date evaluation of the subject.

Review articles of this kind individually cover one facet of the whole study, each is intended to stand in isolation; it is possible, of course, that there may be some overlap with another review especially when more basic details are discussed. It is difficult to arrange them in logical order, there is no conformity of thought as is provided in a text book, rather it is an anthology. No attempt has been made, therefore, to adopt a uniform style of presentation, each of the invited authors is an eminent expert in his own field and he has tackled the subject in his own way.

Each volume will include a short review of the whole field of radiotherapy and oncology. It will point out advances, highlight problems, report pertinent news which is of interest to oncologists, raise questions, criticise, possibly give opinions and will try to indicate ways in which future progress will, or may, develop.

Immunology has seen tremendous growth in recent years. There is much speculation and little factual knowledge and at present it is not clear what role the subject will eventually play in the whole field of malignant diseases. Immunological investigations may help us to detect tumours, to assess the body's response to the tumour, to follow the response to treatment and to detect the occurrence of metastases. Further, this immunological response may be stimulated to such a degree that it can take part in the annihilation of the tumour. A rapidly developing field, incompletely understood, the chapter by Dr Pritchard throws light on this fascinating subject and helps us to illuminate the path of study.

Some thirty years ago the treatment of cancer of the breast appeared to be relatively simple and straightforward: the breast was removed, if nodes were involved radiation was given to the appropriate areas, if the primary tumour was near to the chest wall this was also treated. Recurrences were treated with appropriate hormones, depending on the age of the patient. Then doubt arose: should the operation be a radical or a simple mastectomy? The importance of the hormone-dependent tumour was appreciated, biochemical tests attempted to rationalize the response, newer, more powerful hormones were developed, and the responsible endocrine glands were ablated. More recently a whole battery of cytotoxic drugs has been shown to influence the growth, and very sophisticated techniques of administration have been developed. The literature abounds with advice on how to treat, but conflicting results are reported from similar controlled clinical trials. The average oncologist is at a loss to know what is best; it seems almost as if some tumours do well and some do badly, whatever the treatment employed. Dr Edelstyn reviewed this very difficult subject and sorted out some of the existing problems. Though fully aware of the prognosis of his illness he laboured to complete the task. The whole of the text was completed before death brought an end to his brilliant career.

Cancer of the oesophagus is showing an increasing incidence in recent years. The method of spread, along the length of the oesophagus among the loose submucosal tissues, often means that the patient with very early symptoms is found to have enlarged nodes in the neck or around the stomach. The results of treatment have not been encouraging; this is a site where careful assessment of the tumour size and extent is essential, correct alignment and coverage by the fields of irradiation mandatory and where the results of treatment reflect the care taken in all aspects of its administration. Professor Pearson, looks at this somewhat neglected lesion and points out what can be done.

A malignant tumour is diagnosed, the best known treatment is given and will either be successful or not. As time goes by the probability of recurrence gets smaller. A recurrence of symptoms does not always indicate a poor response, in accessible tumours if there is doubt direct examination and biopsy will usually provide the answer. With cerebral tumours the clinician is often in the dark for a long time, fresh growth or fibrosis or tumour necrosis or haemorrhage into the growth may all produce similar appearances. Professor Nordman and Dr Rekonen have investigated the possibility of obtaining information by repeated isotope studies, illustrating basic studies which may be applicable to other sites.

In recent years much has been written about radiosensitizers, a generic term which implies that the abnormal cell can be made more sensitive to the effects of radiation upon it. Realization of the effects of radiation on anoxic cells suggested radiation treatment under hyperbaric oxygen and controlled clinical trials have been in progress for many years. An alternative was to use a form of radiation which is less dependent on the cell oxygenation – neutron therapy – again some work has been done over a long period of time but the results are far from conclusive. More recently a new group of drugs has become available which increases cell sensitivity, and new trials are projected. The time is opportune for Dr Dische to look back on what has been achieved, to assess the results of any trials completed and to speculate on possible new trials.

The importance of accuracy in treatment planning, calculation of dose, set-up and day-to-day management, is appreciated by all radiotherapists; checks are made and mistakes are few. Mr Sutherland has assiduously set out to monitor every stage of the progress from initial planning to final calculation of dose given. Risking some resentment in a busy department he has checked every prescription, irrespective of who prescribed it; in this way it was possible to determine where errors could occur and to take practical steps to prevent them. The resultant article is provocative but points out that careful checking and rechecking can improve accuracy. One by-product of the checking system has been the development of a computer which checks and verifies all aspects of treatment.

Chemotherapy has had a chequered career. Given as a single agent it had somewhat limited application, but combinations of drugs made it possible to hit the malignant cells at differing times in the cell cycle and in addition to select drugs which whilst synergistic in their tumour response affect differing normal tissues. Newer, more sophisticated drugs have called for complex systems of administration. They may be used alone or be given as adjuvants to surgery and radiotherapy. There is voluminous literature on the subject – confusing, misleading, contradictory. Claims are sometimes exaggerated, based on very few patients, unsupported by statistical analysis, and frequently estimates of efficacy are assessed mainly on immediate response. Practising clinicians need an authoritative review of the whole subject, such as that given by Professor Carter.

Finally, the editor must explain his own contributions. It may justly be claimed that he has 'hogged' the work but this was not the original intention. Regrettably at a late date one of the invited authors was unable to prepare his work, but no editor undertakes his tasks without he is prepared for such a catastrophe. Written initially as one chapter it lacked cohesion because it covered two extremes, that for the expert and that for the general public; these are two distinct approaches and so they have been separated.

This first volume covers, therefore, a small portion of the field of radiation therapy and the much wider field of oncology; other volumes will cover other subjects. The editor would welcome suggestions about topics which should be covered in future reviews.

It is a pleasure to thank the authors for the chapters they have contributed, their willingness to undertake the task within a specified period of time is commendable. The publishers have been particularly helpful and I am grateful to them for their considerable assistance. In particular I would thank Mr Roy Baker, Managing Editor of John Wright & Sons.

Dr George Edelstyn died during the production of this book after a distinguished career in Oncology. We are grateful to his wife for giving us permission to publish this, his last work, a chapter to which she too contributed.

April 1980 Thomas J. Deeley

Contributors

S. K. Carter MD
Director, Northern California Cancer Program, 1801 Page Mill Road, Building B, Suite 200, Palo Alto, CA 94304

T. J. Deeley FRCR
Director of the South Wales Radiotherapy and Oncology Service, Velindre Hospital, Whitchurch, Cardiff CF4 7XL

S. Dische MD, FRCR
Marie Curie Research Wing for Oncology, Regional Radiotherapy Centre, Mount Vernon Hospital, Northwood, Middlesex HA6 2RN

George A. Edelstyn MD, FRCR, DMRT
Late Consultant Radiotherapist, Northern Ireland Centre for Radiotherapy and Oncology, The Belvoir Park Hospital, Belfast BT8 8JR

E. M. Nordman MD
Department of Radiotherapy, University of Turku 20520, Turku 52, Finland

J. G. Pearson FRCS, FRCSE, FRCR, FRCP(C)
Director of Radiation Oncology, University of Alberta, Cross Cancer Institute, 11560 University Avenue, Edmonton, Alberta, T6G 1Z2, Canada

J. A. V. Pritchard MSc, PhD, MIBiol
Principal Scientific Officer, South Wales Radiotherapy and Oncology Service, Immunology Department, Velindre Hospital, Whitchurch, Cardiff CF4 7XL

A. H. Rekonen MD
Department of Radiotherapy, Central Hospital of Middle Finland, SF. 40620, Jyvaskyla 62, Finland

W. H. Sutherland BSc
Chief Physicist, Velindre Hospital, Whitchurch, Cardiff CF4 7XL

Contributors

Contents

Contents

Thomas J. Deeley

1 A Review of Radiotherapy and Oncology

In this first review it is difficult to know what to cover. Should it be confined to the past two, three, four years or so, or take in a wider overall view of say ten or twenty years? Should it go back to a definite milestone, the development of megavoltage X-ray therapy, the genesis of radiobiology, the use of chemotherapeutic agents, radiosensitizers, and so on? Perhaps it should take the term 'oncology' and cover the years when this has been used to describe all aspects of tumour.

> 'Where shall I begin, please your Majesty?' he asked.
> 'Begin at the beginning' the King said, gravely, 'and go on till you come to the end: then stop.'
> *Alice in Wonderland.* Lewis Carroll (Charles Lutwidge Dodgson 1832–1898).

Regrettably it is not possible to start at the beginning, but there is a great need for such an historical account of radiotherapy. Already it is difficult to obtain details of past techniques: old machines have been replaced by more sophisticated and complex apparatus, articles mislaid or forgotten, photographs destroyed, all in the progress of the specialty. The generation of early workers is rapidly being decimated, but while some remain their experience and reminiscences should be recorded. Such a project should be multi-author work and it is to be hoped that someone will undertake the mammoth task of collating the history of our specialty.

Whatever this present review covers it must be limited to certain aspects of the whole specialty, highlighting some parts and omitting others. It is, of necessity, biased.

Definition of Oncology

The universal acceptance of a definite term for the study of tumours brought about some problems. If there was a new study, with new exponents, was this to become a new medical specialty with a career structure? The term means no more than a study, it is not a medical specialty but a concept. An examination of the subjects involved in the study indicates the catholic view it takes; epidemiology, aetiology, symptomatology, cancer detection, diagnosis, treatment, surgery, radiotherapy, chemotherapy, immunology, aftercare and follow-up, rehabilitation, terminal care, cancer information and public education—and that list is not comprehensive. The disciplines involved include doctors, scientists, biologists, radiobiologists, biochemists, physicists, statisticians, radiographers, mould room technicians, nurses, social workers, rehabilitationists, and so on. Many branches involving many disciplines, it must be concluded, therefore, that it is impossible for any one man to cover the whole or for there to be such a medical specialty.

The term can be applied in conjunction with a medical specialty indicating that the holder has a particular interest in the study of tumours within that specialty, thus surgical oncologist, paediatric oncologist, pathological oncologist, radiation oncologist, and so on. What the concept does imply is that all work together with no single individual, medical specialty or discipline claiming to be the only one in the field. Oncology is a good term, it acknowledges that individual specialties are merely a part of a large 'jigsaw puzzle' making up a field of study which includes all those concerned with tumours.

Basic Information

Considerable advances have been made in recent years through certain biological investigations. The work of the radiobiologist is still mainly concerned with the response of the cell or tissue, either malignant or normal, to irradiation. Not only has basic knowledge been increased but new clinical techniques proposed and tested. An important line of research enquires into methods of improving the radiosensitivity of the tumour cell, a first study which has already resulted in some clinical improvements and offers more for the future.

Immunology has explained many of the confusing aspects of tumour growth, host response and normal tissue reaction. The work is so absorbing and logical that there is a danger of falling into the trap that all is known, or of adapting the facts or observed responses to fit pet theories. Much of the knowledge is speculative, unsupported by test, and at a preliminary stage only and much work remains to be done. Work to date is concerned with cancer detection, assay of tumour response and the prospects of immunotherapy, all still very much at an experimental stage.

Early cancer detection, before clinical signs and symptoms develop, has proposed new approaches to clinical management. Instead of a presenting patient being investigated over a period of weeks, each test adding to the probability that he has a malignant lesion until finally the diagnosis is confirmed, a single test may indicate that a cancer is present or even determine where the cancer is. If this test is negative there is no problem about delay in making a definite diagnosis and there is no possibility of spread of cancer cells if the lesion is not malignant.

In recent years the value of tumour markers, which show variations during the natural life cycle of the tumour during growth, treatment and at follow-up after therapy, has been recognized. Whilst still at an early stage of development it is to be expected that they will enable the clinician to monitor tumour changes during treatment and at follow-up. There are several excellent reviews and publications, all neatly summarized in the proceedings of a recent symposium [14].

Prevention

Some tumours are preventable, the prime example being lung cancer caused by smoking; but there are others also. Cancer of the cervix is a sexually transmitted disease and changes in sexual habits have resulted in younger patients presenting with growths. Such knowledge is available for only a few malignancies and considerable epidemiological and aetiological research remains to be done. To date there has been insufficient collaboration between the clinician and the epidemiologist. Furthermore, improvements need to be made in the dissemination of epidemiological knowledge to the clinician and to the general public.

Detection and Diagnosis

It seems quite logical to suggest that many tumours are unifocal in origin and that dissemination occurs from this one focus. It would therefore be reasonable to suggest that the tumour can be permanently controlled, if it is sensitive to radiation and if it remains at the primary site. This theory is confirmed in such an unpromising lesion as oat cell carcinoma of the bronchus where 6 per cent 3-year survival rates have been reported.

Delay in diagnosis increases the probability of dissemination but this probably depends to a large extent on the blood and lymphatic supply to the organ concerned; for example, both are prolific in the lung hence a high frequency of metastases. It is essential that diagnosis is made at the earliest possible time and treatment started immediately. Thus, any test which reduces this time is important and research should aim at establishing such tests. A growth found on routine clinical examination may preceed patient awareness, examination of secretions may demonstrate malignant cells shed from an area of metaplasia or intra-epidermal growth long before it has penetrated to the deeper tissues served by blood vessels and lymphatics, routine chest radiographs may reveal asymptomatic masses, but, most exciting of all, recent work suggests that an immunological test carried out on the patient's blood may indicate tumour formation many years before other tests or examinations. There can be little doubt about the need for 'well person clinics', and ways must be found of financing them and of inducing fit people to attend.

Delineation of Tumour

One of the intrinsic problems of treatment is that of defining the extent of the local tumour. Clinical examination, endoscopic viewing, radiological techniques and surgical operation are employed to assist the clinician whose knowledge of tumour spread, infiltration into normal tissues and the probabilities of adjacent lymph node metastases, enable him to apply a radiation field of sufficient size to cover the tumour and any possible local spread. But 'geographical misses' still account for a proportion of failures and increased impetus needs to be given to studying improved methods of tumour demarcation using all available modes, diagnostic radiology, isotope studies, thermography, ultrasonics and computerized tomography.

Improvement of Treatment Results

Every clinical oncologist searches for ways of improving the results of treatment in his patients. There seems little doubt that there are many differing types of malignancies and that treatment will involve many modes. Surgery, the earliest weapon in the battle, has reached its peak over the years, rationalization may provide some improvements with emphasis being laid on selection of suitable patients for this attack. Radiotherapy, initially lagging behind because of inadequate methods of measurement and insufficient voltage for penetration to deep seated tumours, is now becoming rationalized. Instead of an infinite number of variables there is a distinct possibility of optimization of radiation techniques which, together with improvements in the selection of suitable cases for the treatment will enable the clinician to make a determined attack on some lesions.

The therapist is beginning to take a rational view of the whole problem and to realize that some hoped for improvements are impossible. Optimism alone is responsible for such illogical acts as seeking to cure more than a handful of lung cancers by local irradiation, a disease where some ninety-two per cent of tumours have already metastasized when the patient presents. The therapist has been encouraged by radiobiological research to expect improvements with hyperbaric oxygen, neutron therapy and radio-sensitizers. The former has produced limited improvements but many workers remain unconvinced about the value of neutron therapy and recently a new impetus has been given to drug sensitizers.

Recent work on the effects of heat on malignant cells raises two possibilities; one of improvements in the local effects of radiation or cytotoxic drugs, the other, perhaps less encouraging, of the effects on micrometastases by raising the whole body temperature.

Wide field irradiation has shown some encouraging results but much work needs to be done to establish its place. Chemotherapy, at first encouraging, went through a slack period to be restimulated by the advent of multiple drug techniques and later by a whole range of new agents, hopefully produced by expectant drug firms. Great advances have been made in the treatment of certain less common tumours, but there has been little impact so far on the solid tumours. Chemotherapy, adjuvant to local treatment by surgery or radiotherapy, offers distinct possibilities for dealing with occult metastases. Immunotherapy is still in the early stage of investigation.

Selection of Patients

There can be little doubt that the clinician needs some method of selecting his patients for radical therapy. Deterioration in a patient's general condition during treatment and the appearance of metastatic deposits a few days after starting indicate poor selection; that patient should not have been subjected to active measures at that time and such failure does little to establish the role of this method of treatment or to induce earlier referral.

One fruitful line of research is the detection of occult metastases using radioactive isotopes. Vigorous local treatment is given if the disease is localized. Evidence of dissemination demands a different approach involving either chemotherapeutic agents, immunotherapy or whole body irradiation.

Radiotherapy Equipment

It is important that the design of radiotherapy apparatus keeps pace with other developments in the specialty, there is no room for sitting back and hoping that a new machine design will last for many years to come. Regrettably, this hope is fostered by the present economic situation; each major machine must serve its full expectation of life, many exceed this, and there are insufficient funds to scrap a serviceable machine merely because it has been superseded by a more efficient up-to-date one. Improvements are essential and we have seen many examples over the past few years. New apparatus has been expertly surveyed in two articles, linear accelerators by Sutherland [17] and other equipment by Aird and Evans [1]. Both articles give references for further reading, and a reminder of the necessity to develop new machines and to review existing ones. Sutherland points out that there has been a swing from cobalt machines to linear accelerators, he reviews the machines available on the market, giving very useful criticisms and including current prices. Dual purpose machines giving electrons and X-rays raise problems of possible hazards and special safeguards are suggested. Aird and Evans look into other therapy apparatus, low and medium energy X-ray machines, cobalt machines and a brief account of linear accelerators. Their article also includes simulators, CT scanners, computer treatment planning, automation and afterloading techniques. For the future neutrons and *pi*-mesons need careful assessment.

The Radiotherapy Apparatus Safety Measures Panel (RASMP) has been active in recent years in suggesting measures to be incorporated in the design of new machines. These recommendations also advise a careful look at the machines installed in departments, of methods of bringing them up to current standards and suggest conditions indicating that they should be replaced [9].

Controlled Clinical Trials

In the late 1940s the present author thought that he was helping, in a small way, to pioneer a new field comparing the results of treatment in similarly composed groups of patients. For many years there were only sporadic articles suggesting the use of controlled clinical trials and the application of medical statistics to cancer studies. At first there was criticism, almost scorn: 'you can prove anything by statistics', to be followed by growing enthusiasm, until the present period of rationalization where only the very brave or naive would consider presenting an article for publication without statistical support. Controlled clinical trials are an essential feature of the management of malignant diseases and organized work of such bodies as the Medical Research Council in the UK and similar bodies overseas has resulted in large trials on a scale which was never dreamed of some twenty to thirty years ago. Small trials demand dramatic differences in results, large co-operative trials can detect smaller variations but demand very careful control, agreement by participators and the development of a relatively simple protocol which can be accepted and carried out by busy clinicians.

Presentation of Results

The presentation of the results of treatment has caused concern for some years. Death, like virginity, is absolute and forms a very definite end-point. Morbidity is not so clearly defined; to do so requires a statement of criteria and acceptance by all participating workers and usually such definitions apply only to a particular clinical trial. There have been several attempts to define an assessment which is universally accepted, notably by Karnofsky and Burcheral [12] and more recently by Priestman and Baum [15].

In recent years workers have been more concerned with tumour response and many oncologists are convinced that this is related to cure, but we all have seen tumours respond whilst the patient dies. In cytotoxic therapy an assay of response has been the 50 per cent regression. If pure tumour doubling alone is considered and other factors such as necrosis, effects on blood vessels, repopulation and all the factors which affect response discarded, the 50 per cent regression effectively means that the tumour has been put back one doubling time in its life-cycle. If the other factors given above are included it may be a little more than one doubling. But, by the time a tumour presents it has already undergone many doublings and cure is only effected if this is taken right back to zero, i.e. no tumour. Radiotherapy attempts to do this, the last few stages probably being brought about by fibrosis and strangulation of the remaining cells. Fifty per cent regression gives no more than an indication that the tumour shows some sensitivity to the therapy used and as such it is a pretty inadequate index on which to assess tumour response.

Economies

In recent years it has been necessary to take a look at the cost of treating a cancer patient. New complex machinery, new drugs, increasingly sophisticated combined methods of treatment have meant a greater burden on an already overloaded health service. The average clinician resents the need to study the cost effectiveness of his patient management, he takes the view that he will advise the best and that it is not his responsibility to provide the finance nor to limit his patient care to what can be afforded. Regrettably it is only in Utopia that such reasoning can be countenanced. In practice, at least at the present time, we must attempt to give the best to as many as possible within the financial limits laid down.

Calman [5] introducing a series of articles entitled 'Can we afford to treat cancer?' pointed out the paucity of information that was available on which to assess the cost of cancer detection and treatment. Various authors considered specialized techniques. In the same journal Bleehan [4], discussing the cost of radiotherapy, suggests that it is unlikely that many economies can be made in this specialty without detriment to the patient. Soukop [16] reviews chemotherapy; whilst noting the high cost of cytotoxic drugs, he points out that many of the patients do not need expensive in-patient care. McKillop [13] looks at isotope scanning of breast cancer and provides a comparative price list of studies, the most useful bone scan being the most expensive. Back further in the history of the disease Husain [11] discusses screening programmes and covers the five main sites: cervix, bladder, breast, lung and stomach, while George [10] adds further information on breast cancer screening. Whitehouse [19] estimates the average cost of treating a patient with acute myelogenous leukaemia and points out that the drug bill is small when compared with the cost of in-patient care. This series is an interesting brief introduction to the economics of cancer therapy and serves to make the clinician critical of expensive treatments which are of doubtful clinical value. Berry [3] takes it further concluding the 'maximum cost-effectiveness is most likely to be achieved in the use of cytotoxic drugs if they are prescribed largely by staff in oncological centres (and by well-trained specialists) where properly designed prospective clinical studies will be carried out and the experience gained will be pooled most efficiently.' He condemns the widespread and casual use of cytotoxic drugs by doctors with a limited interest as being costly and potentially dangerous. Bagshawe [2] pointed out the savings that could be made by routine screening for hydatidiform moles. The early detection of malignancies, for example, carcinoma of the cervix by cervical smears, could mean that less intensive methods of treatment may be used; there is an added advantage, also, that survival rates are likely to be improved. Thus, on economic grounds, also, the emphasis is pushed away from treatment towards early diagnosis, detection and prevention.

Specialty of Radiotherapy and Oncology

The standing of radiology in the UK was recognized when Her Majesty the Queen, at a meeting of the Privy Council, approved the Petition seeking Collegiate status. Permission had already been received to use the title 'Royal' and so the Royal College of Radiologists came into being in 1974.

The Charter recognized the establishment of the Faculty Board of Radiotherapy and Oncology, which would promote the views and interests of those members and fellows concerned with the treatment of disease, particularly malignant diseases. Consultants in radiotherapy and oncology have a responsibility in consultation with the family doctor and other medical and paramedical colleagues for the clinical care of patients with malignant diseases using radiation, cytotoxic chemotherapy, hormone therapy and other therapeutic measures and for the care of the patient after treatment, during rehabilitation and in the terminal stages of the disease.

Recruitment into the Specialty

A survey was carried out to determine the factors thought to influence recruitment into the specialty and the two most important factors were undergraduate training and the academic status of the specialty [6]. Many undergraduates are not introduced sufficiently to radiotherapy during their training and consequently have little, if any, idea of its potential and little chance of subsequently becoming interested in it. In some places the specialty enjoys the reputation of being somewhat second-rate and has little support from medical schools, as is evidenced by the small number of academic units in the UK. Other factors were considered to play only a subsidiary part in the problems of recruitment, in decreasing order of importance there were, heavy service commitments, too much physics, little medical interest to attract keen students, the feeling that the specialty is depressing, few facilities for private practice, long periods of training and a curriculum which is too all-embracing.

It is disappointing to see that there has been little or no improvement in the academic status in recent years. It is imperative that sufficient postgraduates of the right calibre are attracted to raise the standard of the work and to replace the deficiencies which will occur when the large number of elderly radiotherapists retire within the next ten years or so.

The Public and Cancer

The word 'cancer' has been a taboo term for many years; not openly mentioned in public conversation it is often whispered only at the demise of the sufferer. There is every need to inform the public about this disease, to examine what accounts for their current attitudes to the subject, to determine what information needs to be given and the methods to be adopted. Mystery, shame, despair, must be replaced by a rational approach which presents the public with open discussion, based on easily simulated facts. An attempt has recently been made [7] and it is hoped those more erudite will continue their effort so that cancer becomes accepted as any other disease which can be cured in a proportion of patients, diagnosed earlier and even prevented.

The clinical oncologist has a responsibility to study all aspects of the subject from prevention, detection, diagnosis, treatment, aftercare, rehabilitation, to terminal care. It is encouraging to see that all over the world they are accepting responsibility for terminal care; at one time therapists preferred not to mention it and affected disinterestedness; now a new approach has enabled several hospices to be established where people may die in peace, with dignity and usually free from pain and suffering.

The radiotherapist and oncologist with his unique knowledge of malignant diseases has an obvious duty to inform the public of the facts about this disease in an attempt to improve the existing attitudes.

Directories of Research

The research worker is plagued with the problem of communication. Should he announce his research interests? Will others take up his ideas, rush manpower into the project and publish before him, or should he keep his work to himself until the profession are presented with the final *fait accompli* beautifully presented in a learned article? In the past few years the researcher has been encouraged to share his knowledge and enthusiasm and to provide details of his work to others in the same field. Thus 'there is obviously a great need for the exchange of information between laboratories working on cancer research' [20] and 'it is hoped that the directory will open up lines of communication between cancer related establishments' UICC [18], and again 'a single volume listing most of the cancer information sources around the world' [8] – three of the leading directories.

The Future

It is possible to hazard a mere guess only on the lines of future developments. Of prime importance is the need for early diagnosis so that the therapist is presented with an early confined growth instead of the large number of 'too late' advanced malignancies that he now sees. This demands improvements in early diagnosis and detection and an increase in public education. But, if possible it is better to prevent, thus more effort needs to be expended on aetiological investigations and also determination of the individual susceptibility to cancer – again there is a need for public education.

For localized disease the first priority would appear to be improved selection of patients, followed by an optimization of existing treatment modalities. Disseminated disease constitutes the biggest obstacle to successful treatment and calls for improvements in systemic drug administration or stimulation of host response. An evaluation of the possible permutations of treatment techniques is time consuming and will take several years to achieve by controlled clinical trials.

The co-operation of many different disciplines has already resulted in advances being made. The whole concept of oncology demands co-operation and a knowledge of the work of others, who may be closely allied but may at first appear unrelated. The vast output of relevant literature imposes a considerable burden on the oncologist, first to read what is pertinent but also to find out where it is. It is hoped that reviews of this kind will help to disseminate such knowledge.

Finally, the possibility of future success depends on the calibre of the workers that can be recruited into the specialty. In the past radiotherapy has not enjoyed the popularity status of other medical specialties and every attempt must be made to remedy this. The problems of cancer are immense, the rewards of seeing successful treatment and control leaves little to be desired.

REFERENCES

1. Aird E. G. A. and Evans R. G. B. (1978) Modern radiotherapy equipment. *Br. J. Clin. Equipment* **3,** 260–270.
2. Bagshawe K. D. (1977) Choriocarcinoma. Walker Prize Lecture. Royal College of Surgeons Report. *Cancer Topics* **1,** No. 7, 5.
3. Berry R. J. (1978) Dare we count the cost of cancer chemotherapy? *Lancet* **2,** 516–618.
4. Bleehen N. M. (1977) The cost of radiotherapy. *Cancer Topics* **1,** No. 7, 4.
5. Calman K. C. (1977) Can we afford to treat cancer. *Cancer Topics* **1,** No. 7, 1–2.
6. Deeley T. J., Baker J. and Brindle J. (1976) Recruitment in radiotherapy. *Med. Ed.* **10,** 313–314.
7. Deeley T. J. (1979) *Attitudes to Cancer,* London, SPCK.
8. DHEW United States (1977) *Directory of Cancer Research Information Resources.*
9. DHSS (1975) *Recommendations of the Radiotherapy Apparatus Safety Measures Panel.* London, HMSO.
10. George W. D. (1977) Breast cancer screening. *Cancer Topics.* **1,** No. 8, 8.
11. Husain O. A. N. (1977) The cost of screening programmes. *Cancer Topics.* **1,** No. 8, 4–5.
12. Karnofsky D. A. and Burcheral J. H. (1948) In: McCleod M. (ed.), *Evaluation of Chemotherapeutic Agents.* New York, Columbia University Press.
13. McKillop J. H. (1977) Isotope scanning of breast cancer patients. *Cancer Topics.* **1,** No. 8, 1–5.
14. Neville M. (1978) In: Griffiths K., Neville M. and Pierepoint C. G. (ed.), *Tumour Markers.* Cardiff, Alpha Omega Publishing Co. 6th Tenovus Workshop.
15. Priestman T. and Baum M. (1976) Evaluation of quality of life in patients receiving treatment. *Lancet* **1,** 899–901.
16. Soukop M. (1977) The cost of chemotherapy. *Cancer Topics.* **1,** No. 7, 4–5.
17. Sutherland W. H. (1978) Standard equipment–the linear accelerator. *Br. J. Clin. Equipment* **3,** 197–209.
18. UICC (1976) *International Directory of Specialised Cancer Research and Treatment Establishments.*
19. Whitehouse J. M. A. (1977) Cost of A.M.L. therapy. *Cancer Topics* **1,** 8–9.
20. WHO (1977) *Directory of Laboratories Working on the Biology and Biochemistry of Tumour Cells in Asia and Europe.*

J. A. V. Pritchard

2 Immunological Aspects of Malignant Disease

The subject of tumour immunology over the last decade has mushroomed to such an extent that the newcomer or casual reader to the subject can be excused initial confusion. A cursory glance at the literature will also show that this branch of science has developed an extensive vocabulary consisting of numerous, difficult to decipher abbreviations. Although the existence of tumour immunity has been extensively documented and established for animal systems the same cannot be said for man where dependence on clinical features of malignancy has suggested that host defence mechanisms must play a part in the course of the disease. This can be illustrated by the documented cases of spontaneous regression of disease and the direct observation that components of the immune system such as lymphocytes, macrophages and plasma cells can be found in close association with tumour masses [6, 7, 8, 36, 48, 52]. Cell mediated immune reactions in man, where cells of the immune system can be shown to have a direct effect in immunological responses to tumour material have been extensively documented [3, 26, 87]. The establishment of laboratory tests for demonstrating cell mediated response and humoral immunity in cancer resulted from investigations concerned with transplantation immunology where cell mediated processes are primarily responsible for tumour rejection. Tumour resistance can also be transferred between compatible animals by lymphoid cells [56 or 57]. Ethical considerations make such experiments in man difficult to undertake although an early series of experiments conducted in 1960 using viable tumour cells innoculated subcutaneously showed that a response was dependent upon cell numbers used and numbers in excess of 10^8 tumour cells were required to produce a skin nodule [10, 92]. Delayed hypersensitivity reactions in man to suitably treated tumour extracts also support the existence of host immunological response although the reactions are generally non-specific and difficult to evaluate because of the lack of suitable controls [37, or 38, 60, 61]. The majority of investigations, designed to illustrate cell mediated response in neoplastic disease have been directed towards animal systems where tumours have been shown to express strong transplantation antigens of chemical or viral origin [3 or 4, 56 or 57].

It has long been considered that the immune system in neoplastic disease has the ability to recognize that the disease is present but that some defect within the system allows the tumour to escape elimination. A survey of the literature reveals a considerable number of laboratory tests which have claimed to monitor the immune response in cancer, and that adoption of these tests can provide meaningful information pertinent to the clinical status of the patient. It is not the intention of this chapter to review all these tests but to concentrate on two which have been and still are controversial, and at the same time pointing out some of the pitfalls likely to be encountered with the immunological detection of malignant disease.

Immunodiagnosis

The term 'immunodiagnosis' is one that has been extensively cited in the literature to describe *in vitro* tests, having some immunological basis, designed to establish the presence of a host immunological response in relation to possible tumour burden and clinical status of the patient, and perhaps provide some index as to the state of the disease. This terminology is open to criticism in that laboratory tests in their own right cannot diagnose but only measure a reaction between components which may or may not be meaningful in the clinical diagnosis of the disease or state of advancement of the disease; the term 'immunodetection' is more desirable.

Table 2.1. Possible Use of Immunological Tests for the Detection of Cancer

Screening – detection of disease
As an aid to clinical diagnosis
Tumour localization – by specific cell mediated reaction to tumour extract or demonstration of tumour markers
Assessment of prognosis
Monitoring the course and extent of disease

Table 2.2. Characteristics of an Immunological Cancer Test

Must effectively and reproducibly differentiate between benign and malignant disease of the same site
False positive rate should be low – specificity of response
False negative rate must be low – sensitivity of response
Anatomical site specificity for tumour location

In general terms, the immunodetection of malignant disease can have several important clinical applications. Firstly as a general screening technique, either for whole populations or more realistically for those at high risk, such as heavy smokers. Secondly, for the site localization of tumour, the monitoring of therapy, and the pre-clinical detection of metastases with some prognostic index (Table 2.1).

Any test aimed at the detection of malignant disease, whether based on immunological principles or not, must also satisfy certain criteria, as shown in Table 2.2. For any system to satisfy all these conditions is extremely difficult. Whereas it is more convenient to have a test which does not give a high rate of false positive results, problems can arise if a proposed test has high sensitivity, since the screening of a normal or ill population, not known to have malignant disease, should statistically give rise to false positive results at the time of the test. This does not mean that the test results may be wrong [98]. However, a high rate of false negative results in proven cases of the disease is not acceptable. It is also extremely important to design the correct clinical trial for the test in question. There is no value in attempting a clinical assessment of a test claimed to have a potential for cancer detection unless the test can be reproducibly operated in the laboratory and all the factors likely to influence the result are thoroughly understood. It is also essential to incorporate some control system to check that during the operation of a trial the technique has not failed due to some unknown factor. The population under study also needs to be chosen carefully with adequate documentation and possible follow-up facilities, so that any false positive results can be evaluated in case a 'lead time' may result from the investigation.

Although there is a need for a simple cancer detection test that is both sensitive and specific and can be readily applied to a large number of samples, the indications are that at present the available immunological techniques are more suitably directed towards the identification of the tumour and anatomical site location once some clinical symptoms occur, such as a lump in the breast. In this instance a simple test to distinguish between benign or malignant would be extremely useful, without immediately resorting to biopsy. From an operational point of view the adoption of an immunodetection technique is greatly facilitated by the examination of samples of serum or plasma for some immunologically related component since these can be readily acquired, stored and transported. The use of cell mediated techniques, requiring the interaction of a viable white cell population with a tumour component, imposes severe operational limitations as the test invariably has to be done on the day the sample is taken, and more often than not, in close proximity to the laboratory operating the test. This limitation should not, however, exclude a test from acceptance, providing that it is both specific and sensitive in response.

During the growth of a tumour there is the probability that a finite size is reached after which metastases may occur, and that by the time a tumour is sufficiently large enough for a test to give a meaningful result, the tumour will have metastasized with associated patient symptoms [5]. The proportion of patients developing metastatic disease from primary breast lesions has been shown to be closely related to the initial tumour size [33]. The incidence of distant metastases increased with tumour size up to a maximum of 6 cm. In this series the mean time from first treatment to the demonstration of metastases was 10·2 years for patients with tumours of 1 cm or less. This was significantly longer than for all other groups, and suggested that the early detection and diagnosis of primary cancers is of prime importance in obtaining high survival rates and minimizing the risk of death from breast cancer. In another analysis it was suggested that patients with early treated breast cancer (Stage 1) only show a 10 per cent 'cure' rate when analyzed on a 25-year basis rather than the conventional 5-year period [59]. It has also been argued that the early detection of cancer does not greatly influence eventual patient survival figures for a particular site under investigation, but merely gives the patient more years of disease [88]. Opinions vary widely as to the benefit of the early detection of cancer, and are as controversial as the many varied treatment regimens for the disease itself.

A consensus of opinion, however, would suggest that the early detection of malignant disease can influence the eventual survival of the patient, where the screening by cytological techniques for cervical cancer and fibreoptic gastroscope examination for early gastric cancer are two prime examples [13]. Cost effectiveness has also been implicated and it has been suggested that using conventional radioimmunoassay techniques to mass screen once a year, for cancer of the lung, gastrointestinal tract and breast, in some fifteen million people would require an outlay of some £45 million plus recurring additional costs [59]. Should such screening be possible it is a further challenge to recruit and maintain the most vulnerable members of the population into the programme, since it is the least vulnerable that use any such facility [58].

In the context of cancer detection two controversial *in vitro* tests have been proposed within the last eight years. Initially the results appeared to fulfil the criteria considered essential for their role as cancer screening tests, and by examining these two systems in more detail, many of the aspects previously mentioned can be expanded in the light of experimental data, to illustrate these points.

THE MACROPHAGE ELECTROPHORETIC MOBILITY (MEM) TEST

This test procedure was first described as the 'lymphocyte sensitization: an *in vitro* test for cancer' by Field and Caspary in 1970 [40], and became universally known as the Macrophage Electrophoretic Mobility (MEM) test [78]. This title originated from the procedure and describes the essential features of the test, that is, the measurement of a change in the electrophoretic mobility of guinea pig macrophages by a soluble product of a lymphocyte antigen interaction. The technique of cell electrophoresis for the measurement of cellular changes is not new. The theoretical foundations were formulated as early as 1879 by Helmholtz [55], but not until 1967 was there documented evidence that the technique had a use in immunological methodology, where the interaction of bacterial antigen with lymph node cells was demonstrated by a change in their electrophoretic mobility [97]. Hypersensitivity reactions in the guinea pig by measurement of changes in the electrophoretic mobility of antigen-treated peritoneal exudate cells was also demonstrated [31]. Adopting this technique Field and Caspary initially set out to investigate lymphocyte sensitization in neurological disease, and were able to establish that the cell electrophoresis technique could demonstrate lymphocyte sensitization in neurological disease. It was an extension of this investigation involving neuropathy in malignant disease that showed lymphocyte sensitization could be demonstrated in all cancer patients, irrespective of tumour type or anatomical origin. The results suggested some common antigenic response for all human cancers and immediately created controversy.

The basic technique of the MEM test is shown in *Fig. 2.1,* and is not unlike that of the established Macrophage Migration Inhibition (MMI) test

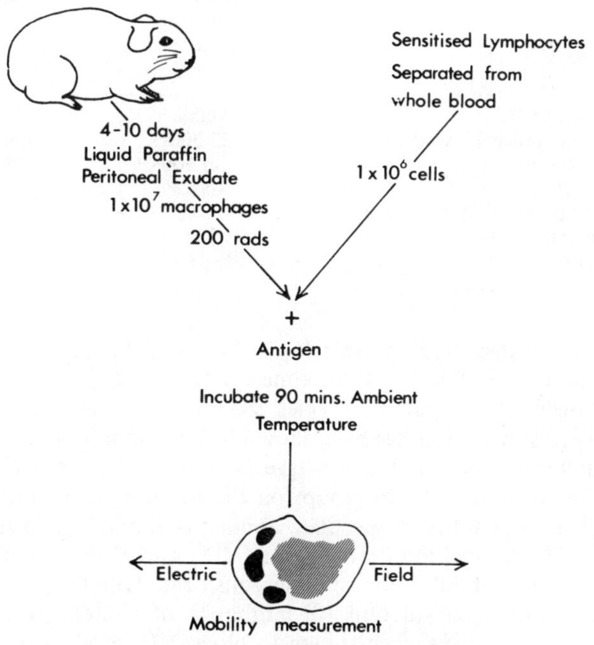

Fig. 2.1. Principal features of the MEM Test.

[9, 28] except that incubation times of test lymphocytes and antigen are considerably shorter than the 18–48 hours normally quoted for incubations in the MMI technique. The two test techniques differ in respect of the method of assaying macrophage function in response to a soluble product of the lymphocyte–antigen interaction. Whereas in the MMI test response is evaluated by the inhibition of macrophage migration from a small capillary tube, response in the MEM test is directly a measure of altered charge characteristics of individual macrophage cells by electrophoretic

mobility determinations. Both the soluble components of the lymphocyte–antigen interaction have been partially chemically defined (Table 2.3). In an attempt to establish the molecular weight of the soluble mediators, Sephadex chromatography has been used to separate the fractions which contain biological activity. Encephalitogenic factor (EF) derived macrophage slowing factor (MSF), the soluble mediator of macrophage slowing in the MEM test has been shown to have two active fractions of approximate molecular weight 20 000 and 8000, whereas two separate laboratories

Table 2.3. Comparison of MIF and MSF Characteristics

	Macrophage inhibitory factor (MIF)	*Macrophage slowing factor (MSF)*
Temperature 56 °C	stable	stable
Approximate molecular weight	23 000	8000 – 23 000
Dilution activity	1 in 100	1 in 10 000
Storage – 10 °C	stable	stable
Blocking of production by protein synthesis inhibitors	Yes	No
Time for production	18 – 48 hr	60 – 90 min

suggest that cancer basic protein (CaBP) derived slowing factor exhibited activity in a single fraction approximately to 20 000 [75, 79, 80]. Macrophage slowing factor is not species specific. MSF derived from human lymphocyte stimulation has been shown to interact in mouse macrophages and lymphoma cells and this suggests a simple non-specific chemical interaction with the charge groups on the surfaces of the indicator cells. Although it is possible to speculate about the similarities in the mode of action of Migration Inhibition Factor (MIF) and MSF on indicator cells, the production of MSF by suitable sensitized lymphocytes, cannot be blocked by the introduction of inhibitors of protein synthesis [80]. Similar inhibitors have been shown to block MIF production [27]. MSF has also been shown to retain activity when diluted to a greater extent than MIF. This may not necessarily suggest that there is more MSF produced than MIF for a particular lymphocyte–antigen interaction but that in the MEM assay, the macrophage cells are very sensitive and have an in-built biological amplification capability manifest by a change in their cell surface charge characteristics, which attains a maximum level and cannot be increased by addition of excess MSF.

Experimental Technique

An early problem that affected the operation of the MEM test was one associated with the contamination of the peritoneal macrophages by guinea pig lymphocytes. The resultant mixed lymphocyte reaction between guinea pig lymphocytes and human test lymphocytes was overcome by irradiating the peritoneal exudate with 100 rad of gamma radiation [4]. The technique can be simply described as follows.

Test lymphocytes are incubated with appropriate antigen, normally encephalitogenic factor (EF) and irradiated guinea pig macrophages at ambient temperature for 90 minutes. After this period the sample is introduced into suitable equipment capable of measuring the electrophoretic mobility of selected macrophage cells. The results are expressed as a percentage reduction in mobility using the formula

$$[(t_a - t_c)/t_c] \times 100$$

where t_c is the time taken for selected macrophages in the absence of antigen to transit a calibrated distance in the presence of an electric field and t_a the time for similar cells in the test sample in the presence of antigen.

Although the description of the essential techniques does not suggest difficulties these can easily, and have in many laboratories, caused considerable problems. Several areas where difficulties in the operation of the MEM test can be identified are as follows.

Lymphocytes

The response of the MEM test does not increase with increased numbers of test lymphocytes. The effect reaches a plateau with 5×10^5 cells per 3 ml test sample [11, 76] as shown by *Fig. 2.2.* The method of separation

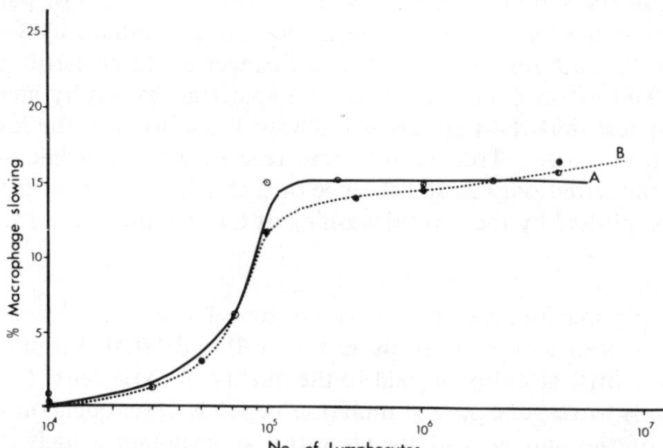

Fig. 2.2. Dependence of MEM Test response on lymphocyte number (semi-log plot). Lymphocytes incubated as indicated with 33 μg/ml EF and 10^7 irradiated guinea pig macrophages in 3 ml tissue culture medium for 90 min. Solid line Carnegie et al. [11], dotted line Pritchard [76]. (Reproduced by courtesy of Alpha Omega.)

from whole blood does not appear to markedly affect the result. Defibrinated blood followed by a carbonyl-iron/methyl cellulose sedimentation technique was favoured by the original test described by Field and Caspary [4]. Several subsequent investigations have used the Ficoll/Triosil density gradient technique with equal effect. Cells with the maximum activity were found to be collected from a gradient where the density was between 1·070 g/ml and 1·080 g/ml [66]. This separation contained small lymphocytes whose immunological functions have been established in transformation experiments, mixed lymphocyte reactions, graft versus host responses and stimulation by antigen studies. Although the use of density gradients for the separation of white blood cells from whole blood is common laboratory practice, it is often the case that the lack of adherence to established and documented methodology may result in the inability to successfully reproduce a published technique. The use of density gradients for the separation of white cells from whole blood is often badly controlled with little attention being paid to maintenance of centrifuge and solution temperatures. Density gradients are susceptible, by definition, to temperature and lack of control over these important parameters can often result in the incorrect cells being separated (*see* SCM technique). Serum in many immunological tests can be shown to have an inhibitory effect. Lymphocyte suspensions used in the MEM assay must be well washed to ensure removal of a factor known to depress lymphocyte response to antigen [41, 42, 43].

The blocking or depressive effect of serum and dilutions of serum on the lymphocyte–antigen reaction in the MEM test was first observed in an investigation associated with multiple sclerosis, but also found to be present in the serum of cancer patients [44]. The serum of patients with advanced cancer had considerably higher titres of inhibitory factor and a weak test result for cases of advanced cancer could be attributed to this effect. This effect could be overcome to a certain extent by increasing the cells per test, but the response was always found to be at the lower end of the 'cancer range'. True lymphocyte reactivity to antigenic stimulation can be measured only in the absence of such inhibitory factors, which can be accomplished by the careful washing of test cell preparations.

Macrophages

Guinea pig macrophages raised by peritoneal injection of liquid paraffin B.P. have been used extensively in the MMI and MEM techniques and all too often little attention is paid to the quality of these cells. The ability of these cells to respond to a stimulation depends a great deal on the general health of the animal, and the necessity to maintain a high standard of animal husbandry has been persistently suggested [47]. There is no need to resort to specific pathogen free (SPF) conditions, but animals should originate from a closed colony maintained under clean conditions. Guinea pigs are susceptible to many sub-clinical infections and these can be avoided by the addition of vitamin C to the drinking water, or by daily supplement of fresh washed vegetables. Since the 'positivity' of the MEM test is considerably dependent upon the effect of slowing factor on the macrophage cells it is essential that these cells are in good physiological and immunological condition. Macrophages from an infected animal may already be incapable of response to slowing factor if the animal has responded immunologically to any infection. Macrophage cells to be used in the MEM test should also be checked for any unpredicted response to the antigen in use. A further check can be made with a standard preparation of slowing factor before embarking on any large series of tests. The reliance on guinea pig macrophages in the MEM test can be also considered a disadvantage should the test have any potential for the screening of malignant disease, since large animal facilities would be required by all laboratories attempting to operate the technique.

Macrophage Mobility Measurement

One of the major obstacles that has prevented the adoption of the technique of cell electrophoresis for the routine measurement of immunological reactions is the lack of a well designed reliable apparatus. Neither the Zeiss Cytophorometer nor the Rank Cylindrical Cell apparatus are completely suitable for the measurement of macrophage cells, although various modifications have been incorporated into their basic designs to facilitate measurements [50, 74].

Macrophages suitable for measurement are selected on their size and oil droplet content [90]. These cells should be 12–16 μm in diameter and contain more than two or three oil droplets. Larger or smaller cells appear to be unresponsive to slowing factor, and give rise to erratic results. Mobility determination must be made under drift-free conditions over a calibrated distance, usually 16 μm, since this aids selection of cells of the correct size. The applied current is reversed and the same cell timed over the same distance to obtain a pair of readings. Under ideal conditions these readings should not differ by more than 10 per cent. Ten pairs of readings are accumulated and the mean calculated and expressed as a percentage slowing according to the formula previously described.

Antigens

A considerable number of antigens have been shown to be reactive in the MEM test, although the most commonly used have been encephalitogenic factor (EF), myelin basic protein (MBP), cancer basic protein (CaBP) and purified protein derivative (PPD). A variety of extraction techniques have also been documented [12, 30]. Human chorionic gonadotrophin (HCG) and carcinoembryonic antigen (CEA) have also been shown to be active in the MEM assay [44, 102].

Most antigen preparations are crude and polyacrylamide gel electrophoresis can demonstrate as many as 20–30 major bands for preparations of encephalitogenic factor. The quality of the extract does not appear to impair the test response and over-purification can be disadvantageous. Crude 3M KC1 extracts of tumour tissue have been shown to result in reproduceable and anatomically site specific responses [68].

The amount of antigen to be used in an individual test is best found by experiment and a titration curve obtained for each antigen in use. A typical curve is shown in *Fig. 2.3.*

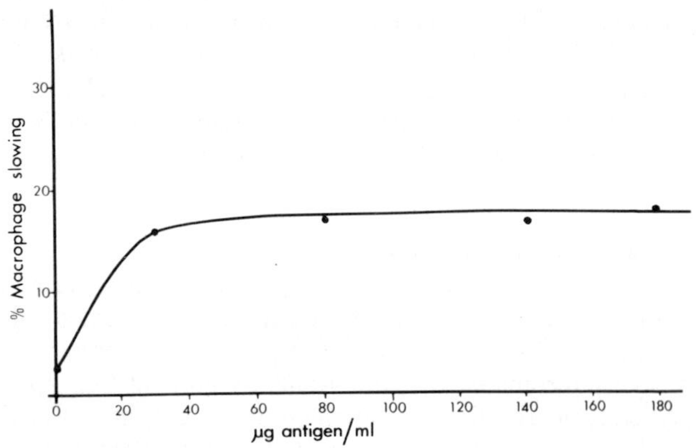

Fig. 2.3. Effect of antigen concentration (EF) in the MEM Test. (Reproduced from Pritchard [76], by courtesy of Alpha Omega.)

MOD–MEM Technique

As previously mentioned the peritoneal exudate of the guinea pig containing test macrophages was treated with 100 rad of gamma radiation to suppress the possibility of a mixed lymphocyte reaction occurring between the human test lymphocytes and guinea pig lymphocytes present in the exudate. The effect of an increased dose of radiation was found to increase the degree of 'positivity' that could be achieved in the MEM technique (*Fig. 2.4*). The use of any dose of radiation in a technique can be considered a limiting factor due to the availability of suitable facilities; this is especially so if large doses are to be considered necessary. To remove any effect of guinea pig lymphocytes in the MEM technique the MOD–MEM technique was proposed which, in effect, kept the macrophage cells isolated from the human test lymphocyte–antigen incubation. Since macrophage slowing factor had been shown to be a soluble factor, the lymphocytes could be simply removed by centrifugation after the incubation had been completed (*Fig. 2.5*) [79, 80].

Two factors emerged from the adoption of the split incubation technique. Firstly, an increase of temperature to 37 °C for the second stage of the test, that is, the incubation of supernatant containing slowing

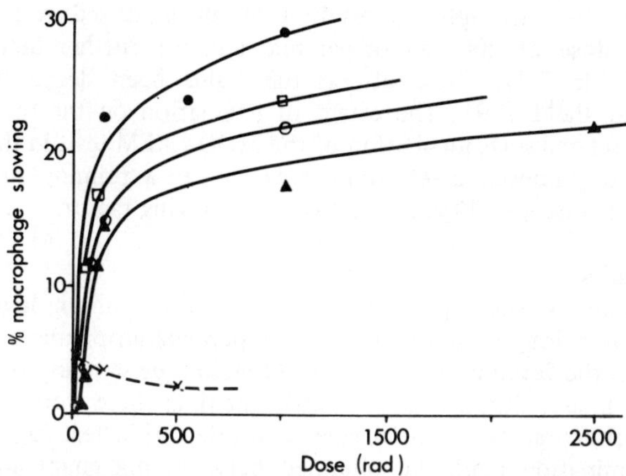

Fig. 2.4. Effect of radiation dose to guinea pig macrophages in the MEM Test for 4 cancer patient samples (solid lines) and 1 healthy donor (broken line). (Reproduced from Pritchard et al. [79] by courtesy of 'British Journal of Cancer'.)

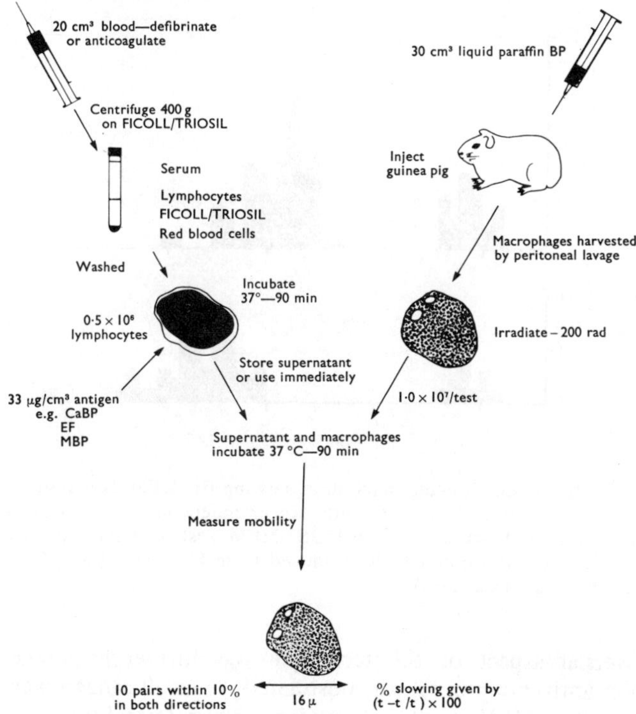

Fig. 2.5. Principal features of the MOD–MEM Test.

factor with the macrophages resulted in an increased response, and secondly, a dose of 200 rad of gamma radiation further increased the response (Table 2.4). These effects have also been demonstrated by Shenton and Field [89]. The effect of irradiation on the macrophages prior to the second stage incubation of the MOD–MEM test, in the absence of any mixed lymphocyte reaction is suggestive of a 'priming' process that increases their susceptibility, or reactivity, to slowing factor.

Clinical Results

The technique of electrophoresis in the study of immunological phenomena has been long established, and it is perhaps unfortunate that at an early stage in the development of the MEM technique so many presumptive claims were made, although at the particular time these were founded on sound experimental data. Initial claims for the MEM test suggested that good discrimination could be obtained between malignant and control samples with a remarkable lack of overlap, when lymphocyte response to encephalitogenic factor was measured. This discrimination was further improved with the adoption of the MOD–MEM procedure (*Fig. 2.6*). The

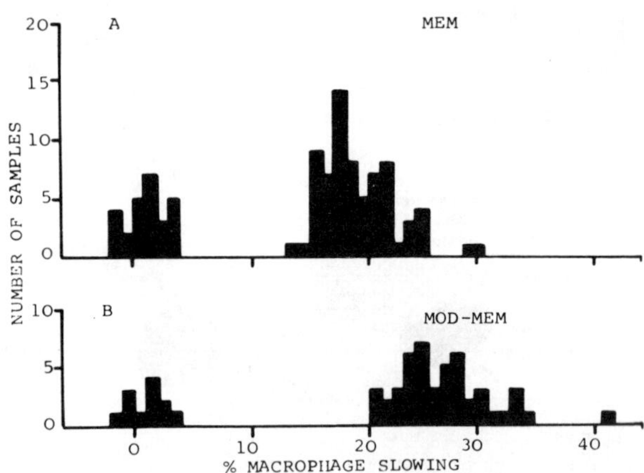

Fig. 2.6. a, Histogram showing percentage slowing for MEM Test results on samples from healthy donors and patients with cancer independent of histological type or anatomical site. *b,* Results with the MOD–MEM Test on similar groups illustrating the greater separation obtained. (Reproduced from Pritchard et al. [80] by courtesy of 'British Journal of Cancer'.)

controversial aspect of the technique was further heightened when a common antigenic process was postulated, since all cancers were found to give a positive MEM result, independent of histological type of anatomical origin. Furthermore, sensitization was found to persist for long periods, up

Table 2.4. Effect of Radiation Dose and Incubation Regimen on Macrophage Percentage slowing in the MEM Test (Reproduced from Pritchard et al., [79 or 80] by courtesy of *Br. J. Cancer*)

	Single stage incubation at:			*Split incubation: lymphocytes + EF at 23°C: supernatant + macrophages at:*			
Sample No.	*23°C 0 rad* A	*23°C 200 rad* B	*37°C 200 rad* C	*23°C 200 rad* D	*37°C 0 rad* E	*37°C 200 rad* F	*37°C 2500 rad* G
'Malignant'							
1	–	21·0	–	24·0	–	40·0	–
2	–	16·8	15·0	17·0	–	27·0	–
3	–	18·4	17·0	17·9	–	30·5	–
4	–	18·3	18·9	18·2	–	32·3	–
5	–	17·3	–	–	–	25·8	–
6	1·8	16·6	–	–	21·4	25·1	25·8
7	0·5	17·2	–	–	18·2	29·0	28·6
8	1·0	16·6	–	–	18·6	22·6	22·8
9	–	15·6	–	–	–	30·0	–
'Normal'							
10	–	0·1	–0·1	–1·0	–	0·7	–
11	1·8	2·0	–	–	0·2	1·3	1·8

to 30 years in one instance, after successful 'cure' of the tumour [39]. This suggested however, that the technique would have little value in the monitoring of disease, if sensitization to antigen persisted for such a long time.

The assessment of the MEM technique during its early phases of development depended upon those centres which were able to demonstrate a difference between groups of normal controls and subjects with malignant disease (*Fig. 2.6*). Whilst it is necessary to adopt this approach to establish the technique in the laboratory, the results do not necessarily establish the test to be of clinical value. This can be assessed only by a rigorous, carefully controlled clinical study designed to establish whether the technique can differentially detect cancer when contrasted with patients who have benign disease of the same or different sites. It is further essential that different laboratories can successfully reproduce the technique. Since 1970 when the technique was originally published eleven centres around the world have published confirmatory data which support the general principle that the MEM test could discriminate with reasonable accuracy between cases with proven malignant disease and normal subjects (Table 2.5).

Table 2.5. Centres Successfully Operating the MEM or MOD–MEM Test

Location	*Confirmed cancer cases tested*	*MEM/MOD–MEM positive > 10 %*	*Reference*
Newcastle	296	295	[39]
Cardiff	104	104	[79]
Edinburgh	13	13	[51]
Bristol	36	36	[74]
Rostock (DDR)	33	30	[67]
Italy	18	14	[100]
London (Charing Cross)	41	39	[86]
Dresden (GDR)	76	57	[68]
W. Germany (Leibig University)	105	96	[64]
Tokyo	115	82	[69]
USA (Roswell Park)	44	37	[50]

However, failure to obtain any separation between cancer and control subjects has also been documented [1]. It was also suggested that there was no evidence for sensitization by guinea pig lymphocytes to tuberculin in guinea pigs sensitized *in vivo,* although in a separate study of murine neoplasia where tumour-bearing animals with distinct tumour-associated transplantation antigens (TATAS), the MEM technique could demonstrate that lymphocytes from such mice reacted strongly to KCl extracts of the same tumour, unrelated tumours and rabbit myelin basic protein [70]. In a further study patients with ocular neoplastic disease could not be clearly separated from those with inflammatory disease although there was evidence for some discrimination between choroidal melanoma and ocular inflammation [85]. In this particular trial there was a large variation in the timings quoted for the macrophage cells and substantially beyond that considered acceptable for the successful operation of the MEM technique [90]. Although it has been considered essential to adhere to the basic principles of the technique no significant reactions could be observed in a series of 42 patients with proven malignant disease [49]. However, an overview of the literature does support the fundamental hypothesis that stimulation of sensitized lymphocytes by specific antigens does result in a soluble mediator which is able to modify the surface characteristics of guinea pig macrophages, as measured by the MEM technique.

Clinical Relevance

Whilst it is possible to establish demarcation between normal and cancer populations with the MEM or MOD–MEM techniques, the clinical usefulness of the test can only be truly evaluated in conjunction with established clinical diagnosis. This has been undertaken in two anatomical sites – prostate and breast. Lymphocytes from 113 preoperative patients admitted for transurethral resection of enlarged prostate were assayed for reactivity to encephalitogenic factor with the MEM technique. Eighty-three were reported as histologically non-malignant and 80 of these cases gave negative MEM values; the remaining 3 cases were positive. The remaining 30 cases were reported as histologically positive and 24 of these gave positive MEM responses, but the remaining 6 cases gave negative MEM values, and as such were considered as false negative results [46]. The data relating to breast disease is not so convincing and there is a large variation in the data reported (Table 2.6). It has been suggested that because of the fairly high false positive and false negative rates the technique has little value in this area as a screening test. The high false negative rate for proven cancer reported by Lewkonia et al. [65] may have been due to technical troubles in the operation of the MEM technique, since the same laboratories had previously reported good discrimination for the same technique [51]. For any screening test to be adopted in clinical practice it must retain a low false negative rate coupled with ease of operation and reproducibility of results. If a test is shown to be particularly sensitive then, within limitations, a false positive rate may be acceptable – false negative results are not acceptable. A survey of the literature during 1976 revealed that a very low false negative rate of 1·2 per cent could be claimed for the MEM test in proven cancer [81]. This suggested that a

Table 2.6. The MEM/MOD–MEM Test in Breast Disease

Centre	*No. of cases*	*MEM result*		*% False results*		*Reference*
		(+)	(–)	(+)	(–)	
Charing Cross						
Malignant	19	15	4	10·8	9·0	[86]
Benign	27	5	22			
Edinburgh						
Malignant	9	2	7	0	41·0	[65]
Benign	8	–	8			
Cardiff						
Malignant	3	1	2*	29·0	2·1	[77]
Benign	91	19	72			

*Subject had negative thermogram, mammogram and biopsy. Primary lesion not localized.

negative MEM result might be more useful for the exclusion of malignant disease, rather than use a positive result to indicate its presence. Since this date further centres have recorded data which has shown an overall increase in the false negative rate to 9·5 per cent. This is consistent with the false negative rate shown for breast disease by the Charing Cross group, and those of West and East Germany [64, 68, 86]. The Cardiff data concerning breast disease (*see* Table 2.5) showed an artificially low false negative rate because of the low numbers of proven cancer cases in the study. This was not by design but a result of investigating a group of females with localizing symptoms who were referred for thermography and mammography where there was an extremely low incidence of malignancy.

For a cancer test to have any clinical value it must be specific in response. Before any claims can be made for test specificity it must be evaluated in disease conditions other than cancer, so that resultant positive results can be attributed only to malignancy. The MEM test has been shown to be non-specific for cancer, because a large number of disease conditions can give a positive test response (Table 2.7) [39, 46, 81 or 83, 86]. Thus if the MEM test in its present form were to be used as an aid in the differential clinical diagnosis of malignant disease, a large number of disease conditions would have to be excluded – a clinically unacceptable task at the present time. However, the use of the MEM test in the clinical detection of disease has been suggested in establishing diagnosis before operation, especially in patients with abdominal masses [64]. A further optimistic report has also demonstrated specific tumour extract responses, especially in breast cancer. Lymphocytes from 18 out of 19 women with breast cancer were shown to respond to a KCl extract of breast tumour tissue and not to similar extracts derived from other tumours [68]. However, a recent double blind trial with 210 coded samples showed that the MEM technique as a routine laboratory test had little value in the detection of malignant disease because of unacceptably high false positive (34 per cent) and negative results (43 per cent) [84].

Table 2.7. Diseases Other than Cancer Shown to give Positive MEM or MOD–MEM Results

Asthma	Farmer's lung	Peripheral vascular disease
Asbestosis	Influenzal infections (transient)	Pulmonary tuberculosis
Acute appendicitis	Hypertension	Rheumatoid arthritis
Cerebral arteriosclerosis	Leukoplakia	Sarcoidosis
Cerebrovascular attack	Liver cirrhosis + ascites	Subarachnoid haemorrhage
Collagen disease	Myocardial infarction	Tylosis
Dermatomyositis	Pneumonia	Ulcerative colitis/Crohn's disease

Early Warning Hypothesis

From a study of the MEM test in a series of patients with non-malignant disease 13 positive test results were found for which no clinical explanation was apparent, and as such, could be considered true false positives. It was suggested that such a result may be due to preclinical malignant disease, undetectable by conventional techniques [45, 81 or 83]. A model was proposed, developed from Cancer Registration returns, which attempted to predict the number of false positives that might be expected in a control series if a test was to give an average of 'x' years of 'early warning' regardless of histological type or anatomical site, and that a minimum number of malignant cells are required to give a positive test result. This is referred to as the 'detection threshold' (*Fig. 2.7*) [98]. A sample of 100 000 subjects of the same age and sex was scaled down to give the statistical result expected from one individual of that age and sex in the actual test series. Subjects who exceed the detection threshold at age A − (x − 1) will appear in Registration records N at age (A + 1) one year after they have given a positive test result. Subjects whose cancer was clinically detected at age A would be excluded as controls since they would already appear in the Registration records at the time of the test. At the other extreme, a subject who passes the 'detection threshold' in the year of the test will not appear in the registration records until age (A + 1). The number of 'unexplained positives' to be expected from 100 000 cases is equal to $(N_1 + N_2 + \ldots N_x)$ and when this is scaled down it gives a fractional false positive contribution from a single individual tested at age A. This calculation is done for each subject with the aid of age and sex related registration returns appropriate for the area, and the sum of the

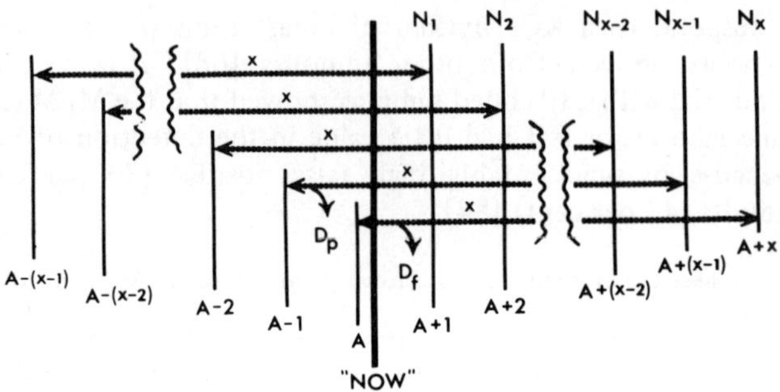

Fig. 2.7. Schematic representation of the hypothetical model used to estimate a false positive rate that might be expected from a control population if a cancer test gave 'x' years of early warning. (Reproduced from Sutherland et al. [98] by courtesy of 'Annals of Clinical Research'.)

individual fractional contributions finally gives the total number of false positives that might be expected in a particular series.

Although the 13 false positives fitted a curve which would predict an early warning period of approximately 15 yr, there are many assumptions in such a model and this figure is likely to be an overestimation, as discussed by Sutherland et al. [98]. Whilst such an hypothesis is considered unacceptable by some, it does draw attention to one very important fact. It has been previously stated that any cancer test must be both sensitive and specific. If a proposed test is shown to be highly sensitive then the testing of any healthy population with a reasonable age spectrum must be expected to produce false positive results. It is also likely that a highly sensitive test which depends on a small number of tumour cells in the body to evoke a response is unlikely to be specific and that a much larger tumour mass will be necessary before tumour specific responses can be demonstrated.

Conclusions and Future

In its present form the MEM and MOD–MEM test does not warrant routine use in the detection of cancer. The technical difficulties associated with electrophoretic mobility measurement of guinea pig macrophage cells impose severe restriction on the operation of the technique. It has also been suggested that there is too much subjective bias in the selection of macrophages for measurement but in the majority of centres cited samples have been measured 'blind' to remove any operator bias.

Present day assessment of *in vitro* tests seem to be preoccupied with the use of double blind protocols, and quite often these are advocated too early in the development of the technique. Providing the operator of a technique handles a coded sample of unknown origin, objections to subjective measurement of calculation of data should be overcome. The more blind a series becomes the greater the chance of error in coding, especially when several investigators are involved. The MEM technique, like many other immunologically based tests, depends upon the physiological condition of separated test lymphocytes from whole blood. Blood sampling techniques vary considerably between institutions and individuals. Such factors and the importance of sample transport must be taken into account when organizing a trial, upon which the fate of a particular test may be decided, particularly when short periods of travel have been shown to impair human macrophage function, and blood sampling techniques can impair lymphocyte response to antigen [35, 71].

Although many objections have been raised to the use of the MEM technique as a screening procedure, it is now possible to purchase a complete laboratory system designed around the MEM test for the detection of cancer. The problems of suitable indicator cells and their mobility measurement have attracted considerable attention. The routine use of guinea pig macrophages limits any test procedure where large numbers of samples can be anticipated because of the considerable animal facilities that are required. To overcome this problem alternative indicator cells have been suggested. Autologous granulocytes have been used as indicator cells for slowing factor derived from myelin basic protein stimulation of sensitized lymphocytes [75]. The mobility of the autologous granulocyte was reduced for patients with proven malignancy, but those from control samples were not affected. Although this technique has the advantage that the blood sample contains its own test indicator cells, the technique has not been adopted by other centres.

Ideally indicator cells should be homogenous, stable and readily available so that data between centres can be easily compared. Sheep red blood cells, used widely in rosetting techniques for establishing T and B cell ratios in blood preparations, have been used as alternative indicators for the presence of lymphocyte mediated factors which alter surface charge effects [72, 73]. Sheep red blood cells have to be treated with tannic acid and stabilized with sulphosalicylic acid before use and are referred to as SETS. Such cells can be prepared in large batches and have been found to remain stable over long periods. They are also extremely homogenous. The clinical data also suggests that SETS can be used in place of guinea pig macrophages for the operation of this modified MEM test, when 87 per cent of patients with cancer could be distinguished from normal subjects and patients with other diseases. In pre-cancerous disease, the MEM test result using SETS as indicator cells, correlated with subepithelial lymphocytic infiltration and histological evidence [72, 73]. The difference between a group of 84 patients with pulmonary disease and 20 controls was also statistically significant. The use of SETS as alternative indicator cells in the MEM test was also confirmed by Jenssen and Shenton [62]. The MEM test using SETS, was also shown to discriminate between patients with proven malignancy and those with diagnosed benign and inflammatory disorders [32]. A comparison of guinea pig macrophages and SETS as indicator cells in the MEM test showed that the kinetics and mechanisms associated with the interaction of slowing factor and indicator cells was remarkably similar [91]. It has been suggested however that the tanning and fixing procedure used in the method of preparation can influence SETS' response to slowing factor [94].

In a clinical study Harlos and Weiss [53] showed a measure of agreement between MEM test results using macrophage and sheep red blood cells as indicator cells. Their method of preparation of the red blood cells was different from that previously reported since 40 per cent formaldehyde was used as the fixative. They concluded, however, that neither system inspired much confidence for the initial detection of cancer, whether guinea pig macrophages or sheep red blood cells were used as indicators of slowing factor, since 32 out of 42 correct results were obtained using macrophages and 28 out of 42 with tanned and fixed sheep red blood cells. However Dyson and Corbett [34] have shown that providing the experimental conditions are thoroughly investigated and the effects of antigen concentration on erythrocytes established, these alternative indicator cells can be used with confidence in the MEM assay. Once the experimental conditions were optimized, 43 out of 51 cancer patients gave 'unequivocal positive' test results whereas 22 out of 22 healthy donors gave clear negative values. There were no false positive results in the 73 samples tested.

The results also suggested an alternative interpretation from the affect of antigen, in this instance crude brain extract, on lymphocytes derived from cancer patients and healthy donors. Whereas a positive value in the original MEM assay was dependent on the release by sensitized lymphocytes of a soluble mediator which resulted in a decrease in electrophoretic mobility of the macrophages, an opposite effect has been postulated for the erythrocyte model. Reduction in the electrophoretic mobility of sheep erythrocyte (EME) was shown to be attributed to the brain extract (BE) alone, but the effect of incubation with lymphocytes from cancer patients was to decrease the slowing capacity of the brain extract. As such the technique does not appear to be founded on immunological principles, but the results do indicate that the technique may have some relevance in the detection of malignant disease.

The use of a homogenous suspension of sheep red blood cells (SETS) as indicator cells in the MEM test has also helped to resolve one of the major problems of the technique, i.e. that of subjective measurement. Development of automated measurement technique has followed two major trends. Firstly the adoption of a technique known as 'cell partition'. This does not depend upon actual mobility determinations under the influence of an electric field, but the counting of indicator cells once they have separated in an aqueous two phase polymer system [101]. Aliquots from two separated phases can be simply taken and the cell numbers enumerated by particle counters such as the Coulter Counter, thus removing any subjective bias. Initial results using this procedure but with guinea pig macrophage cells, showed that the cell partition technique produced a significant difference between a group of 14 cancer patients and 9 normal subjects [96]. Such differences can also be observed using SETS [95].

The second approach has been to retain the electrophoresis technique and hence the mobility measurement aspect of the technique, but to automate the measurement of the indicator cells. This can be accomplished in two ways: by utilizing Döppler principles incorporating laser optics and by electronic particle correlation technology involving specially designed microprocessors. Both systems have been shown to have some success and they have the advantage that large numbers of cells can be measured in a short time, with a resultant distribution plot of cell mobilities. To observe any change simply requires the comparison of two charts.

The initial suggestion that the MEM test was a unique test for cancer, its development, and its clinical appraisal have been so controversial and intermingled with emotion that it is difficult to arrive at an unbiased assessment. Although there are convincing published reports that the test has little value in the detection of malignant disease, there are equally valid and convincing reports to the contrary. That the technique can measure a lymphocyte–antigen interaction is not in doubt. Its relevance to the cancer problem is yet to be resolved. Considerable attention in the literature has been directed towards the technique and its pitfalls: the same degree of attention has not been paid to a most important aspect of the test, that of the antigens and extracts used to elicit a response from the 'sensitized' lymphocytes. Where attempts have been made to tackle this problem both cancer and site-specific response have been documented. Careful selection of the correct extraction procedure for antigens may well resolve some of the high false negative rates that have been experienced in some centres, and at the same time reduce the false positive rate for the test. Whether or not the test ever gains clinical acceptability it will be remembered as controversial.

At the height of the MEM test controversy, data was published concerning a test, the results of which suggested none of the disadvantages of the MEM test and was both cancer and site-specific in measuring lymphocyte response to antigen. This technique has become known as the Structuredness of Cytoplasmic Matrix (SCM) test and has succeeded in maintaining the controversy of *in vitro* tests for cancer when the MEM test was beginning to suffer from the trauma of modern day clinical science.

THE STRUCTUREDNESS OF CYTOPLASMIC MATRIX (SCM) TEST

Whereas the MEM technique measured a soluble product of lymphocyte stimulation the Structuredness of Cytoplasmic Matrix (SCM) test measured lymphocyte response to antigen directly thus eliminating the need for any identification procedure requiring indicator cells. The test developed from a study of changes in cell cycle parameters using a fluorescence polarization technique [14, 15, 25]. The SCM was adopted to describe the biophysical state at a molecular level of the cytoplasmic matrix of a cell. The organization and interaction of macromolecules within a cell are normally in a state of equilibrium and this can be readily influenced by changes in osmolarity, concentration of ions, ATP and cyclic AMP. Changes at a molecular level can be detected by the introduction into the cell of a non-fluorescent probe, fluorescin diacetate (FDA). Enzymatic hydrolysis results in free fluorescin being produced and changes in fluorescence characteristics in terms of emission spectra and emission polarization spectra can be detected in a suitable apparatus [16, 19].

From the observation that lymphocytes from healthy human subjects and chronic leukaemic patients could be differentiated on the basis of SCM changes induced by the mitogen, phytohaemagglutinin (PHA), it was a short step to investigating the effect of tumour antigens in the same technique, following the much documented MEM test [24]. The initial results of a study of the SCM technique in a series of 41 patients with proven cancer, 17 cases with non-malignant disease and 71 healthy subjects was extraordinary. Lymphocyte response to either PHA or tumour antigen enabled complete separation to be obtained between the cancer group and those patients with non-malignant disease and healthy subjects [23]. However, before embarking on an examination of the clinical relevance of the SCM test it is useful to discuss the technique since this, as with the MEM test technique, has a direct influence on the results, and thus the discrimination that can be obtained with the test.

SCM Test Technique

The performance of the SCM test depends upon the separation from whole blood of a particular fraction of lymphocytes referred to as 'SCM responding lymphocytes'. These can be obtained from heparinized blood, preincubated with carbonyl-iron and finally separated on a modified Ficoll/Triosil gradient. The density of this gradient should be 1·0810 g/cm^3 at 25 °C [20]. Extreme care must be exercised in the removal of the separated lymphocytes and only those found floating as an indistinct band at the interface should be collected. These are then carefully washed once in normal physiological saline and twice in Dulbecco's phosphate buffered saline (PBS). Both solutions should be pre-warmed to 37 °C before use. Such SCM responding cells are kept at 37 °C until use at a concentration not exceeding 6×10^6/ml. The stimulation of aliquots of lymphocytes by either PHA or tumour extract is carried out at 37 °C for periods of 30–60 mins, dependent on the extract activity, and as assessed by experiment.

The fluorescein diacetate (FDA) substrate is not very soluble in water, and must be either dissolved in spectroscopic grade acetone or high purity acetic acid. The final FDA concentration in PBS should be 2·5 μM, with an osmolarity of 0·330 osmol/ kg and pH 7·4. For a detailed review of the procedures and precautions to be taken with the SCM technique reference should be made to two comprehensive reviews by Drs L. and B. Cercek [20, 21]. The principal features of the technique are shown in *Fig. 2.8.* The essential measurement required in the SCM technique is the Index of

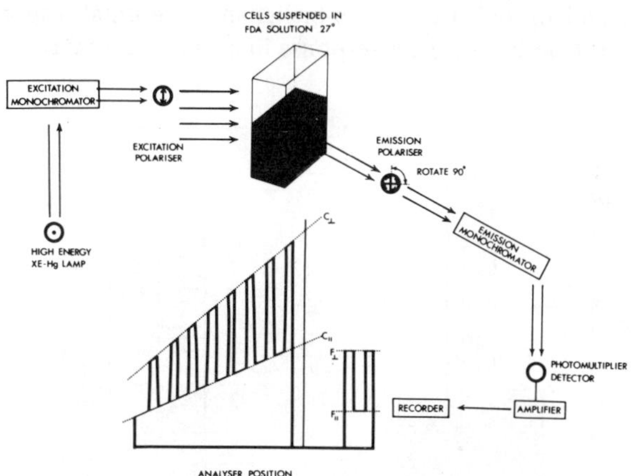

Fig. 2.8. Principal features of the Structuredness of Cytoplasmic Matrix (SCM) Test.

Polarization (P) for the test lymphocytes which is calculated from data derived from a recorder chart. The Index of Polarization (P) is given by –

$$\frac{I_{11} - I\perp G}{I_{11} + I\perp G}$$

where the intensity of fluorescence (I) is calculated from I parallel (I_{11}) and I perpendicular ($I\perp$) emission from the chart recorder. $I_{11} = C_{11} - F_{11}$ and $I\perp = C\perp - F\perp$ where C is the chart intensity and F the filtrate intensity. G is a machine constant, experimentally derived.

Clinical Data

The clinical data first published suggested that the SCM test was cancer specific and that many of the non-malignant conditions shown to give false positive MEM test results gave SCM responses in the normal range. What could not be anticipated was the finding that lymphocytes from patients with malignant diseases did not respond to PHA, but did so to cancer basic protein (CaBP) similar to that originally used in the MEM test. To clarify the pattern of response the term 'SCM response ratio' (RR_{SCM}) was devised. This is the ratio the degree of fluorescence polarization obtained after CaBP stimulation (P_{CaBP}), divided by that obtained for a similar stimulation for PHA, (P_{PHA}),

$$\text{thus } RR_{SCM} = P_{CaBP}/P_{PHA}.$$

The use of this ratio artificially created the value of 1 as the dividing line between a cancer or non-cancer response, as shown by a decrease in P values. (*Fig. 2.9*) [23]. SCM responses <1·0 are more indicative of malignancy and those >1·0 of non-malignant or normal responses. It was thus possible to define a cancer response in a single test by two parameters.

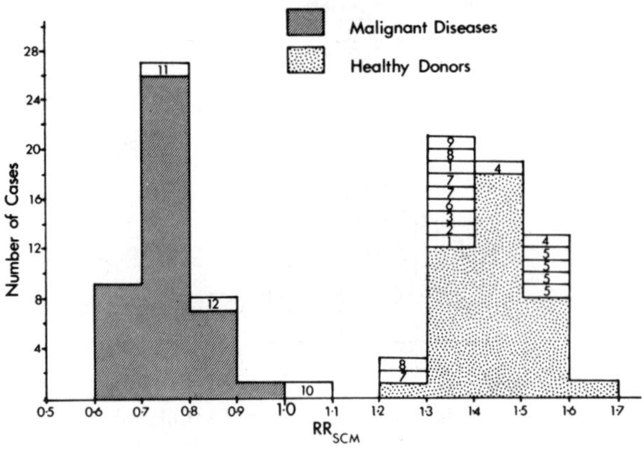

Fig. 2.9. Distribution of the SCM Response (RR_{SCM}) of lymphocytes from healthy donors and patients with cancer. Numbers in histogram indicate following diseases: 1, multiple sclerosis; 2, infective hepatitis; 3, Crohn's disease; 4, cirrhosis of liver; 5, pregnancy; 6, ulcerative colitis; 7, chronic bronchitis; 8, rheumatoid arthritis; 9, peptic ulcer + benign enlargement of prostate; 10, hyperkeratosis of skin; 11, polyposis coli; 12, 'false positive' – normal donor. (Reproduced from Cercek et al. [23] by courtesy of 'British Journal of Cancer'.)

Firstly, by negligible or no response to PHA, and secondly, by response to CaBP or related tumour extracts. From this initial series (*Fig. 2.9*) only 1 out of 71 of the control subjects showed a cancer type response, but clinical examination did not reveal any obvious malignancy. It was further shown that lymphocytes from subjects with multiple sclerosis could be identified as different from those of cancer origin by their ability to respond to both PHA and EF. Such differentiation was not possible with the MEM test. In a later comprehensive summary of data (Table 2.8) the false negative rate for 316 cases of cancer was 1·26 per cent and remarkably similar to that initially claimed for the MEM technique [77]. However the false positive rate was also extremely low (1·32 per cent) unlike that of the MEM technique. Further studies showed that after surgical removal of malignant tissue the RR_{SCM} changed and lymphocyte response to PHA

Table 2.8. Summary of SCM Responses of Lymphocytes from Patients with Cancer, Non-malignant Diseases and Healthy Donors to PHA and CaBP Stimulation (Reproduced from Cercek and Cercek, [21], by courtesy of Alpha Omega)

		Cases with RR_{SCM}				
	No. of cases	< 1·0		> 1·0		*Mean* RR_{SCM}
Diagnosis		0·5–0·9	0·9–1·0	1·0–1·1	1·1–2·0	
Healthy donors:	304	2/304	2/304	2/404	300/400	1·46
Non-malignant disease:	30				30/30	1·36
Benign or pre-malignant growths:						
Thyroid adenoma	1				1/1	1·25
Verrucae vulgaris	2				2/2	1·32
Lipomas	5				5/5	1·41
Pituitary tumour	2				2/2	1·33
Prostate enlargement	2		1/2		1/2	0·95/1·35
Dysplasia cervix uteri	14	1/14	7/14	6/14		1·00
Breast disorders	22	8/22	5/22	9/22		0·98
Hyperkeratosis	1			1/1		1·05
Polyposis coli (familial cancer)	1	1/1				0·75
Malignant:						
37 different cancer groups	316	198/316	14/316		4/316	0·75

was restored within two weeks [17]. It thus appeared that the SCM technique had the capacity to monitor the presence of tumour tissue but whether the technique could be used clinically in this role remains to be resolved. A site-specific response was also demonstrated by 'baiting' test lymphocytes with small pieces of well washed tumour tissue. For example, autologous breast tumour tissue was found to cause an SCM change in lymphocytes obtained from a patient with breast cancer but not in lymphocytes from patients with cancer of other anatomical sites [18].

Although many of the early claims for the MEM test had been considered unacceptable, those for the SCM technique did nothing but add to the controversial aspects that lymphocyte function can demonstrate cancer specific responses *in vitro*. The SCM technique satisfies many of the criteria required of a test for the detection of malignant disease. The false positive and negative rates are extremely low, and the results give both cancer and anatomically site-specific responses. In the face of such claims numerous centres embarked upon programmes designed to confirm or refute the acceptability of the technique, and as such, continued to fuel the fires of scepticism. For any cancer test to be 'acceptable' it must be easily reproducible in many laboratories. Both the MEM and SCM techniques have had in common the misfortune to be introduced as tests for the detection of cancer at too early a phase in their development and before the techniques have been fully understood and all technical parameters identified.

It was not until three years after the original article on the SCM test had been published that confirmatory evidence was forthcoming establishing the usefulness of the SCM test in the detection of gastric cancer (*Fig. 2.10*) [99]. The results showed that there was very good separation between all cancer cases investigated and non-malignant disease incorporating some healthy donors. It was further suggested that the test had

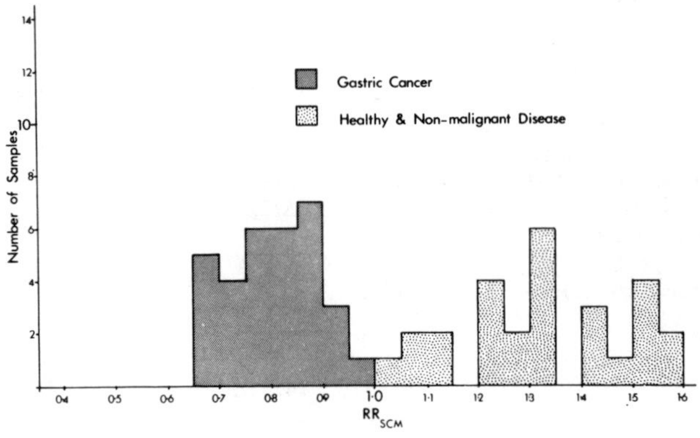

Fig. 2.10. RR_{SCM} differentiation for gastric cancer, non-malignant disease and healthy donors. Gastric cancer group includes both early and advanced disease. Non-malignant diseases included Shilder's disease, acute hepatitis, lymphadenitis, systemic lupus erythematosus, rheumatoid arthritis and iron deficiency anaemia. (Adapted from Takaku et al. [99].)

potential in the early diagnosis of gastric cancer with tumours as small as 0·8 × 1·4 cm being detected by a change in the RR_{SCM} ratio. During 1976, and as a result of a workshop held on the SCM technique it became apparent that there were certain technical parameters associated with the SCM test which, unless carefully adjusted and controlled, would considerably influence the operation of the test [2]. It is extremely important to maintain precise temperature control for the gradient used in the separation of SCM responding lymphocytes, and the density of this gradient should be 1·081 g/cm^3 at 19 °C, and must have an osmolarity of 0·320 osmol/kg. Good control should also be maintained over the pH and osmolarity of the substrate, which must have a pH of 7·4 and osmolarity of 0·330 osmol/kg. Attention was also drawn to the unsatisfactory quality of polarizers used in conjunction with the spectrophotometer in many of the centres attempting to reproduce the technique. The polarizers must have precision optical surfaces and have no polarization defects. The extinction of light in the crossed position should be better than 1 per cent. Similar criticism was also extended to the incorrect use of fluorescent spectrophotometers. In order to accurately measure SCM changes it is necessary to have a sensitive and stable machine, free of fluorescence contamination, and which uses a xenon light source. Particular emphasis was also placed on the necessity to use pure chemicals for solutions and all glassware must be scrupulously clean.

The awareness and adoption of the technical parameters likely to affect SCM responses in lymphocytes has led to other centres publishing SCM data which has been essentially confirmatory but cautious in conclusion. One of the main problems that has been resolved is the influence of separation gradient density and its effect on the SCM's response to recovered lymphocytes (*Fig. 2.11*) [82]. The maximum decrease in the

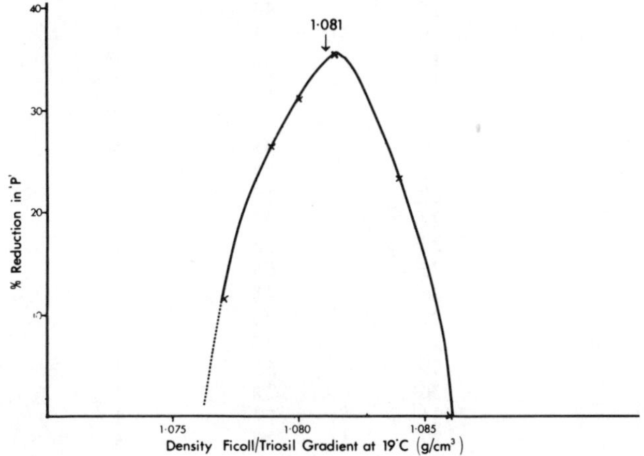

Fig. 2.11. Effect of separation medium density on lymphocyte response to PHA as determined by a reduction of the index of polarization (P). (Reproduced from Pritchard and Sutherland [82] by courtesy of 'British Journal of Cancer'.)

polarization index (P) for PHA stimulated cells was found when lymphocytes were carefully removed from a Ficoll/Triosil gradient of density 1·081 g/cm^3. It was then possible to obtain SCM results which differentiated a group of patients with breast cancer from normal healthy donors, with respect to lymphocyte response to breast tumour antigen (Table 2.9). In three cases (Nos. 10, 14 and 15), response to breast tumour antigen could not be detected, but neither could response to PHA stimulation be detected. Only one of the healthy donors (No. 33) responded to breast antigen. In this instance a reduction in the polarization index of 21 per cent was also obtained for PHA stimulation.

Table 2.9. Response of Lymphocytes from Patients with Breast Cancer and Healthy Donors to Breast Tumour Extract and PHA

	Case No.	*Age*	*Sex*	RR_{SCM}
	1	47	F	0·62
	2	87	F	0·59
	3	37	F	0·84
	4	63	F	0·75
	5	53	F	0·82
	6	76	F	0·74
	7	70	F	0·65
	8	46	F	0·77
Breast cancer	9	51	F	0·69
	10	72	F	1·00
	11	46	F	0·86
	12	44	F	0·90
	13	47	F	0·84
	14	81	F	0·98
	15	46	F	1·00
	16	51	F	0·81
	17	53	F	0·74
	18	84	F	0·84
	19	67	M	0·81
	20	35	M	1·20
	21	23	F	1·26
	22	18	F	1·34
	23	23	F	1·42
	24	36	F	1·82
	25	56	M	1·22
	26	41	F	1·42
	27	30	F	1·21
Healthy donors	28	47	F	1·45
	29	55	F	1·21
	30	22	F	1·08
	31	27	F	1·23
	32	28	M	1·24
	33	39	F	0·71*
	34	54	F	1·34
	35	27	F	1·32
	36	57	F	1·46
	37	27	F	1·56 +

* 21 per cent reduction in 'P' value with PHA stimulation.
+ 12 weeks pregnant

A concensus of the four published reports from independent centres concerning the successful operation of the SCM test supports the original SCM data regarding the non-responsiveness of lymphocytes from cancer patients to PHA stimulation and some degree of site specificity with tumour antigens [54, 63, 82, 99].

The immunological basis of the SCM test, like the MEM technique is difficult to establish and define at the present time. Lymphocytes separated for use in the MEM test have been shown to be similar to those implicated in transformation reactions and delayed hypersensitivity responses. The enriched 'SCM responding cells' separated on a modified gradient constitute about 10–25 per cent of the total peripheral blood leucocyte population. Providing that care is taken with the separation procedure there is minimal contamination by erythrocytes, granulocytes and monocytes in the SCM lymphocyte suspension. Approximately 85 per cent of the SCM responding cells have been estimated to be 'T' cells [21]. Until both techniques have been applied to established animal models it is unlikely that any solid immunological basis for either test can be put forward.

The future of the MEM test depends a great deal on whether the use of more chemically defined antigens and homogenous indicator cells will reduce the false positive and false negative results obtained in the clinical evaluations so far undertaken. At the present time the use of the technique as originally published does not have much clinical relevance. That the technique can measure lymphocyte response to antigen has been established in many laboratories. It is perhaps possible that some of the problems encountered in the SCM test with regard to the separation of responding lymphocytes might well resolve some of the MEM test difficulties. Measurement of the mobility of indicator cells should not present problems with the advancement and development of laser and electronic measurement techniques. Any future developments must be tested thoroughly in the laboratory before any move is made regarding finite clinical assessment, so that the results can be judged objectively in the absence of controversy. A similar approach will benefit the development of the SCM test. Much remains to be resolved with respect to the biophysical changes of lymphocytes found with stimulation by antigens. At the present time the extracts used in both the MEM and SCM tests are little more than 'soups' containing a variety of ill-defined chemical substances. Although much attention has been paid to lymphocyte populations and the choice of indicator cells, it is equally important to define the nature of the substances eliciting the responses upon which the fate of the technique depends.

REFERENCES

1. Arvilommi H., Dale M. M., Desai H. N. et al. (1977) Failure to obtain positive MEM results in either cell mediated immune conditions in the guinea pig or human cancer. *Br. J. Cancer* **36**, 545–549.
2. Bagshawe K. D. (1977) Workshop on Macrophage Electrophoretic Mobility (MEM) and Structuredness of Cytoplasmic Matrix (SCM) Tests. *Br. J. Cancer* **35**, 701–704.
3. Baldwin R. W. and Embleton M. J. (1977a) Demonstration by colony inhibition methods of cellular and humoral immune reactions to tumour specific antigen associated with animoazodye induced rat hepatomas. *Int. J. Cancer* **7**, 17–25.
4. Baldwin R. W. and Embleton M. J. (1977b) Assessment of cell mediated immunity to human tumour associated antigens. *Int. Rev. of Expl. Pathol.* **17**, 49–95.

5. Berlin N. (1974) Early diagnosis of cancer. *Prev. Med.* **3,** 185–186.
6. Black M. M. (1973) Human breast cancer – A model for cancer immunology. *Isr. J. Med. Sci.* **9,** 284.
7. Black M. M. and Speer F. D. (1958) Sinus histocytosis of lymph nodes in cancer. *Surg. Gynecol. Obstet.* **106,** 163–175.
8. Black M. M. and Speer F. D. (1959) Immunology of cancer. *Surg. Gynecol. Obstet.* **109,** 105–116.
9. Bloom B. R. and Bennett B. (1966) Mechanisms of a reaction *in vitro* associated with delayed type hypersensitivity. *Science* **153,** 80–82.
10. Brunsehing A., Southam C. M. and Levin A. G. (1965) *Ann. Surg.* **162,** 416–423.
11. Carnegie P. R., Caspary E. A., Dickinson J. P. et al. (1973a) The Macrophage Electrophoretic Migration (MEM) test for lymphocyte sensitisation: A study of the kinetics. *Clin. Exp. Immunol.* **14,** 37–44.
12. Carnegie P. R., Caspary E. A. and Field E. J. (1973b) Isolation of an 'antigen' from malignant tumours. *Br. J. Cancer.* **28,** Suppl. I. 219–223.
13. Carter S. K. (1978) *The Multidisciplinary Approach to Cancer Therapy.* Montedison Pharmaceuticals Ltd.
14. Cercek L. and Cercek B. (1973a) Relationship between changes in the structuredness of cytoplasm and rate constants for the hydrolysis of FDA in saccharomyces cerevisiae. *Biophysik* **9,** 109–112.
15. Cercek L. and Cercek B. (1973b) Effect of centrifugal forces on the structuredness of cytoplasms in growing yeast cells. *Biophysik* **9,** 105–108.
16. Cercek L. and Cercek B. (1974) Involvement of cyclic-AMP in changes of the structuredness of cytoplasmic matrix (SCM). *Radiat. Environ. Biophys.* **11,** 209–212.
17. Cercek L. and Cercek B. (1975a) Changes in the SCM response ratio (RR_{SCM}) after surgical removal of malignant tissue. *Br. J. Cancer* **31,** 250–251.
18. Cercek L. and Cercek B. (1975b) Apparent tumour specificity with the SCM test. *Br. J. Cancer* **31,** 252–253.
19. Cercek L. and Cercek B. (1976) Effects of osmolarity, calcium and magnesium ions on the structuredness of cytoplasmic matrix (SCM). *Radiat. Environ. Biophys.* **13,** 9–12.
20. Cercek L. and Cercek B. (1977) Application of the phenomena of changes in the structuredness of the cytoplasmic matrix (SCM) in the diagnosis of malignant disorders. A review. *Eur. J. Cancer* **13,** 903–915.
21. Cercek L. and Cercek B. (1978a) Detection of malignant disease by changes in the structuredness of cytoplasmic matrix of lymphocytes induced by phytohaemagglutinin and cancer basic proteins. In: Griffiths K., Neville A. M., Pierrepoint C. G. (eds.), *Tumour Markers – 6th Tenovus Workshop.* Cardiff, Alpha Omega.
22. Cercek L. and Cercek B. (1978b) Effects of osmolarity and density of gradients on the isolation of SCM responding lymphocytes. *Br. J. Cancer* **38,** 163–165.
23. Cercek L., Cercek B. and Franklin C. I. V. (1974b) Biophysical differentiation between lymphocytes from healthy donors, patients with malignant disease and other diseases. *Br. J. Cancer* **29,** 345–352.
24. Cercek L., Cercek B. and Garrett J. V. (1974a) Biophysical differentiation between normal human and chronic lymphocyte leukaemia lymphocytes. In: Lindahl-Kiessling K. and Osoba K. (eds.), *Lymphocyte Recognition and Effector Mechanisms.* London, Academic Press, p. 553.
25. Cercek L., Cercek B. and Ockey C. H. (1973) Cell membrane permeability during the cell generation cycle in Chinese hamster ovary cells. *Biophysik.* **10,** 195–197.
26. Cochran A. J. (1978) In: *Man, Cancer and Immunity.* London, Academic Press, p. 5–66.

27. David J. R. (1968) Macrophage migration. *Fed. Proc.* **27** (1) 6–12.
28. David J. R., Al-Askari S., Lawrence H. S. et al. (1964) Delayed hypersensitivity *in vitro.* 1. The specificity of inhibition of cell migration by antigens. *J. Immunol.* **93**, 264–278.
29. Dickinson J. P., Caspary E. A. and Field E. J. (1972) Localisation of tumour specific antigen on the external surface of plasma membranes. *Nature* (*New Biol.*) **239** (93) 181–183.
30. Dickinson J. P., Caspary E. A. and Field E. J. (1973) A common tumour specific antigen 1. Restriction *in vivo* to malignant neoplastic tissue. *Br. J. Cancer* **27**, 99–104.
31. Diengdoh J. V. and Turk J. L. (1968) Electrophoretic mobility of guinea pig peritoneal exudate cells in hypersensitivity reactions. *Int. Arch. Allergy Appl. Immunol.* **43**, 297–302.
32. Douwes F. R., Hütteman U., and Mross K. (1977) Immundiagnostik maligner erkranbungen. *Dtsch. Med. Wochenschr.* **102**, 419–422.
33. Duncan W. and Kerr G. R. (1976) The curability of breast cancer. *Br. Med. J.* **2**, 781–783.
34. Dyson J. E. D. and Corbett P. J. (1978) Effect of lymphocyte supernatants on the electrophoretic mobility of erythrocytes: Significance in cancer diagnosis. *Br. J. Cancer* **38**, 401–410.
35. Dyson J. and Dickinson J. P. (1978) Personal communication.
36. Everson T. C. and Cole W. H. (1966) *Spontaneous Regression of Cancer.* Philadelphia, Saunders, pp. 1–487.
37. Fass L., Heberman R. B. and Ziegler J. (1970a) Delayed cutaneous hypersensitivity to autologous Burkitt lymphoma cells. *N. Engl. J. Med.* **282** (14), 776–789.
38. Fass L., Ziegler J. L., Herberman R. B. et al. (1970b) Cutaneous hypersensitivity reactions to autologous extracts of malignant melanoma cells. *Lancet* **1**, 116–118.
39. Field E. J. (1973) Macrophage electrophoretic migration (MEM) test in cancer. In: Björklung B. (ed.), *Immunological Techniques for the Detection of Cancer.* Sweden, Bonniers, p. 79.
40. Field E. J. and Caspary E. A. (1970) Lymphocyte sensitisation: an *in vitro* test for cancer. *Lancet* **2**, 1337.
41. Field E. J. and Caspary E. A. (1971a) Inhibition of lymphocyte response by serum. *Lancet* **2**, 95–96.
42. Field E. J. and Caspary E. A. (1971b) Lymphocyte response depressive factors in multiple sclerosis. *Br. Med. J.* **4**, 529–532.
43. Field E. J. and Caspary E. A. (1972a) Lymphocyte sensitisation in advanced malignant disease: A study of serum lymphocyte depressive factor. *Br. J. Cancer* **26**, 164–173.
44. Field E. J. and Caspary E. A. (1972b) Lymphocyte sensitisation to carcinogenic antigen (gold) with special reference to multiple sclerosis. *Br. Med. J.* **4**, 261–263.
45. Field E. J., Caspary E. A. and Shepherd R. H. (1972) Immunodiagnosis of cancer. *Br. Med. J.* **3**, 641–642.
46. Field E. J., Caspary E. A. and Smith K. S. (1973) Macrophage electrophoretic mobility (MEM) test in cancer: A critical evaluation. *Br. J. Cancer* **28** Suppl. 1, 208–214.
47. Field E. J. and Shenton B. K. (1975) Macrophage electrophoretic mobility (MEM) test for lymphocyte sensitisation: Importance of macrophages from healthy animals. *I.R.C.S. Med. Sci.* **3**, 154.
48. Foley E. J. (1953) Antigenic properties of methylcholanthrene induced tumours in mice of the strain of origin. *Cancer Res.* **13**, 835–837.

49. Forrester J. A., Dando P. M., Smith W. J. et al. (1977) Failure to confirm the macrophage electrophoretic mobility test in cancer. *Br. J. Cancer* **36**, 537–544.
50. Glaves D., Harlos J. P. and Weiss L. (1977) The macrophage electrophoretic mobility test: Results of carcinoma of the colon and rectum. *Int. J. Cancer* **19**, 474–481.
51. Goldstone A. H., Kerr L. and Irvine W. J. (1973) The macrophage electrophoretic migration test in cancer. *Clin. Exp. Immunol.* **14**, 469–472.
52. Gross L. (1943) Intradermal immunisation of C3H mice against a sarcoma that originated in an animal of the same line. *Cancer Res.* **3**, 326–333.
53. Harlos J. P. and Weiss L. (1978) Comparison between the macrophage electrophoretic mobility (MEM) and Fixiell tanned erythrocyte electrophoretic mobility (FTEEM) tests in the detection of cancer. *Int. J. Cancer* **21**, 413–417.
54. Hashimoto Y., Yamanada T. and Takaku F. (1978) Differentiation between patients with malignant diseases and non-malignant diseases or healthy donors by changes of fluorescence polarisation in the cytoplasm of circulating lymphocytes. *Gen.* **69**, 145–149.
55. Helmholtz H. (1879) Studien iiber electrische grenzschichten. *Ann. Physik* **7**, 337–341.
56. Hellström I. and Hellström K. E. (1969a) Studies on cellular immunity and its serum mediated inhibition in Moloney-virus induced mouse sarcomas. *Int. J. Cancer* **4**, 587–600.
57. Hellström K. E. and Hellström I. (1969b) Cellular immunity against tumor antigens. *Adv. Cancer Res.* **12**, 167–223.
58. Henderson M. (1976) Validity of screening. *Cancer* **37**, 573–581.
59. Hobbs J. R. (1974) Laboratory monitoring and screening for cancer. *Lancet* **2**, 1305–1307.
60. Hollinshead A., McWright C. G., Alford T. C. et al. (1972) Separation of skin reactive intestinal cancer antigen from carcinoma-embryonic antigen of gold. *Science* **177**, 887–889.
61. Hughes L. E. and Lytton B. (1964) Antigenic properties of human tumours: Delayed cutaneous hypersensitivity reactions. *Br. Med. J.* **1**, 209–212.
62. Jenssen H. L. and Shenton B. K. (1975) Electrophoretic mobility test for lymphocyte sensitisation using tanned sheep erythrocytes. *Acta Biol. Med. Ger.* **34**, 29–33.
63. Kreitzmann H., Flieder T. M., Galla H. J. et al. (1978) Fluorescence polarisation changes in mononuclear blood leucocytes after PHA incubation: Differences in cells from patients with and without neoplasia. *Br. J. Cancer* **37**, 797–805.
64. Lampert F., Mitzschke U. and Zwergel T. (1977) Lymphocyte sensitisation in childhood solid tumours and lymphoblastic leukaemia, measured by electrophoretic mobility test. *Br. J. Cancer* **35**, 844–849.
65. Lewkonia R. M., Kerr E. J. L. and Irvine W. J. (1974) Clinical evaluation of the macrophage electrophoretic mobility test for cancer. *Br. J. Cancer* **30**, 532–537.
66. Minderhoud J. M. and Smith J. K. (1972) Immunological activity of blood lymphocyte fractions: A study by the macrophage electrophoretic mobility method. *Clin. Exp. Immunol.* **10**, 571–579.
67. Meyer-Reinecker H., Jenssen H. L., Köhler H. et al. (1975) Zur Bedentung des Makrophagen-Elektrophorese-Mobilitätstests für die Diagnostik de geschwülste des Zentralrowensystems. *Dtsch. Med. Wochenschr.* **100**, 538–543.
68. Müller M., Irmscher J., Fischer R. et al. (1977) Immunological tumour profile: Organ-specific carcinoma diagnosis in patients employing the Macrophage Electrophoretic Mobility Test. *Cancer Letters* **2**, 139–146.

69. Nakajima T., Chikamori M., Isojima K. et al. (1977) Lymphocyte reactivity to allogenic tumours antigens and myelin basic protein in gastric cancer patients. *Gen.* **68,** 449–457.

70. Pasternak L., Jenssen H. L., Köhler H. and Pasternak G. (1976) Cross reactions among mouse tumours of different etiology as detected by Macrophage Electrophoretic Mobility (MEM) Test. *Eur. J. Cancer* **12,** 389–393.

71. Pentycross C. R. (1968) Personal communication. PhD. Thesis University of London.

72. Porzsölt F., Mühlberger G. and Ax W. (1975a) Electrophoretic mobility Test (EMT). II. Is there a correlation between the clinical diagnosis and immunologic test for pre-cancerous disease? *Behring Inst. Mitt.* No. 57. 137–145.

73. Porzsölt F., Tautz Ch. and Ax W. (1975b) Electrophoretic mobility test. 1. Modifications to simplify the detection of malignant disease in man. *Behring Inst. Mitt.* No. 57. 128–136.

74. Preece A. W. and Light P. A. (1974) The Macrophage Electrophoretic Mobility (MEM) test for malignant disease. Further clinical investigations and studies on macrophage slowing factor. *Clin. Exp. Immunol.* **18,** 543–552.

75. Preece A. W. and Light P. A. (1976) The granulocyte electrophoretic mobility (GEM) test for malignant disease. *I.R.C.S. Med. Sci.* **4,** 201.

76. Pritchard J. A. V. (1978) The MEM Test. In: Griffiths K., Neville A. M. and Pierrepoint C. G. (eds.), *Tumour Markers – 6th Tenovus Workshop.* Baltimore, University Park Press, Cardiff, Alpha Omega, p. 199.

77. Pritchard J. A. V., Davies D. K. L. and Preece P. (1977) Unpublished data.

78. Pritchard J. A. V., Moore J. L., Sutherland W. H. et al. (1972) Immunodiagnosis of cancer. *Br. Med. J.* **3,** 823.

79. Pritchard J. A. V., Moore J. L., Sutherland W. H. et al. (1973a) Evaluation and development of the Macrophage Electrophoretic Mobility (MEM) test for malignant disease. *Br. J. Cancer* **27,** 1–9.

80. Pritchard J. A. V., Moore J. L., Sutherland W. H. et al. (1973b) Technical aspects of the Macrophage Electrophoretic Mobility (MEM) test for malignant disease. *Br. J. Cancer* **28,** Suppl. 1, 229–236.

81. Pritchard J. A. V., Moore J. L., Sutherland W. H. et al. (1976) Clinical assessment of the MOD-MEM cancer test in controls with non-malignant disease. *Br. J. Cancer* **34,** 1–6.

82. Pritchard J. A. V. and Sutherland W. H. (1978) Lymphocyte response to antigen stimulation as measured by fluorescence polarisation (SCM) Test. *Br. J. Cancer* **38,** 339–343.

83. Pritchard J. A. V., Sutherland W. H. and Deeley T. J. (1976) Cancer detection. *Lancet* **1,** 637.

84. Pritchard J. A. V., Sutherland W. H., Teasdale C. et al. (1978) The Macrophage Electrophoretic Mobility (MEM) Test – an investigation of its value as a routine laboratory test in the detection of malignant disease. *Ann. Clin. Res.* **10,** 71–74.

85. Rahi A. H. S., Otiko G. and Winder A. F. (1976) Evaluation of Macrophage Electrophoretic Mobility (MEM) Test as an indicator of cellular immunity in ocular tumours. *Br. J. Ophthalmol.* **60,** 589–593.

86. Rawlins G. A., Wood J. M. F. and Bagshawe K. D. (1976) Macrophage Electrophoretic Mobility (MEM) with myelin basic protein. *Br. J. Cancer* **34,** 613–618.

87. Ristow S. and McKann C. F. (1977) Tumour associated antigens. In: Green I. Cohen S. and McLuskey C. F. (eds.), *Mechanisms of Tumour Immunity,* New York, Wiley, pp. 109–145.

88. Sackett D. L. (1975) Screening for early detection of disease: To what purpose? *Bull. NY. Acad. Med.* **51** (1), 39–52.

89. Shenton B. K. and Field E. J. (1975) The Macrophage Electrophoretic Mobility (MEM) test. Some technical considerations. *J. Immunol. Methods* **1,** 149–162

90. Shenton B. K., Hughes D. and Field E. J. (1973) Macrophage Electrophoretic Migration (MEM) test for lymphocyte sensitisation: Some practical experience in macrophage selection. *Br. J. Cancer* **28** Suppl. 1, 215–218.
91. Shelton B. K., Jenssen H. L., Werner H. et al. (1977) A comparison of the kinetics of the Macrophage Electrophoretic Mobility (MEM) and Tanned sheep Erythrocyte Electrophoretic Mobility (TEEM) tests. *J. Immunol. Methods* **14,** 123–139.
92. Southam C. M. (1967) Evidence for cancer specific antigens in man. *Prog. Exp. Tumour Res.* **9,** 1–39.
93. Southam C. M. (1973) Effects of malignant tumours on immune response. In: *Immunology and Cancer.* Ottawa, University of Ottawa Press, p. 45.
94. Smith J. J. (1977) Personal communication.
95. Smith J. J. (1978) Personal communication.
96. Smith J. J. and Dickinson J. P. (1976) Cell partition: A simple test for lymphocyte sensitisation. *Lancet* **2,** 1336–1337.
97. Sundaram K., Phonke G. and Sunderesan P. (1967) *In vitro* studies in antibody production by lymph node cells using cells electrophoresis. *Immunology* **13,** 433–439.
98. Sutherland W. H., Pritchard J. A. V. and Smith C. W. (1977) The clinical assessment of cancer tests: A statistical approach to the production of false positive rates from controls. *Ann. Clin. Res.* **9,** 45–51.
99. Takaku F., Yamanaka T. and Hashimoto Y. (1977) Usefulness of the SCM test in the diagnosis of gastric cancer. *Br. J. Cancer* **36,** 810–813.
100. Tognella S., Mantovani G., Floris C. et al. (1975) Test Citroferometrico per l'evidenziazone di cinofociti sensibilizzati ad antigeni neoplastici (MEM Test). *Tumori* **60,** 203–210.
101. Walter H., Krob E. J. and Ascher G. S. (1969) Separation of lymphocytes and polymorphonuclear leucocytes by ionic current distribution in aqueous two polymer system. *Exp. Cell Res.* **55,** 279–283.
102. Wass M., Pentycross C. R., Rawlins G. A. et al. (1977) Response of lymphocytes from cancer patients to human chorionic gonadotrophin. *Lancet* **1,** 181–172.

George A. Edelstyn

3 Breast Cancer

INTRODUCTION

To write a chapter on breast cancer integrating the various disciplines involved with their multiple, conflicting approaches to virtually every aspect of the disease whilst doing justice to all is an impossible task, so there is no apology for what many will judge a lamentable failure. To further confuse matters, strongly held views alter with time, sometimes rapidly and often profoundly.

Probably each generation tackling this problem feels its contribution to be the most important yet to emerge, and no doubt we are as guilty of such intellectual conceit as our bygone colleagues. Nevertheless, certain important matters are for the first time gaining general acceptance. Thus, the acquisition of reliable cancer statistics indicates that despite improvement in surgical and radiotherapeutic technology, mortality rates have not improved as might logically have been expected. A clinico-pathological appraisal of the reasons underlying this situation has led to an increasing appreciation that the cause of failure commonly lies beyond the scope of these local treatments, namely in microscopic dissemination of disease far from the primary growth and originating at some ill-defined time prior to clinical diagnosis. Hence come arguments for systemic treatment hopefully capable of reaching and eradicating this widespread disease. The emergence of the anti-oestrogens and of combination chemotherapy, now developed to a point at which it would be inappropriate to be considered as just a progression of original single drug treatments, have given clinicians possible tools for this purpose. Such developments could mean that the next decade will unveil real achievements in the century's old battle to reduce mortality rates from this disease.

History

It is fascinating and informative to consider the history of breast cancer treatment, though 5000 years of evolution affords little ground for satisfaction. Some of the ancient remedies may have been little less effective than certain current practices though possibly giving the patient more support and inflicting less undesirable sequelae. Thus, the Ebers medical papyrus of 3000 BC mentions calamine, caul of ox, flies' dirt and yellow ochre, mixed together and rubbed on the breast for four days. An Indian writing about 2000 BC describes surgical extirpation, cautery and arsenical ointments. Celsus (25BC–50AD) believed treatment could be damaging and that surgery should be limited and used only in the earliest cases whilst extensive operations involving removal of the pectoral muscles were not indicated. Relatively major surgery was common at the time and continued for a thousand years until 1162 when Church authorities at the Council of Tours declared against such practices. Whilst this may have been for reactionary reasons, the decision would seem reasonable to many today. Perhaps however the Council were better informed than we know, for an Arabian surgeon Abu 'el-Quasim had written with rare objectivity a few years before that he had never been able to cure a case of breast cancer nor did he know of anyone who had.

In the nineteenth century Robert Liston (1794–1847) commented: 'No one could now be found so rash or cruel as to attempt the removal of (axillary) glands thus affected whether primarily or secondarily.' About the same time Sir James Paget (1814–99) wrote: 'We have to ask ourselves whether it is probable that the operation [mastectomy] will add to the length or comfort of life enough to justify incurring the risk of its consequences.' He went on: 'In deciding for or against the removal of the cancerous breast in any single case we may I think, dismiss the fact that the operation will be the final remedy for the disease.' Another surgeon Hayes Agnew could not claim one single cured case amongst his own series: 'I do not despair of carcinoma being cured in the future, but this blessed achievement will never be wrought by the knife of the surgeon.'

Up to this time local mastectomy had been commonplace, but increasing awareness of the high incidence of local recurrence led towards more radical surgery in the hope that residual cancer tissue left by the simpler procedure might be removed and cure achieved. A number of nineteenth century surgeons accepted this philosophy and indeed the basic foundations for the classical radical mastectomy ascribed to Halstead were laid by others some years earlier. There can be little doubt that results obtained represented an improvement on those which had gone before, though current developments in asepsis and anaesthesia reduced immediate postoperative mortality and allowed surgery to be more thorough. These factors, associated with an increasingly informed approach to operability criteria based on the clinical extent of the disease, also made an important contribution and still does to the subsequent gradual improvement in results though the technique itself has remained largely unchanged.

The mid-twentieth century initiated the 'era of the pendulum' with opinions on appropriate treatment for primary disease moving increasingly apart. One extreme advocated removal of the lump alone, usually followed by radiotherapy to the breast residue. The other extreme advocated extended or even supraradical mastectomy, sometimes with contralateral mastectomy on the grounds of disease multifocality. One description of such approaches was 'the contemporary consummation of somatic reduction, limited solely by the ability of the human remnant to survive.'

Somewhere between these limits presumably rests appropriate local treatment, i.e. the least disturbing procedure compatible with commonly accepted 10-year survival figures. This implies minimal mortality and morbidity, both immediate and delayed, physical and psychological. Just what constitutes such a procedure, a matter of considerable importance, remains in dispute. Reliable answers to such questions can only be obtained by prospective clinical trial and had this approach been adopted earlier, the medical profession would have been saved much inconclusive argument based on dogma deriving from superstition, myth, and other human frailties. Facts upon which progress could be built or at least a realization of shortcomings might have emerged and many patients would have avoided considerable suffering which contributed little or nothing to their ultimate well-being.

Magnitude of the Problem

In western society 1 in 15 women will contract breast cancer. Britain experiences approximately 12 000 deaths annually; in the USA the figure is almost three times greater whilst the global total is perhaps a quarter of a million. These figures make breast cancer the commonest fatal malignant disease amongst women. More sadly still is its social significance, for in the age group 35–54 years it is the commonest cause of all deaths, four times that of bowel cancer, six times that due to accidents, and thirteen times more frequent than cervical cancer. It is just in this age group that woman's role within the family and society is at a maximum so that disruption of life, distress and economic repercussions of such an event are enormous.

Basic Issues

Surprisingly with so many patients available for study, basic issues about disease behaviour and treatment have remained obscure. A few observers have long doubted traditional concepts but these have only lately come under serious debate. This questions the standard view that if only the correct loco-regional treatment, some undefined combination of surgery and radiotherapy, could be devised and promptly applied so as to eradicate disease in breast and glands then cure would result. Certain questions which had never been answered, let alone asked, now seem clear, e.g. what is the genuine cure rate in breast cancer and how is it related to treatment? Consideration of these points results not from some fundamental breakthrough in knowledge, but rather a gradual realization of facts long available yet poorly appreciated.

The Probable Cure Rate

The potential for cure inherent in local treatment has been well reviewed (Baum [14]). Thus the Brinkley and Haybittle study [23] probably the most accurate of its type suggests that at 20 years, an overall 18 per cent of patients are cured, the figure rising to 30 per cent for those presenting with early cancer. Other series range from almost 40 per cent (Adair [1]) to the gloomy view (Bond [19]) that virtually none are cured. From these and other studies Baum concludes that between 20 and 30 per cent of women treated for early breast cancer enjoy a normal life expectancy. However this figure is not necessarily wholly ascribable to treatment, because some women survive untreated for many years. The influence of this fact could only be determined by a controlled prospective study in which half the patients received no active treatment. As this is impossible, evidence has to be historical, based on more or less comparable groups of patients who for some reason remained untreated. Considering available information, Baum concludes that the closest approximation to such a study is that of MacKay and Sellers [114]. From a rather small series of patients with apparently early disease they demonstrate a 68 per cent 5-year survival rate, a figure comparable to that obtained in many treated series. The possible influence of such facts upon commonly claimed cure rates, merits reflection. Relationships between the time of diagnosis, its influence on treatment outcome and prognosis will be discussed later.

ROLE OF CLINICAL TRIAL: TREATMENT TYPE AND RESULTS

A *British Medical Journal* Editorial [57, 58] observed that the major problems in breast cancer treatment resulted from the fallacy of clinical staging, long survival of untreated patients, and the dearth of controlled studies. However, although the first problem may make it difficult to assess the individual patient, it is the second two that make this field so uncertain. It is a widely accepted truism that adequate assessment of any treatment requires patients and patience. Patients, should present no problem if trial recruitment is on a multicentre basis. Patience is more of a problem, as long follow-up times are required, 10 years being a realistic minimum and 20 years more desirable. This clearly presents problems for individual doctor's careers, as the fruits of their labours and subsequent publications are long in coming. The lack of controlled studies is surprising, though the randomized controlled trial is a relatively recent development. Barnes [11] illustrates how medical knowledge was acquired as recently as the early 20th century by discussing surgery for visceral ptosis; for example, when the kidney was supposed to be too low, the patient's neurosis, back pain, constipation, etc. were all explained. Operations were performed, and repeated if judged necessary. Although the concept underlying such treatment is now believed incorrect, the unfortunate aspect is the length of time this idea was accepted, and was probably due to the lack of control experience, a concept which was unknown at that time.

A control allows a valid comparison to be made between one treatment and an alternative treatment policy which may be nothing, a placebo, or another active treatment. In the recent past, attempts have been made to use historical controls, or results in one centre with a particular treatment have been compared with results in another centre with an alternative treatment. Byar et al. [33] have written an excellent critique of such practices, arguing that by far the most useful method of comparison is randomization, by which patients considered as being suitable for study are randomly allocated to one of the alternative treatments. Randomization has three major benefits, all essential for obtaining clear unequivocal answers in clinical research. First, allocation bias is removed, by ensuring that choice, conscious or unconscious, does not give rise to different sorts of patients in the two treatments. Secondly, the two treatment groups will tend to become balanced in terms of covariates, or predictive factors. Thus, even if cancer staging is difficult, this error will be applied in an equal and unbiased manner to both treatments and will not give rise to a systematic difference between the two groups. Thirdly, randomization validates statistical tests of significance. The theory underlying the statistical analysis of a treatment comparison is based on calculating the probability that apparent differences will occur in a trial even when no difference between the treatment exists. Randomly occurring differences are assumed to be the only sort present, and if the apparent difference shown in the data is so large that it would be extremely unlikely if there was no true difference, it is concluded that the difference is statistically significant. 'Extremely unlikely' is usually taken as being 5 per cent, or preferably 1 per cent or less.

The need for controls, and for randomization, has been long appreciated, but a further problem exists, namely the amount of data available. In order to be reasonably certain (95 per cent) that a trial will detect an improvement in efficacy from a success rate of 50 per cent to a rate of 55 per cent the two treatment groups each need 2590 patients. The largest trial of local treatment in breast cancer to date, that sponsored by the Cancer Research Campaign [102], had a total usable recruitment of over 2200 patients, enough to be 95 per cent confident of detecting an improvement in success rate of from 50–57·5 per cent. The next largest trials are the two from Manchester [54] each with over 700 patients. Taken separately each can detect (at a 95 per cent confidence) a 13 per cent improvement (i.e. from 50 per cent to 63 per cent). Viewed as one trial, by combining results the difference detectable would be about 10 per cent. Other trials have reported results in about 400 cases [8, 27, 94], a number capable of detecting an improvement of about 18 per cent. Some even smaller trials have been reported; Brinkley and Haybittle [22] having about 200 cases in all, and Turnbull et al. [162] reporting 150 cases. The former is capable of detecting a 25 per cent, and the latter a 28 per cent difference. Not surprisingly, few significant differences have been found in the trials mentioned, as these would have had to be very large to have had a reasonable chance of detection. The main conclusions that seem to emerge are that (a) radical surgery, with or without radiotherapy, does not appear to offer any major benefit over conservative surgery plus radiotherapy, (b) radiotherapy added to simple mastectomy may reduce the incidence of local recurrence, and (c) if radiotherapy is delayed until a recurrence is observed instead of being given routinely postoperatively no worsening of prognosis appears to occur.

INVESTIGATION OF THE PATIENT WITH A POSSIBLE CLINICAL CANCER

Differentiation between benign and malignant breast lesions is a surgical matter and will not be discussed in detail here. Apart from the clinical impression, needle aspiration and radiology repeated at regular intervals if need be, can be of considerable help, but if doubt persists then biopsy is required. Assuming a histological report preferably obtained by paraffin rather than by frozen section confirms carcinoma, then thorough and rapid investigations are required before treatment is undertaken. Symptoms which might indicate distant metastases must be carefully evaluated. Local findings will have been noted, particular attention being paid to the situation, size and fixation of the primary and related glands. Clinical examination may exclude grosser metastatic disease such as pleural effusion, hepatic enlargement and, by pelvic examination, sizeable ovarian deposits.

First investigations are commonly radiology of chest and skeleton. Standard X-ray however fails to detect bone metastases until 75 per cent of cancellous bone has been destroyed, thus in the lumbar vertebrae a defect of up to 2 cm can escape detection [55]. Despite this limitation occult metastases are demonstrated in from 2 to 5 per cent of 'early' patients. Radioisotope scanning using a variety of technetium phosphorus compounds and either a gamma camera or a rectilinear scanner has superior detection potential. Galasko [68] claims positive results in 20 per cent of patients with 'early' disease, stating that focal non-symmetrical uptake unassociated with degenerative or other bone disease is a strong indicator of metastatic cancer. In one series agreement between X-rays and scan findings was noted in 80 per cent of 824 patients (Kirkman and Henk) [103]. However amongst those with any form of clinically local disease, a positive bone scan and negative X-rays were found in 20 per cent, the figure for early cancers being 15 per cent. Of this total 80 per cent were confirmed metastatic within two years. Conversely only 3·7 per cent of patients with normal scans developed metastases within 1 year. The situation is not so clear cut however for in a survey of 8 centres, the British Breast Group [24] found that whilst on average 10 per cent of preoperative bone scans were positive, variations between centres ranged from 2 per cent to 20 per cent. No explanation was found for such discrepancies, but there must be serious inconsistencies in technique and interpretation needing clarification before results can be uniformly accepted. In addition as there must be a minimum finite though unknown size for detection, the earlier the patient is diagnosed the more deposits will be missed. One series [159] demonstrated that amongst patients presenting with diagnosable metastatic disease, bone scans failed to correlate with necropsy findings in approximately one third of instances yet such metastases must have been considerably larger than when the patients had originally been diagnosed with 'early' cancer. This is not surprising when it is remembered that the overall detection rate quoted above was 10 per cent, whilst bony metastases were probably present in at least two-thirds.

Urinary hydroxyproline levels related to creatinine excretion are also of value. Disadvantages are that values may be elevated by non-malignant bony disease and that for three days prior to urine collection the patient must avoid gelatine-containing foods. Under the optimal circumstances most patients with elevated levels and negative X-rays will ultimately demonstrate bony metastases [47 or 48]. Information may also be obtained by simpler means, e.g. serum alkaline phosphatase and urinary calcium levels, but abnormalities are not necessarily diagnostic of metastatic bone disease. Liver metastases are even more difficult. Thus, the Merion-Thomas study demonstrated a poor relationship between non-invasive liver assessment by radioisotope scanning, ultrasound and liver function tests as compared with laparotomy. Less than one-third of patients shown to have hepatic involvement had this suggested by preoperative assessment. Even in the presence of obvious metastatic disease, correlation with autopsy findings was poor.

Lymph Node Status

Closely related to prognosis, nodal status remains the most important single factor in deciding the management of 'early' cancer currently being the determinant for systemic treatment. Incidentally, as chemotherapy is most effective in the presence of minimum residual cancer tissue, nodes should not only be sampled but also eradicated, though not necessarily by the same procedure. There is no problem if a radical mastectomy has been performed but more conservative surgical procedures require separate diagnostic action. Random axillary biopsy is convenient but gives 20 per cent erroneous results [65]. Formal axillary dissection may be associated with conservative surgical procedures. Combined with local mastectomy it is termed a 'Patey' mastectomy, and gives reliable information about the axilla, whilst itself constituting a therapeutic measure may avoid the need for irradiating that region.

Internal Mammary Nodes

It is illogical to assume that internal mammary nodes are less significant than axillary nodes though their evaluation attracts less attention. Caceres [34] has shown such involvement in 13 per cent of outer half, 21 per cent of central, and 28 per cent of inner half tumours. With a negative axilla, internal mammary nodes were involved in 7 per cent of patients, rising to 29 per cent when the axillary nodes were positive, irrespective of primary site. In these circumstances figures for medial tumours were 44 per cent, central tumours 33 per cent, whilst outer half tumours had 19 per cent. Information about internal mammary nodes is less important with positive axillary nodes as these will dictate treatment. In an individual patient problems arise when the axilla is negative though internal mammary nodes are probably uninvolved when the growth is in the outer half. They are however more likely to be involved in inner half tumours unless there is contrary evidence obtained by node dissection or more simply by biopsy, though neither procedure finds much favour. The CT scanner seems of limited value, and perhaps the best method is isotope lymphography. Ege [60] reporting over 1000 results found that amongst patients with a negative axilla 16 per cent have clearly abnormal findings with a further 16 per cent designated suspicious. Over three years he claims that the treatment failure rate experienced is similar to that amongst patients with a positive axilla and negative internal mammary scan. This suggests that the investigation might be incorporated in the routine evaluation of patients with negative axillae.

THE CLINICAL RELEVANCE OF TUMOUR MARKERS IN MANAGEMENT

There has been considerable interest for several years in the determination of substances that are characteristic of cancer cells, i.e. tumour markers. Since the ultimate purpose of developments in tumour detection is to provide useful clinical information the areas where biochemical monitoring of these substances may be of value and should first be considered are:

1. Early diagnosis of breast cancer and its distinction from benign disease.
2. Provision of a better prognostic index than axillary node involvement, thereby facilitating prediction of the necessity for adjuvant chemotherapy or immunotherapy.
3. Detection of relapse at an early stage as systemic cancer therapy is more effective in the presence of a small tumour burden.
4. More sensitive indication of response to treatment than radiological or other similar changes.
5. Recognition of drug resistance.
6. Localization of tumour metastases.

At present, biochemical monitoring can indicate overt metastatic disease, but ideally it should be possible to detect abnormal levels in the presence of micrometastases. The ideal marker should also be specific and its concentration in plasma or urine should be proportional to the tumour burden.

The object of this section is to review the available markers for breast cancer and to evaluate their usefulness and limitations in the context of their clinical application.

CLASSIFICATION AND CHARACTERISTICS OF TUMOUR MARKERS

The biochemical alterations that can be associated with cancer cells are of three types:

1. *Cell-associated components.* These include cell-surface antigens, which it is suggested exist on the tumour cell membrane. Hormone receptors should also be considered in this category of breast tumour markers.
2. *Secreted tumour markers.* These products, which are mainly specific proteins, including hormones, enzymes and antibodies, have been studied most widely. Tumour proteins may be adult or embryonic in type; the latter may be classed as fetal or placental. The observation of embryonic substances suggests that genetic depression is a common and possibly universal phenomenon in cancer cells. A further indication of this feature is the appearance of 'inappropriate' or 'ectopic' products in neoplastic tissue.
3. *Biochemical response to tumour.* Serum constituents normally present may undergo a change in the cancer-bearing patient.

Cell-associated Components

Cell Surface Antigens

Identification of these markers has been based on evidence that they provoke a humoral or cellular immune response in the host. Some *in vitro* tests of cell-mediated immunity have been established on the finding that peripheral blood lymphocytes from cancer patients respond to crude extracts of myelin basic protein [62] or a tumour extract called 'cancer basic protein' [49]. These methods involve tests of macrophage electrophoretic mobility [62] and structuredness of cytoplasmic matrix [37]. The sensitization of lymphocytes has been shown more directly by simple histone micro-agglutination [151] and more recently a poly-L-lysine-induced agglutination assay has been described by Bauer and Ax [13]. A range of other methods encompassing intradermal sensitization tests [86], cytotoxicity assays [9], tests of leucocyte adherence [74] have also been assessed for a variety of malignant disease types, including breast cancer. None are clinically applicable, however, in their present form, as considerable uncertainty exists concerning their specificity, reproducibility and interpretation.

Hormone Receptors

The measurement of cytoplasmic oestrogen (ER) protein in biopsy specimens is a useful marker of hormone dependence of a breast tumour [111]. Tumours containing ER have a 50–55 per cent response rate to endocrine therapies, whereas less than 10 per cent of ER negative tumours are sensitive. It has been noted that the presence or absence of ER is the single most important prognostic factor of early disease relapse in primary breast cancer [106]. Eighteen months after mastectomy, recurrence occurred in 34 per cent of 54 ER negative cases and in only 13 per cent of 91 ER positive patients. This pattern was independent of other known prognostic variables. It is suggested that ER negative tumours have a higher growth fraction [120] and cytotoxic agents are known to be more effective in rapidly proliferating tissues. Detailed studies of response to chemotherapy and correlation with ER status are now emerging, but the results are conflicting. Allegra et al. [5] and Jonat and Maass [93] reported that the response rate to chemotherapy is significantly higher in receptor-poor tumours, whereas contradictory results have been obtained by Frenning et al. [67], Kiang and Kennedy [102].

The subdivision of mammary carcinomas into ER positive and negative categories is an oversimplification. Recent studies have demonstrated a correlation between the amount of receptor and an increased probability of response to hormone therapy [112]. This quantitative approach can help to determine whether ablative treatment or a less aggressive endocrine therapy should be used in the first instance. In an effort to determine which ER positive tumours will not respond to hormonal therapy, additional markers of the oestrogen response pathway have been suggested. These include progesterone receptor and nuclear oestrogen receptor [111] and oestrogen-inducible enzymes [52, 53]. Androgen [87, 167] and glucocorticoid [87] receptors have also been demonstrated. While the significance of these additional steroid receptors is not clear, it is probable that simultaneous assays of hormone receptors in human breast tumours would provide greater correlation with therapeutic results. There are several sources of error in the ER binding assays, the major complication being that oestrogen binds unspecifically the albumin and specifically the sex hormone binding globulin [128]. Improvements in methods for separating steroid-bound ER have provided better data, but more important progress may depend on the purification of ER and the development of antisera to ER for the establishment of radioimmunoassays.

Secreted Tumour Products

The products involved include:

Fetal and Placental Antigens

Several fetal antigens are recognized but only carcinoembryonic antigen (CEA), α_2-H-foetoprotein (ferritin) and DNA-binding protein have proved to be of practical value in management of breast cancer.

CEA

Since CEA was first described by Gold and Freedman [71], elevated plasma levels have been observed in a variety of malignant and non-malignant states [124]. Several studies of CEA levels encountered in breast cancer [21, 38, 109, 123, 157, 161, 170] lead to the conclusion that plasma CEA is not an efficient indicator of primary disease or early metastases. It can be of some use, however, in prognosis and clinical monitoring of disseminated disease, although some conflicting data exist in the literature. The importance of CEA determinations in prognosis is unclear. Post-mastectomy values have been correlated with recurrence rate [170], but this finding has been disputed by Tormey and colleagues [161]. These authors observed good correlation of CEA levels with response to chemotherapy: less meaningful results, however, have been reported by Steward and his coworkers [157]. In general, CEA levels paralleled patient response to chemotherapy [157, 161] and hormonal therapy [157], but Chu and Nemoto [38] found clinical improvement with chemotherapy sometimes to precede fall in CEA levels. Also, Borthwick et al. [21] showed monitoring of anti-oestrogen therapy using CEA determinations was not always accurate. It is obvious that more detailed studies are required before the role of CEA in assessing the treatment of breast cancer is established.

Ferritin

A significant increase in the ferritin content of several mammary carcinomas suggested its possible use as a marker [117]. Elevated levels of serum ferritin have been found in 41 per cent of 38 preoperative patients and in 67 per cent of 97 women with locally recurrent or metastatic disease [117]. Patients with initial circulating ferritin concentrations above 200 μg/l have a higher recurrence rate during the subsequent 4 years [90]. Elevated ferritin levels have obviously some clinical significance.

DNA-binding Protein

A human serum DNA-binding protein, C3DP, has been associated with various neoplastic disorders [85, 131]. Unlike other tumour markers, it appears to be present regardless of the type of cancer or tissue of origin; also, C3DP levels are normal or only slightly elevated in various non-malignant conditions. In monitoring the response of a variety of tumours to chemotherapy, Parsons et al. [130] found serum C3DP values declined abruptly in 89 per cent (25 out of 28) of patients showing favourable clinical responses, of which 10 out of 13 were cases of breast carcinoma.

Placental Antigens

A secondary category of substances secreted by the cancer cells are placental antigens. Human chorionic gonadotrophin (HCG), found in the serum of all trophoblastic tumours, has been studied in relation to breast cancer by Tormey et al. [160, 161], and placental alkaline phosphatase has also been investigated [35, 91]. Both of these antigens, however have found only little application to breast cancer studies.

Hormones

Numerous studies clearly demonstrate that, between them, all the types of tumour are capable of secreting virtually all of the polypeptide hormones. Ectopic production of both calcitonin and prostaglandins have been associated with mammary carcinomas.

Calcitonin

High plasma levels of immunoreactive calcitonin have been found in a number of advanced non-thyroid tumours, particularly in breast cancer [41]. Increased serum values were observed in 8 per cent of 13 patients with localized disease and in 82 per cent of 28 cases with metastatic disease, and so calcitonin levels may be useful in staging.

Prostaglandins

Breast tumours can produce materials that mediate bone destruction and there is considerable evidence that the prostaglandins are implicated in this respect [17, 51, 133]. Prostaglandin metabolites in urine [152] and in plasma [134] have been measured, but their significance in management of the disease has yet to be established.

Milk Protein

Clinical samples of human tumours and plasma from patients with mammary carcinoma show differences in the levels of certain milk proteins, particularly casein-K and α-lactalbumin.

Casein-K

Measurements of casein-K in plasma have been correlated with recurrence and metastatic extension, and surgical removal was found to produce a decreased incidence in elevated values if nodes were not involved [84, 176]. Casein-K is also a useful marker in staging and monitoring the breast cancer, but its role as a screening agent seems limited by the relatively high number of positive values for benign disease and also due to the large number of false negative results [175]. Also, casein-K is not specific for breast carcinoma, as elevated levels are found associated with pulmonary and digestive cancers [84, 176]. Reports on the production of casein-K by human breast carcinomas have been disputed by Monacco et al. [121], who found serum casein-K levels to be no higher in breast cancer patients than in controls. The conflicting data may arise from differences in specificity of the antibodies used in the casein-K radioimmunoassay.

α-lactalbumin

Normal circulating levels of α-lactalbumin in patients with mammary carcinoma have been reported by Kleinberg [105]. The radioimmunoassay of α-lactalbumin in serum, however, is subject to error due to the presence of antilactalbumin antibodies [175]. Using a modified procedure to prevent interference, Woods and Heath found that in women of reproductive age, the presence of α-lactalbumin is common; the protein is undetectable in normal post-menopausal women, but is present in the sera of breast cancer patients. There is some indication that the occurrence of α-lactalbumin in human breast tumours is related to the presence of oestrogen receptors but controversy exists [32, 175].

Enzymes and Metabolic Products

There are a number of enzymes which may originate directly from neoplastic tissue of which the glyocosyltransferases have received considerable attention [18, 83, 100, 101]. Sialyltransferase has been shown to be most sensitive for measuring the extent of neoplastic disease in breast cancer patients [89]; 42 per cent of 12 patients with benign disease, 67 per cent of 15 with primary breast cancer and 100 per cent of 24 with metastatic disease had elevated levels. Oddly, an apparent inverse relationship between serum sialyltransferase and lymph node involvement was noted and the cause of elevated levels associated with benign disease is unclear; sialyltransferase, however, is undoubtedly a useful tumour marker.

Polyamines have attracted interest in view of their probable function in regulating nucleic acid synthesis and consequently as possible indicators of malignancy. Increased amounts of putrescine, spermidine and spermine in the urine of cancer patients was reported originally by Russell and Russell [150] and it was proposed later that spermidine correlates with tumour cell kill, whereas putrescine reflects the growth fraction of the tumour [149]. Consequently pre- and post-treatment values could be useful in prognosis. Polyamines are not good indicators of disease stage in breast cancer, although the ratio of the pre- and post-treatment differences in spermine and spermidine correlate better with disease status than other possible combinations of the polyamines [173]. Attempts are being made to refine polyamine determinations in order to improve the significance of assay data [28, 147].

Increased amounts of RNA nucleosides have been observed in the urine of patients with various cancers [165]. In studies of breast cancer (Woo et al. [173]), N^2, N^2-dimethylguanosine levels were most frequently abnormal. Elevated amounts occurred in 57 per cent of 75 patients with metastatic disease. The ratio of the levels of N^2, N^2-dimethylguanosine and pseudouridine correlated better with disease status than the methylated nucleoside alone.

Biochemical Responses to Tumour

There is a vast range of serum protein anomalies that can occur in cancer patients, all of which are entirely non-specific. They can be useful, however, where no acute metabolic or inflammatory disease is present. The factors included below appear to have some potential for monitoring breast cancer.

Acute-phase Reactant Proteins

Plasma profiles of haptoglobin, α_1-acid glycoprotein, α_1-antitrypsin, ceruloplasmin and C-reactive protein have been determined. A disturbed profile is generally only seen in metastatic disease. C-reactive protein and α_1-acid glycoprotein appear to be the most sensitive markers in this group [42, 43, 45].

Protein-bound Carbohydrates

Serum L-fucose is a useful marker in breast cancer [144, 145, 146] and sialic acid is also of importance [165].

Pregnancy-associated α_2-glycoprotein (PAG)

Stimson [158] and Anderson et al. [6] have found good correlation between PAG levels and clinical assessment in patients examined serially and the changes in concentration always showed a preclinical indication of response. The strongly significant differences between the PAG levels of clinically well patients and those with metastatic disease suggest that PAG may have some use in the detection of micrometastases.

The most common site for metastases from breast cancer is the skeleton. Development of tumour deposits in bone may be caused by release from the primary tumour of osteolysins such as the prostaglandins mentioned earlier. These may mediate the degradation of collagen, which is reflected by the extent of excretion of hydroxyproline. The urinary output is usually measured as the hydroxyproline : creatinine ratio; this factor becomes elevated before there is radiological evidence of bone metastases [75]. The prognosis for patients with abnormally high hydroxyproline levels at presentation is poor [47]. The hydroxyproline : creatinine ratio has been found to be of use in monitoring of metastatic disease and appears to provide an early indication of response to hormone therapy [135]. It is doubtful whether hydroxyproline estimation will help to detect bone metastases before they are apparent by radioisotope scanning but when the bone scan is doubtful or when scintigraphy is not available it can prove helpful in disease classification [69].

Other organ-site indicators of metastases are included in the liver enzymes. Elevated levels of γ-glutamyl transferase and alkaline phosphatase can suggest hepatic metastases whereas high alkaline phosphatase and normal γ-glutamyl transferase values are usually found when there is an established metastasis in bone [123]. The acute-phase reactant proteins, α_1-antitrypsin and haptoglobin, appear to correlate with lung involvement.

Multiparametric Analysis

From the present evidence, none of the biochemical tests appear to be specific or absolute markers for breast carcinoma. The question then arises whether the determination of a combination of significantly useful markers could provide more information. Studies of multiple markers in breast cancer have shown that, in metastatic disease, 97 per cent of 60 patients could be detected by measurement of CEA, HCG and N^2, N^2-dimethylguanosine [161]. CEA and the serum fucose-protein ratio were increased in 93 per cent of 147 patients [165]. The coincidental measurement of CEA, casein-K, HCG and β-HCG was more efficient than the single assays for detection of pathological cases [176]. This array of markers has been extended to include the serum enzymes, γ-glutamyl transferase and alkaline phosphatase, and acute-phase reactant proteins [45]. The different combinations of markers examined gave no indication of staging except for metastatic disease, because of overlap between disease groups. In a survey of 19 of the possible markers for breast cancer by Coombes et al., concentrations of the following 7 were raised in over 50 per cent of 17 patients with overt metastatic disease; ferritin (88 per cent), C-reactive protein (87 per cent), CEA (81 per cent), α_1-acid glycoprotein (75 per cent), hydroxyproline : creatinine ratio (73 per cent) alkaline phosphatase (64 per cent) and sialyltransferase (56 per cent). Forty-four per cent of 16 patients with localized disease but a poor prognosis had an elevated level of at least one of these parameters. These tests could therefore specify a set of patients within this group for whom adjuvant chemotherapy may be particularly necessary. In an attempt to optimize selection of combinations of markers in multiparametric analysis, regression analysis has been applied [173] 1978. It is suggested that the whole range of possible markers for breast cancer could be examined in this way, so that less essential tests could be eliminated and the sensitivity of detection increased for metastatic disease and monitoring therapeutic response.

Concluding Remarks

At present there is no specific tumour marker diagnostic of breast cancer but markers such as CEA, ferritin, polyamines and especially oestrogen receptors have considerable potential as prognostic indicators. Calcitonin and sialyltransferase have particular relevance to staging and PAG may be similarly useful. For evaluation of response to therapy, many of the markers described parallel disease activity. The most useful include C3DP, PAG, CEA and urinary hydroxyproline. Multiparametric monitoring is now being evaluated and it is possible that this may be an approach to the major problem, that is, the detection of micrometastatic disease. This method has been applied to the localization of overt metastases. Physical techniques used in the management of cancer, including ultrasonography and isotope scanning, are of limited value at present for early detection of metastases: potentially one of the most sensitive tests is the determination of tumour markers by immunoassay methods.

A limitation to the use of many marker substances is undoubtedly the lack of specificity in their assay. Differences in specificity may be dependent on whether antibodies are raised against normal or tumour antigens and may explain contradictory findings between reports. It is important, therefore, to select specific antigenic groups produced by the cancer cells as a basis for radioimmunoassay of these markers. Other problems of interpretation include the possible effect of treatment on markers and their production. Tumour cell lysis resulting from therapy can produce temporary increases in plasma concentrations of a marker, which may not be associated with tumour progression. Protein synthesis is affected by the different therapies and so levels of protein markers may be influenced. Plasma concentrations may be modified by metabolic and excretory processes and so, for monitoring purposes, clearance rates should be considered.

As well as optimizing the use of known markers, the direction of future research will undoubtedly include a search for new cancer-related substances. Most tumour markers known to date are protein or polypeptide in nature since immunological methods have enabled their identification. However, it is possible that other materials are more specifically secreted by particular tumour cells. Studies with cancer cells *in vitro* appear to be a promising approach to isolation of the substances that may be produced. By combining *in vitro* techniques with biochemical studies hopefully better methods of measuring disease activity will be obtained.

AN ALTERNATIVE STAGING RELATING DIRECTLY TO THE THERAPEUTIC DECISION

Stage IA: Subclinical Cancer

A tumour is commonly impalpable, the condition being demonstrated by mammography as distorted structure with or without microcalcification, findings often benign. Histology is required and the problem is locating and excising such tissue, thus necessitating close collaboration between radiodiagnostician and surgeon. Radio-opaque markers help as does dye injection to the site of the disease. The excised specimen should be radiographed to ensure that the abnormality has been removed prior to pathology. If carcinoma *in situ* is discovered, it is probably sufficient to perform a more generous wedge excision. Should no further changes be demonstrated then subsequent management can be by regular follow up and mammography. If further cancer is found or if histology suggests invasive carcinoma, the patient should be considered as stage IB.

Stage IB: Early Clinical Cancer

Clinical designation is a tumour less than 2 cm, any fixity being compatible with that diameter. Palpable axillary nodes, if present, should be clinically benign. In view of the poor return it is doubtful whether routine radiology and scanning are justified. Precise management of the primary growth remains controversial, but must be 'Radical', a term commonly but mistakingly taken to imply a surgical approach. Whatever the operation, axillary histology is mandatory and when negative, systemic therapy is usually omitted. If positive the patient must be considered as phase IIA.

Stage IIA

These patients present with a situation where metastases are non-demonstrable but considered probable. Designation is presently based in nodal involvement, though tumours larger than 2 cm may well merit such consideration. Lacking information about internal mammary node involvement possibly all medial tumours should be included. Phase II patients need preliminary radioisotope assessment of bone and perhaps liver, with radiology limited to chest and suspicious areas detected by bone scan. Biochemical assessment is also of value. Treatment is based on the probable presence of metastases and involves a radical approach to the breast and glandular areas utilizing such combination of surgery and radiotherapy considered capable of successfully eradicating local cancer, not only to produce local cure but to prepare the way for systemic therapy.

Stage IIB

This includes patients with matted or fixed axillary lymph nodes, palpable supraclavicular nodes or a primary growth unsuitable for surgery because of size, fixity, ulceration, oedema, or satellite skin nodules but no detectable distant metastases. Investigation is as for stage IIA and treatment which can occasionally be curative should be locally radical with the major contribution by radiation. Systemic therapy is also indicated.

Stage IIIA: Overt Metastatic Disease

Patients presenting initially with primary disease and demonstrable distant metastases. To confirm the diagnosis and to aid chemotherapy some local treatment is required. This should be a relatively conservative undemanding procedure, combined with a systemic element.

Stage IIIB: Recurrence after Primary Radical Therapy

Patients returning with distant metastases. In addition many believe that following initial adequate radical treatment, local recurrence is commonly a harbinger of distant disease, and systemic therapy should be considered at this stage in addition to whatever local measures are applied.

THE ROLE OF SURGERY

Surgery will continue for the present as the first approach for the majority of new patients but differences exist in defining what the extent should be. Closely related is the interrelationship between surgery and radiotherapy; there must be an understanding by each speciality of what the other can obtain, and how one may complement the other in achieving an acceptable end result. Certain points may be made. Firstly, some local cancers (stage IB, stage IIAB) are genuinely non-metastatic and radical local treatment has curative potential. Such patients, whilst in a minority, must not be undertreated locally though the majority with stage II disease harbour covert distant metastases.

However, as treatment for this latter group must be aimed at elimination of all local disease, to optimize the setting for systemic therapy it must be of a potentially curable and therefore radical nature for all these cases. It must again be emphasized that radical treatment does not necessarily imply radical mastectomy, possibly with radiotherapy as a lucky penny. Rather it means an approach directed towards eliminating all local disease, recognizing that thoroughly planned, well-executed radiotherapy may be just as radical as any surgery. No one has acceptable evidence to the contrary. Thus a combination of techniques is available which range from more extensive surgery with perhaps limited radiotherapy to more limited surgery with more extensive radiotherapy. Once the term 'radical' is understood then a rational basis exists for the selection of that combination of treatment which stands a maximum chance of local success, but remains compatible with a minimum of local tissue ablation, morbidity and mortality.

It is a fact that as patients will initially be referred for a surgical opinion, save in those centres where joint clinics operate, the surgeon by his primary decision commonly defines succeeding policy. There are a variety of options, and whichever is pursued there must be an inherent nodal diagnostic element. As surgery is the only reliable manner of achieving this, every operation must be accompanied by some form of axillary evaluation as described above.

Lumpectomy

Arguments for removal of the primary tumour alone with preservation of the residual breast structure are based largely on aesthetic considerations, given added force by womens' groups in Europe and the USA. In addition fear of losing the breast may be a factor causing delay in women seeking advice for breast lumps, for undoubtedly mastectomy carries well-known undesirable physical and psychological consequences.

As breast cancer is multifocal, though the precise significance of this is a little uncertain, there is the hazard of residual cancer cells at the incision this procedure requires subsequent further measures.

Local Mastectomy

Going a step further this operation without radiation is associated with a higher incidence of local recurrence. However, subsequent treatment by local radiotherapy does not seem to prejudice the ultimate outcome though the studies on which this finding is based do not include a systemic element. What the relationships between local residual disease and systemic therapy are is another matter, and further work is required. A modification of local mastectomy which involves implantation of a prosthetic replacement can have physical and psychological if not functional attractions.

What influence such a procedure would have upon postoperative radiation remains uncertain as do possible late complications, although these problems would not seem major. Mastectomy has obvious advantages for those women who wish to be rid of the entire breast believing its retention to constitute an added hazard.

Radical Mastectomy

One advantage is that this permits thorough evaluation and clearance of the axilla. This is not to say that it is the only or the most desirable manner of obtaining these objectives. Morbidity both early and late is increased, whilst if radiation is omitted the internal mammary nodes are left untreated. As with local mastectomy the operation alone is attended by a higher incidence of local recurrence which subsequent radiation controls without prejudicing the outcome, though again such studies do not include a systemic element. The incidence of local recurrence however should be lower than after local mastectomy, therefore posing less of a problem.

Supraradical Mastectomy

Results of this procedure which involves internal mammary node dissection are superior to others in preventing local recurrence, and for some patients this must be synonymous with cure. Even more radical procedures are practised which involve the removal of the supraclavicular glands and dissection of the anteriomediastinum. These have rightly been rejected by those involved in the treatment of breast cancer in the UK, and will not further be discussed.

RADIOTHERAPY

As with the other treatment modalities, controversy exists about the role of radiotherapy and the manner of its administration particularly when given with curative intent. Palliatively, in overtly disseminated disease such as painful bony deposits, its obvious and immediate benefit excites little argument. It is also of value in the patient presenting with a tumour too extensive for surgery. The problem is the technically operable growth without demonstrable distant metastatic disease.

In the past many arguments have been put forward by surgeons and radiotherapists based on uncontrolled personal experience masquerading as some form of clinical trial. The conclusions have in general supported the vested interests of the protagonists. Today an overview of most such reports claiming superiority for something or other, based on historical data or a comparison of results between different centres perhaps in different countries, or simply upon blind faith, would conclude that few are reliable and indeed the remarkable conclusion is the overall similarity rather than the differences between the various results.

Today the concept of comparing like with like and the significance of the clinical trial is appreciated. Unfortunately however, none of the generation of clinical trials now coming to maturity included a breast conservative limit relying on truly radical radiation nor did they take account of the disseminated nature of breast cancer. It must be admitted that had the problem of distant metastases been appreciated when those trials commenced the current development of systemic therapy was such that little could have been offered. Accordingly, well-planned meticulous clinical trials were performed comparing one form of local treatment with another, generally radical or local mastectomy either with or without postoperative radiation. Findings as already discussed have in general been similar, namely, that those patients who did not receive postoperative radiation had a higher incidence of local recurrence, that subsequent radiation eradicated this recurrence, and that the experience of local recurrence had little bearing on ultimate survival. As many patients treated by surgery alone did not experience local recurrence, and the minority who did could then be irradiated successfully there seemed little point in routine radiation as it is attended by some morbidity. Incidentally reports suggesting that routine postoperative radiation increases the risk of distant metastases, are retrospective and as it was common practice to give radiation only to more advanced cases, the irradiated group contained a higher proportion of patients with larger primary growths and axillary nodal involvement with consequent greater likelihood of manifesting such disease.

Future trials must study interrelationships between local and systemic treatments which may well have a bearing upon future trends in local therapy and accordingly an already difficult and confused clinical situation has been compounded. The conclusions of the trials mentioned above will again have to go into the melting-pot and the need is now for a new generation of studies designed to investigate such interrelationships. There are sufficient numbers of breast cancer patients to render such trials feasible provided clinicians participate. Accordingly just as some answers seemed to be emerging it again seems impossible to make an authoritative statement on the respective roles of surgery and radiotherapy, particularly when systemic measures are employed. However, current radiotherapy practice as carried out in one centre will be described and this is fairly typical of many in the UK. Some interesting developments in the field will also be mentioned, as these may well merit subsequent clinical evaluation.

One Surgeon's View in 1978

At this point, the views of a well known American surgeon on the respective roles of surgery and radiotherapy are apposite. Urban [163] writing about operable breast cancer defines the objective of surgery as removing all disease from the breast and regional nodes, and describes three methods whereby this may be attained: modified radical mastectomy, radical mastectomy, and extended radical mastectomy. In his summary, 21 lines relate to these approaches, whilst adjuvant radiation therapy is dismissed in 1 line. Such prejudiced and unscientific conclusions arise from a lack of appreciation that other modalities may have a part to play. Radiation therapists may be just as dogmatic. Such attitudes should have no place in our present thinking, any opinions held being based on fact gained from clinical trials rather than simply projecting the vested interest of the author.

OBJECT OF CONVENTIONAL RADIOTHERAPY

This account is based upon patients treated at the Northern Ireland Radiotherapy Centre (NIRC). These patients will have previously received any of a number of surgical approaches, commonly local mastectomy. Objectives are constant, namely to destroy residual cancer by delivering a radical dose to:

1. residual primary tumour in the breast if present, or to the chest wall and;
2. associated lymph nodes in the axillary, parasternal, supraclavicular, and infraclavicular regions.

The parasternal lymph nodes are considered to lie from 3 to 5 cm below the skin surface, the axillary nodes somewhat deeper.

Treatment Methods

Various methods have been used to deal with this difficult dosimetry problem.

Method 1

Common to most is the Parallel Opposed Glancing Field technique for treating the breast or chest wall. Orthovoltage X-rays of approximately

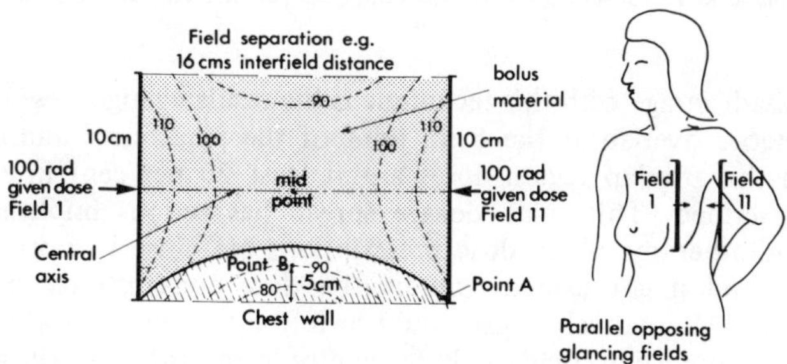

Fig. 3.1. Method 1: Parallel opposed glancing field technique – two glancing fields to chest wall.

3 mm of copper 'half-value thickness' are usual. At the NIRC 3500 rad are delivered to point A in 15 fractions over 21 days. The corresponding dose to point B in this example is 2900 rad (*Fig. 3.1*).

The node areas are irradiated by means of a straight : on parasternal field and two parallel opposed shoulder fields from orthovoltage X-rays of approximately 3 mm 'half-value thickness'. Typical dimensions are 25 X 10 cm for the shoulder fields and 15 X 5 cm for the parasternal field as indicated in *Fig. 3.2.* Doses of 3600 rad to the anterior field entrance point and 3000 rad to the parasternal skin surface have been used at the NIRC as in other centres, in 15 fractions over 21 days.

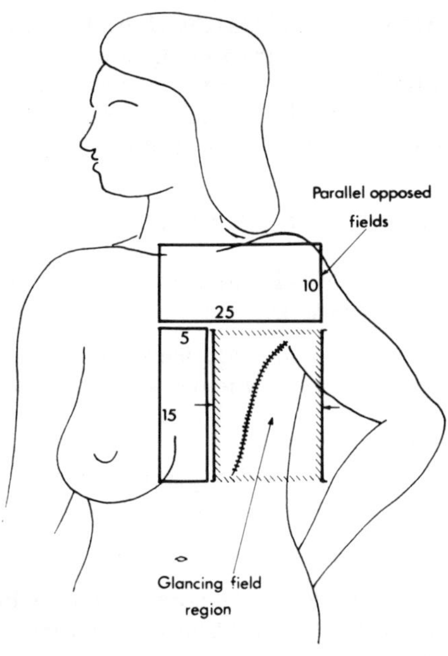

Fig. 3.2. **Method 1: Parallel opposed glancing field technique – fields to node areas.**

The disadvantage with this technique is the resulting high dose region in the geometric overlap at the 5 cm joint of the parasternal and shoulder fields. In this overlap region doses are at least 20 per cent in excess of those prescribed. This wide dosage spread has serious implications in radical radiotherapy where dose prescriptions are close to normal tissue tolerance, and might lead to conservative dose prescriptions to prevent necrosis etc. Alternatively a gap could be left at this junction which could lead to underdosage particularly in proximity to the anterior skin surface.

Method 2

This is a variation of the basic Edinburgh technique using cobalt 60 parallel opposed shoulder fields and an adjoining parasternal field (*Fig. 3.3*). Field dimensions are comparable to method 1. The shoulder fields

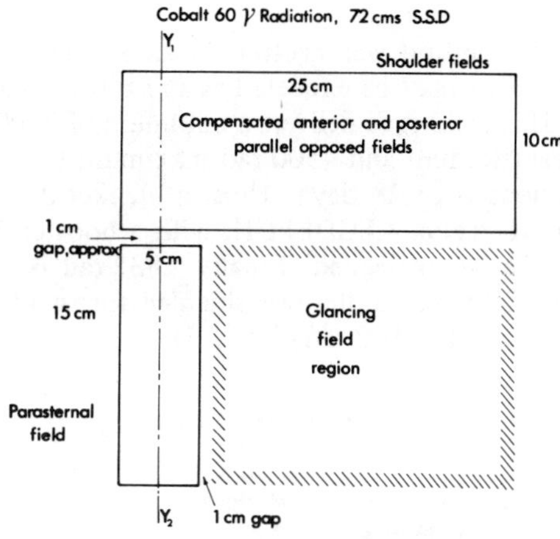

Fig. 3.3. Method 2: Variation of Edinburgh technique.

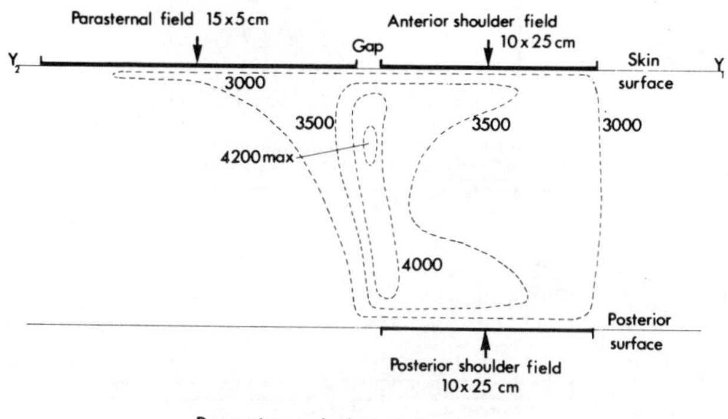

Fig. 3.4. Isodose distribution of method used in *Fig. 3.4.* Section through Y1–Y2.

are compensated to allow for sloping surfaces, while a gap of approximately 1 cm is allowed between the adjoining parasternal and shoulder fields in an attempt to minimize overlap. Dose prescriptions here have been 3000 rad and 3500 rad to subcutaneous tissues in 15 fractions over 21 days. A major weakness in this fairly common technique concerns the matching of the parasternal and shoulder fields. Even with a 1 cm gap there may be considerable overdose (*Fig. 3.4*). It is notoriously difficult to match fields in this manner, as small radiographic set-up errors produce corresponding rapid dosage changes.

Method 3

This L-shaped field method was evolved in an attempt to eliminate the dosage problems which may be expected as a result of combining adjacent cobalt 60 fields. This technique delivers a minimum of 3500 rad to a depth of 5 cm in the parasternum and 4500 rad maximum to the subcutaneous tissue in 12 fractions over 28 days. Thus, a blanket dose of 3840 rad is applied anteriorly to region ABCDEFGH, with a booster dose of 672 rad to ABEFGH, BCDE being leaded. Finally 2832 rad is delivered to the posterior shoulder field. The axilla was shielded for two fractions to limit the skin maximum dose to 4500 rad (*Fig. 3.5*).

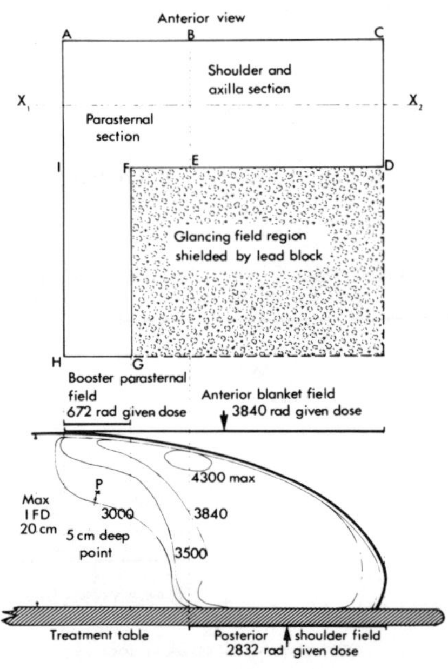

Fig. 3.5. Method 3: using L-shaped field. Isodose distribution through X1–X2.

This was a reasonable approach in solving a difficult dosimetry problem before the availability of a treatment planning computer system. Subsequent computer verification indicates that the 3500 rad isodose line bows inwards towards the maximum dosage point and does not encompass the parasternum to a depth of 5 cm as required. The technique is now being modified to achieve better dosage homogeneity in the parasternal region (*Fig. 3.6*). A single blanket anterior field, suitably modified, will be used as before, with an opposing posterior shoulder field. The computer has been used to design a modifying brass filter for the anterior field, and experimental depth dose and beam profile data will be stored on magnetic tape for this modified field. It will then be possible to use the computer to optimize the dose for distribution for individual patient outline variation. A directly applied electron field for the breast/chest wall region might offer advantages over the orthovoltage glancing fields, particularly when considering the present junctions between the parasternal shoulder, and glancing fields.

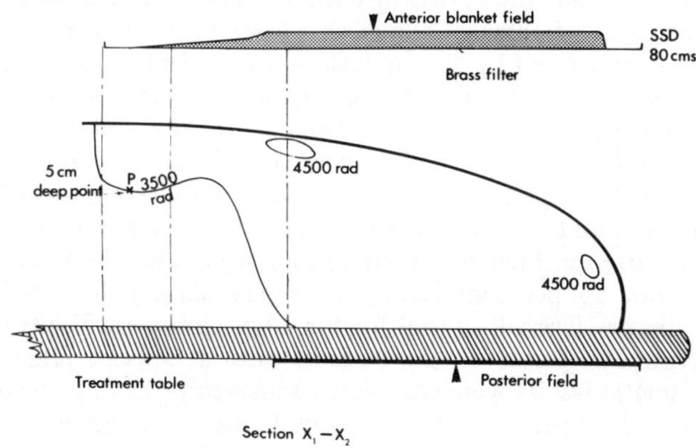

Fig. 3.6. Modification of Method 3 using brass filter.

RADIOTHERAPY AS AN ALTERNATIVE TO MASTECTOMY

The above description is of radiation as broadly used in many UK centres. There is however a small group of radiotherapists who feel that this treatment could have a more significant role and, following conservation surgery, might be as capable of eradicating local disease as is more radical surgery.

As usual there are few, if any, studies to support or refute this view, that by Atkins et al. [8] being the most widely quoted. This indicated that node negative patients treated by wide local excision followed by a radiotherapy schedule which many consider inadequate, carried the same ultimate survival rate but four times the incidence of local recurrence (15 per cent *v.* 4 per cent) when compared with patients treated by radical mastectomy. Mustakallio (19) also experienced more local recurrences in his study, but again radiation techniques can be criticized. Radiation dose and technique must be critical in such situations as is borne out by the studies quoted below which involve considerably higher doses and more elaborate treatment. Veronesi [164] is currently comparing radical mastectomy with simple resection of the breast quadrant plus overlying skin and underlying pectoralis major. An axillary dissection is performed in continuity with the resected quadrant except with a tumour of the lower inner quadrant which requires two separate incisions. Postoperative radiation to a dose of 6000 rad in 5–6 weeks is given, and whilst results are preliminary the cosmetic effect is satisfactory in 70 per cent of women and as yet there is no increased incidence of local or distant recurrence in the conservative group. Further supportive evidence comes from a collaborative study involving six French hospitals currently evaluating similarly intensive radiation therapy following tumour excision. In addition a boost is given to the tumour area by an implant. Unfortunately, this is not a controlled study, but the results in terms of local recurrence and cosmesis support Veronesi's findings. Calle et al. [36] report 10 year's experience on 514 patients treated by similar techniques. Patients with tumours less than 3 cm and without palpable axillary involvement received minimal surgery followed by radiotherapy. Larger tumours and patients with clinically significant lymph nodes received radiotherapy alone without surgery. For the first group 5- and 10-year absolute survival, free of disease, are 85 per cent and 75 per cent with 5 per cent having secondary surgery for local recurrence. Figures for the second group are 68 per cent and 43 per cent with 55 per cent having secondary surgery for persistent or recurrent disease. Overall survival for the whole group are 72 per cent and 51 per cent. Two-thirds of the patients alive at 5 years retained their breast. Cosmetic results were considered satisfactory in 98 per cent of the first group and 85 per cent of the second. Radiation dosage is high by UK standards, thus the lumpectomy patients received a tumour dose of 5000 rad to the entire breast, axillary region, internal mammary lymph nodes and supraclavicular fossa over 5–6 weeks. An additional 1500 rad was delivered to the lumpectomy area through reduced fields and an additional 1000 rad to the lower axilla only, both in one week. Where lumpectomy was not performed a tumour dose of 5000–6000 rad in 5–6 weeks was given to the entire breast and glandular areas. If at the end of this treatment the primary tumour and/or nodes remained unchanged or had reduced by less than 50 per cent radiation was discontinued and surgery performed two to three months later. On the other hand if there had been a significant reduction in size a further 2000 rad was given to the primary tumour with an additional 1500 rad to the lower axilla. The relationship between radiation dose and recurrence has been studied (Bataini et al. [12]) in patients treated by lumpectomy and radiotherapy and those receiving radiotherapy alone. They found that 7000 rad in 7–8 weeks controlled 85 per cent of the first group, whilst 8000 rad in 8 weeks was required to control two-thirds of patients treated by radical radiation alone. Clinically negative axillae were controlled by 6000 rad, whilst if clinically positive 7000 rad were required.

Such results justify further clinical studies provided that (a) the survival figures are comparable to conventional measures, (b) treatment morbidity is acceptable, (c) a satisfactory cosmetic result is obtained, and (d) that salvage surgery for local recurrences is not unduly complicated.

SOME KINETIC CONCEPTS AND THEIR IMPLICATIONS FOR THE DESIGN OF CLINICAL CHEMOTHERAPY SCHEDULES

'Small tumours, due to their large fraction of actively dividing cells, are more 'sensite' to cytotoxic therapy than tumours of equivalent histology but larger size'. This widely held belief has become established as a fact and as such has been incorporated into many treatment programmes. It has often led to the adoption of less intensive chemotherapy. For example, (a) in advanced disease doses are often tapered as the tumour bulk is reduced, (b) schedules chosen to maintain remission are often considerably reduced compared with those used to obtain it, and (c) regimens for adjuvant chemotherapy are frequently less intensive than those used for treatment of a similar but much larger tumour. Unfortunately, clinical results from studies of this kind have often been disappointing; the 'cure' rate for most malignancies is low, the prevention of recurrence after remission often fails and, whilst some preliminary adjuvant studies look promising, the benefit in terms of increased survival is still only a few years.

Norton and Simon [129] suggested that the original premise on which these studies were based may be invalid. They have proposed an alternative hypothesis which can explain many current clinical observations and has implications for altering the design of treatment programmes. Their view is that some tumours may be less sensitive to therapy when they are very small or very large than when they are of intermediate size.

Experimental Details of the Theoretical Concept

This concept is derived from a study of the growth rate of solid tumours, most of which grow in a Gompertzian rather than a exponential fashion. The relationship between tumour size (curve I), 'specific growth rate' (curve II) and growth rate (curve III) is shown in *Figs. 3.7 and 3.8* for unperturbed Gompertzian growth. *Fig. 3.7* shows that while the GF is maximum at the time of initiation of growth, the growth rate is maximum when the tumour is about 37 per cent of its limiting size. The Gompertzian equation used is

$$dN(t)/dt = B.\log\{100/N(t)\}.N(t)$$
$$B = 0{\cdot}4/\log\{100\}$$

Fig. 3.8 shows the relationship in tabular form.

The following points should be emphasized:

1. The 'specific growth rate' which has also been called 'the instantaneous growth fraction', is a complex term incorporating effects of cell birth and cell loss together with alterations in the tumour. It is maximal at the time of initiation of growth of the tumour and decreases as the tumour volume increases (*see also* Table and curves I and II). (*See Fig. 3.8* for Table.)

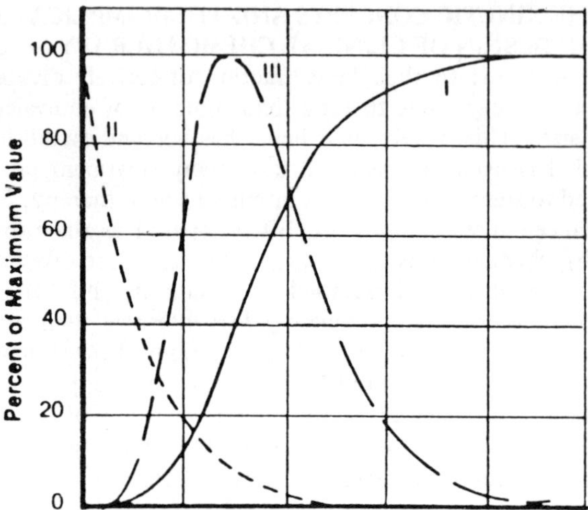

Fig. 3.7. Relationship between tumour size (curve I), instantaneous GF or specific growth rate (curve II), and growth rate (curve III) for unperturbed Gompertzian growth. (Reproduced from Norton and Simon [129] by courtesy of 'Cancer Treatment Reports'.)

2. A large 'specific growth rate' does not necessarily imply a large growth rate (*see the* Table and curves II and III).
3. The growth rate is maximal when the tumour is about 37 per cent of its limiting size (N.B. growth rate does *not* increase in direct proportion to tumour size as in exponential growth).
4. Cell production rate is slowest at either end of the growth curve (*see the* Table and curves I and II).

From these studies it can be shown that the fractional cell kill hypothesis, advocated by Skipper et al. [155], is applicable to exponentially-growing tumours provided treatment goes on long enough, it is *not* appropriate for tumours exhibiting Gompertzian growth. The fractional cell kill hypothesis is based on the proposal that the growth rate inhibiting effect of a treatment is proportional to the size of the tumour, and suggests that tumours will be most sensitive to therapy when the smallest number of malignant cells is present. However, if this is applied to Gompertzian growth then the largest tumours should be the *most* sensitive to therapy, both in terms of numbers of cell kills and rate of regression. Clearly this is not generally found in clinical practice.

Therefore, as an alternative it has been proposed that the growth-inhibiting effect of a treatment is proportional to the growth rate of an untreated tumour. In the opinion of Norton and Simon sensitivity to treatment is a complex function of the interaction between 'specific

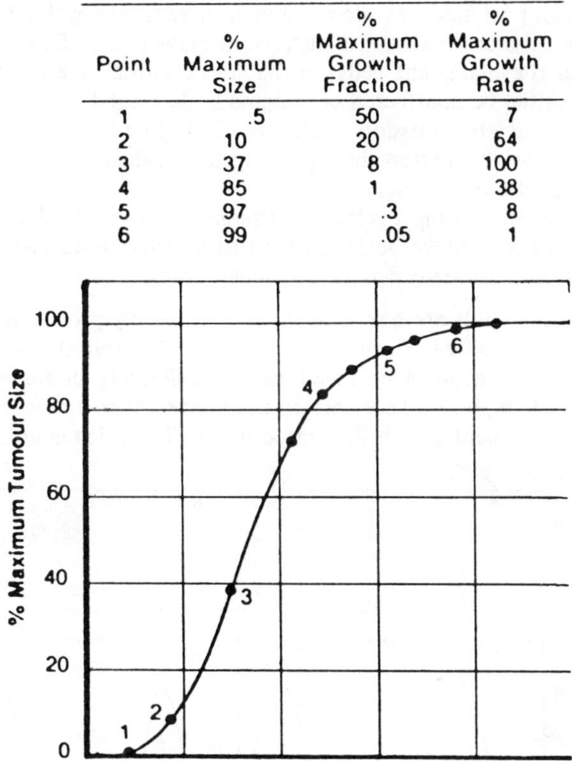

Point	% Maximum Size	% Maximum Growth Fraction	% Maximum Growth Rate
1	.5	50	7
2	10	20	64
3	37	8	100
4	85	1	38
5	97	.3	8
6	99	.05	1

Fig. 3.8. Relationship for Gompertzian growth, between tumour size, instantaneous GF and growth rate presented in tabular form. (Reproduced from Norton and Simon [129] by courtesy of 'Cancer Treatment Reports'.)

growth rate' and 'tumour volume'. When this hypothesis is applied to exponential growth smaller tumours would be expected to be more sensitive than larger ones, in agreement with experience. However, for Gompertzian growth, the rate of regression would be maximal for intermediate sized tumours but would be decreased not only in much larger tumours but also in those of a very small size. This does not necessarily mean that the smaller tumour is also less 'curable' than the intermediate sized one, since it may be closer to a limiting volume beyond which it may be incapable of regrowth.

These concepts have major implications for the clinical managements of malignant disease which are listed below.

1. A protocol which causes a dramatic remission rate in a tumour of intermediate size may be sufficient to cure a small tumour, especially if doses are reduced or given only over a short time.

2. Although prolonged low-dose regimens may lengthen the disease-free interval, the shallow rate of regression may be insufficient to eradicate all the malignant cells, so that the eventual rate of recurrence would either be unaffected or marginally decreased.
3. When 'complete remission' is achieved high-dose therapy over a short period may be better than prolonged low-dose treatment in decreasing rates of recurrence.
4. Intensive alternating cycles of *different* drug combinations in full doses might produce better survival times than using one particular combination of many agents in reduced doses.

These studies also indicate how current chemotherapy protocols might be changed and intensified in an effort to prolong survival. In *advanced disease*, when remission is obtained using moderately intensive chemotherapy, treatment should be escalated in an attempt to eradicate residual disease. This treatment plan is illustrated in *Fig. 3.9* which is simulation of

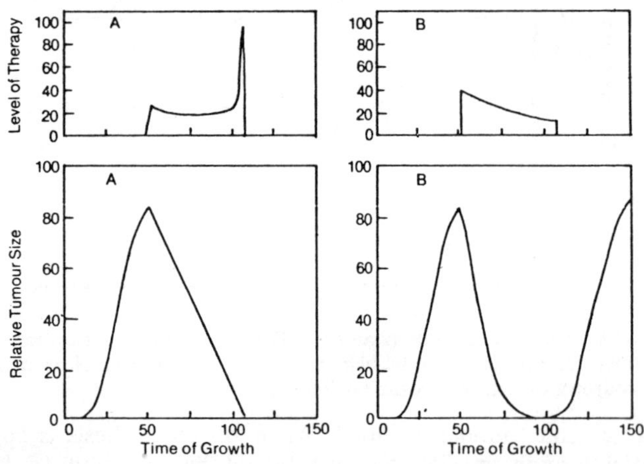

Fig. 3.9. Simulation of the effects of two plans of therapy in causing regression of an advanced tumour. (Reproduced from Norton and Simon [129] by courtesy of 'Cancer Treatment Reports'.)

the effect of two plans of therapy using equation in causing regression of advanced tumour. Plan A applies a therapy level just sufficient to maintain a steady volume regression, saving a 'spike' of intense therapy for late in the course when the small tumour is relatively therapy-resistant; this plan reduces tumour volume below the volume of a single cell resulting in 'cure'. Plan B uses the same total amount of therapy but gives the most intense treatment initially, with tapering of dose levels as CR is induced. When the tumour is small and relatively therapy-resistant, therapy administered is insufficient to reduce the volume below that of a single cell.

Therefore the tumour treated by Plan B regrows after the termination of treatment.

For *adjuvant* therapy, however, intensive schedules using full doses should be employed over a longer period of time. In this respect the approach advocated by Price, Hill and their colleagues [137] which enables intensive chemotherapy to be given safely, may prove most valuable.

Taking into account the above considerations and also various other principles which are at present quite widely accepted, the following additional guidelines are worthy of consideration.

1. Chemotherapy is more effective against smaller total tumour body burdens than larger ones. It should be used at the earliest opportunity in disease management, but only after local measures directed toward reducing the burden have been fully used. The earliest palpable tumour is rarely less than 1 cm in diameter and to achieve this size has undergone 30 tumour cell generations (giving 10^9 tumour cells). Whilst the period in time over which metastases take place cannot be accurately established, evidence suggests that this may be during the 10 generations prior to diagnosis. If for argument it is assumed that a tumour has disseminated 100 metastases at the 20 generation point and that these have grown at a rate similar to the primary tumour, then at the point of primary diagnosis 10 generations later each metastasis will contain 10^3 cells, so the total metastatic tumour burden will be 10^5. Adequate therapy to the primary growth which contains 10^9 cells means that 99·9 per cent of the total tumour bulk will be eliminated by this procedure and indeed if any involved lymph nodes are erradicated this percentage will be greater. Thus chemotherapy is not an alternative to surgery and/or radiotherapy, but an additional weapon.
2. Chemotherapy as pointed out above should be given in full dose even when there is no apparent residual disease. This applies to the adjuvant situation and also to patients with advanced disease in apparent complete drug induced response. Unfortunately, information on therapy duration in the absence of demonstrable disease is not yet available.
3. An individual course of chemotherapy should last between 24 and 36 hr. Longer times will permit normal stem cells to be drawn into cycle and so become susceptible to the cytotoxic drugs with consequent increase in toxicity. This precludes small daily doses of drugs over lengthy periods as has been the practice in the past.
4. Chemotherapy should be repeated as soon as adequate repopulation of the normal stem cell population occurs. This is commonly a three weekly interval though for certain agents it may be as much as six weeks (melphalan, CCNU and hexamethylmelamine).

5. In designing chemotherapy schedules full cognizance should be taken of the kinetic classification of the drugs included. It must be remembered that phase-specific agents are not additively toxic and may be utilized in full dosage provided that overall treatment times fall within the limits specified. Cycle-specific drugs are additively toxic and, if combined, doses should be reduced.
6. When drugs are being selected knowledge of the phase of the cycle during which they are active may be useful. Thus it is theoretically desirable to select phase-specific drugs which operate at different points in the cell cycle, as drugs which operate at the same phase may be of little additional benefit when given together. In this context an agent which arrests cells at a particular stage in the cycle followed by one which kills maximally at the block itself, or at the point immediately following has a certain theoretical appeal though the concept has not been demonstrated as of clinical value.
7. Principal drug toxicities should differ one from another so that should side effects arise they will be disparate rather than cumulative.
8. Drugs selected for inclusion in a combination should previously have been demonstrated as being capable of producing useful response when used as a single agent in a reasonable proportion of patients, for example 20 per cent with that cancer.
9. The possibilities that certain drug comtinations may be synergistic or alternatively antagonistic requires consideration. There is as yet little information on this important point.

MULTIMODAL (ADJUVANT THERAPY) IN THE MANAGEMENT OF 'EARLY' (PHASE II) DISEASE

The past decade has brought an appreciation that, despite technical advances in surgical and radiotherapeutic technique and despite a growing awareness of the importance of public education, genuine cure rates in the treatment of breast cancer have not improved as might have been expected. Mortality is not generally related to local treatment failure but to other factors, and this reasoning has led to a meaningful appreciation of the long recognized fact that haematogenous metastases are the real problem, usually appearing after apparently successful eradication of primary disease. Metastases at this point implies their undetectable presence before the primary growth was removed as this must have been their origin. Opportunities for such dissemination are ample thus an undetectable growth 1·0 mm in diameter contains 10^6 cells whilst the earliest clinical growth, about 1 cm contains 10^9 cells. Such numbers afford opportunity for prediagnostic dissemination and explain how metastases, microscopic in size but abundant in cells, can escape radiological and radioisotope diagnosis.

Consequently, there is now agreement that attempts to reduce mortality must include a systemic element. During the first half of this century only endocrine therapy was available; naturally this was first investigated. Most widely used was surgical and radiotherapeutic oophorectomy, initial reports appearing in the early 1950s.

Their retrospective findings that the procedure was associated with a longer disease free interval (DFI) and indeed improved survival are perhaps questionable. The first prospective trials of castration (Nevinni [125]; Ravdin et al. [140]) indicated that only women with four or more positive axillary nodes benefited in terms of DFI and that this advantage disappeared by 36 months. An early prospective study on radiation oophorectomy, confirmed that (Cole [39, 40]) as did Nissen-Meyer [127] who showed a small advantage in survival at seven years. In Meakin's study [119] pre- and post-menopausal women following mastectomy and radiotherapy, irrespective of axillary status, were randomized to receive either no further treatment or ovarian radiation plus prednisone 7·5 mg daily for up to five years.

Results indicate that in patients under 45 years old there is a statistically insignificant advantage to the oophorectomy group in terms of recurrence and survival although amongst pre-menopausal women over 45 years there was a significant advantage in both these parameters. Post-menopausal women did not benefit. In general ovarian suppression conveys little long term benefit, with the possible exception of the one subgroup mentioned above.

Early efforts with cytotoxic chemotherapy utilized single agents administered for varying periods. Results were unencouraging though the 10-year figures of the National Surgical Adjuvant Breast Project Thiotepa trial indicated lasting benefit to pre-menopausal women with 1–3 nodes positive. In the Nissen-Meyer study over 1000 post-mastectomy patients were randomized to receive either a single 6-days course of cyclophosphamide to a total of 30 mg per kg or alternatively no further treatment. Statistically significant advantages in favour of the treatment group were noted for both recurrences and deaths. These differences increased to the fourth and sixth year respectively, and thereafter remained constant to the tenth year at a level of approximately 10 per cent. Neither menstrual status or node involvement seemed significant, but there was evidence that delaying chemotherapy for three weeks following operation resulted in loss of advantage. Another single agent study (Fisher [64]) utilized phenylalanine mustard orally in regular cycles for two years. Results indicate a greater difference in recurrence rates than with cyclophosphamide, though attended by more morbidity and also the follow up period is shorter. The advantage also seems confined to pre-menopausal women.

Just as single agent chemotherapy for advanced cancer has given way to the combination approach, so has there been a similar move in early disease. This is based on a better understanding of the underlying pharmacological and kinetic principles, and the not unreasonable argument that treatment most likely to be of value in early cancer is that most effective in the later stages. Because of the demands that this treatment makes upon the patient in inconvenience and toxicity, and because of theoretic risks of induction of a second malignancy it is considered at present justifiable to administer it only to patients with a high risk of recurrence, that is nodal disease. Probably primary tumour size might be another selective factor.

The first major study of combination chemotherapy was by Bonadonna [20] with cyclophosphamide, methotrexate and 5-fluorouracil (CMF). The programme commenced in June 1973, patients receiving radical mastectomy without radiation. Those with positive axillary lymph nodes were allocated either to receive CMF for 12 months or no further therapy. Two years later results were statistically in favour of the CMF group so a second trial commenced in which patients were randomized to either six or twelve cycles of CMF. This study was subsequently discontinued in post-menopausal women when the benefit to this group noted in the first study subsequently disappeared by three years. The most recent results indicate a significantly reduced treatment to failure rates for both local and distant recurrence at four years though confined to pre-menopausal women. The second study shows a slight but insignificant advantage in favour of 12 month's treatment though results are preliminary.

In the UK first results came from the British Multicentre Breast Chemotherapy Group. They first designed and evaluated a regimen in advanced patients with the intent that it be suitable for use in early disease. Necessary criteria were that it be therapeutically effective, convenient, and comparatively free from toxic side effects. The group took as their starting point the 5-day regimen commonly used in advanced disease in the early 1970s, and by a series of prospective clinical studies eventually established that similar clinical benefit could be obtained and with less toxicity by a regimen administered on days 1 and 8 of a four-weekly cycle. Three-year results demonstrate a significant advantage to the chemotherapy group, especially marked in post-menopausal patients. Briefly, 277 patients under 70 years of age were included. After primary treatment 126 received no further treatment (controls) and 141 were allocated to receive 2-day chemotherapy for 6 months, beginning within 10 weeks of operation. Patients in whom nodal histology was unknown or negative are excluded from this analysis. The chemotherapy regimen consists of two limbs administered on days 1 and 8 of a four-weekly cycle, with cyclophosphamide 300 mg, vincristine 0·65 mg, and 5-fluorouracil 500 mg on day 1 and cyclophosphamide 300 mg, vincristine 0·65 mg, and methotrexate 37·5 mg on day 8. Ten patients failed to complete six courses, 2 due to toxicity, 4 because of concurrent illness, and 4 defaulted on attendance.

Significant nausea and vomiting were noted in 29 per cent of patients, with one withdrawing. Stomatitis, diarrhoea, neurological disorder, and hair loss were encountered to a moderate or severe degree in under 3 per cent; no patients required a wig. Bone-marrow toxicity has not been a problem. Haemoglobin has remained above 12 g/dl in 89 per cent of patients, and the platelet count above 150 000/μl in 96 per cent. The white blood cell count fell in some patients, counts below 2500/μl being noted in 6 per cent of patients at the mid-point of therapy (3 months). This fell to 3 per cent at 6 months. Whilst treatment was discontinued in 1 patient for this reason no clinical consequences were noted.

These results demonstrate that six courses of adjuvant chemotherapy in breast cancer are associated with a decreased recurrence rate and that the advantage holds constant to 36 months. This advantage has been gained cheaply in terms of immediate toxicity. Delayed complications, such as induction of a further malignancy, are possible but they seem likely to be insignificant when set against the apparent benefits of adjuvant chemotherapy. The group have concluded that it is unethical to continue with a no chemotherapy group, and recruitment to this study has been terminated. In the current trial the 2-day regimen described is being compared with a 1-day system with 12 months tamoxifen as a third limb of the study. Chemotherapy patients are re-randomized after 6 months to an additional 6 months of tamoxifen or no further therapy.

Criticism has been levelled at this study on the grounds that local treatment has been left to the discretion of the participant provided it be considered in the broadest sense as radical. Thus the local treatment should be considered capable of eradicating local disease, that is, in conventional terms 'curative'. Whilst local treatment has a relationship with the incidence of local recurrence, there is no evidence of any influence upon the incidence of distant metastases. As these are the prime targets of adjuvant therapy, this flexibility in entry criteria should not influence results. Standardization of entry whilst statistically attractive would, because of difficulties in obtaining medical participation, restrict the trial to a smaller group of participants, thereby prejudicing a meaningful outcome.

The question of participation in collaborative studies is interesting when one considers the numbers of women developing breast cancer and from the extremely poor and static results of treatment it would seem that the need for collaborative studies was only too clear. Surprisingly and unfortunately, only a fraction (perhaps 10 or 15 per cent) of high risk patients, that is, with positive axillary nodes, are entered into clinical trials in the UK – despite the fact there are 20 or more trials in progress at present. Many will fail because of lack of numbers, and others will take too long to recruit an adequately large sample of patients. It is therefore pertinent to address those surgeons and radiotherapists – the majority who do not participate in any trial. Some of the non-trialists consider that they already know the truth of the matter. Cytotoxic chemotherapy is unpleasant, expensive, has possible long term risks, and should be avoided. Alternatively, in view of the results reported the answer to early breast cancer treatment has been found and all patients can be safely given chemotherapy without further evaluation being necessary. Other non-trialists may not know what the truth is. They are content to rest until the 'facts' emerge and to await a change in 'fashion' before they take action. Finding the facts and leading opinion is for others to do – they are busy enough just treating their patients. For whatever reason, such non-participation has tragic consequences. Answers will take a long time to appear, and every suitable patient not entered into a study adds further to the delay and uncertainty. Whatever our own personal prejudices and doubts, it is only in supporting trials, by joining them oneself, that facts can be substituted for opinion. Non-participation in clinical trials is a decision not to contribute to medical progress and this, surely, is morally, if not professionally, indefensible.

THE MANAGEMENT OF OVERT ADVANCED BREAST CANCER (STAGE III)

Ultimately proving fatal unless another illness or accident intervenes, treatment must have a different objective from that acceptable in 'early' cancer, namely to produce optimum disease regression for the maximum duration, but bearing in mind that undesirable side effects should be compatible with the fact that cure is unattainable. In other words, though radical treatment with its considerable demands is justifiable in phases I and II, where cure is a legitimate goal, this is not the case here. The quality of life experienced by patients with advanced disease undergoing systemic treatment must be the first consideration, therefore unpleasant side effects must be kept to a minimum.

Treatment as usual is enveloped in confusion and argument, principally centring around the relative roles of endocrine manipulation and combination chemotherapy. Non-surgical endocrine therapy is less disturbing than chemotherapy which interferes with the patient's life style by requiring hospital attendance or admission for one to five days per month, and which carries some subjective discomfort, problems dependant upon the regimen utilized. Chemotherapy however produces two or three times more objective responses than endocrine measures, with perhaps a somewhat longer duration.

In one sense current argument about which therapy should come first is academic as all patients will eventually fail on their first treatment irrespective of what it may be, proceeding if well enough to the alternative. Many suggest that endocrine therapy being less distressing should have priority thereby maintaining a superior life quality. Alternatively some argue that preliminary administration of a treatment which proves unsuccessful, adversely prejudices the response to subsequent treatment which would have been more likely to be effective in the first place. This implies that chemotherapy should be given first, but supporting evidence is not well founded. Whilst ineffective chemotherapy (e.g. single agent) may induce drug resistance and so prejudice more effective chemotherapy such interrelationships have not been demonstrated between endocrine and chemotherapy. Indeed Priestman [138] provides in general, contradictory evidence though the number of patients are small. Additionally Nolvadex is as valuable for chemotherapy relapses as when used as first line therapy (Edelstyn et al. [56]). Also relevant is the time which elapses before the outcome of endocrine therapy becomes apparent. Lacking really reliable marker systems to give an early biochemical indication, this is usually about three months. Should response be lacking then the patient will have deteriorated further, subjectively and objectively, and may be less able to tolerate the undoubted greater demands of chemotherapy which because of the greater tumour bulk may be less likely to work. Alternatively chemotherapy response is usually apparent within 4–6 weeks giving a more rapid indication of whether treatment should be changed.

Psychological factors must also be relevant though how is uncertain. Is it better for the patient to first receive a treatment which she quickly recognizes as effective, to be followed later by one more likely to fail? Alternatively what is the impact of giving first a treatment which obviously fails, something which must cause distress, to be followed by one which is beneficial? The answer to such speculation remains unknown but may be important.

Indicators for Selection of Therapy

There are however certain indicators which help in selection between the therapies.

Steroid Receptor Analyses

These are considerd in the section on tumour markers.

If receptor studies are not available or are inconclusive clinical factors alone can help in certain instances but not in others. These are discussed below.

The Disease-free Interval (DFI)

The longer the interval between treatment of the primary cancer and the clinical appearance of recurrence the more likely is a good response to endocrine therapy. An arbitrary period of 24 months is often adopted as the watershed with periods in excess of this being considered as a pointer in that direction.

Visceral Metastatic Disease in Any Age Group

Chemotherapy is the treatment of choice. If for any reason it is not possible, or in the subsequent presence of progressive disease, endocrine therapy is unlikely to work and so should be undemanding, for example, in the younger women oophorectomy or androgens and in the older whichever additive therapy is preferred.

Local Recurrence

In the older age group, especially with a long DFI, endocrine therapy is the treatment of choice. If a response is obtained subsequent relapse is probably best treated by other additive measures with chemotherapy as a last resort. If no response is obtained to the first additive therapy and chemotherapy is feasible then it should be immediately used – if not feasible than an alternative additive therapy can be tried. In the woman less than 5 years past the menopause the choice is more difficult with that not used as first line being used as second. The decision about which to use depends upon the philosophy of the doctor and also upon the condition and attitude of the patient.

Bony Metastases

Many therapists claim that this group respond poorly to chemotherapy, but whilst response rates claimed may be somewhat lower many patients do respond well. This may be explained by an over rigid application of response criteria which whilst suitable for the more readily assessable local and visceral recurrences could well be unsuitable in the more difficult situation presented by lytic disease in bone. Many such patients following chemotherapy may experience great pain relief, a reduction in analgesic requirements, improved mobility (possibly measurable), improvement in local or visceral deposits but show little evidence of radiological bone healing. Such situations are interpreted as a failure in response but this is not necessarily correct for the factors underlying bone healing are poorly understood and have not been related to radiological or histological appearances. Depending upon considerations similar to those for local recurrence the choice again rests between the two modalities. If endocrine therapy is to be used first, present information indicates that 6-amino-glutethimide, preceeded in the younger woman by oophorectomy, may be the treatment of choice. This can serve as an indicator to the likely response from subsequent adrenalectomy or hypophysectomy or may be an end in itself. It is at present unclear whether major endocrine ablation has a role following such therapy and in any case such procedures are more demanding in morbidity than is chemotherapy which can be used after these methods fail. By combing these clinical factors: age, predominant type of recurrence and DFI, further aid in patient selection may be obtained particularly for endocrine therapy. If all factors are favourable to a particular procedure, this will carry a high rate of response. Should all factors be unfavourable there will be no likelihood of endocrine response. The largest group of patients unfortunately possess mixed factors with only intermediate response levels and for them this system is without value.

SPECIFIC ENDOCRINE THERAPIES

Manipulation of the endocrine milieu in breast cancer was predicted by Shinzinger in 1888. The first patients were treated by Beatson in 1896 with surgical oophorectomy, subsequently followed by a range of techniques which fall into two categories, hormone addition and gland ablation. No absolute agreement exists on the precise sequences in which these should be used, individual preference remaining perhaps the most important determinant.

Hormone Administration

Androgens

Even if no response results, a feeling of general well-being is common. Remissions occur in 25 per cent of patients of all ages lasting about 6 months, those with bony metastases showing some response. Occasionally on withdrawal of this and indeed of other hormones further improvement ensues.

Testosterone may produce various side effects including:

1. Masculinization – which causes coarse skin, acne, temporal alopecia, hirsutism, deepening of the voice, clitoral enlargement and increase in libido.
2. Rise in serum calcium usually but not always in the presence of bony metastases. This can cause nausea, vomiting, diarrhoea, weakness, apathy, renal damage and even peripheral circulatory failure.
3. Some fluid retention usually occurs and may be dangerous in patients with cardiovascular disease.

There are three methods of administration, the first two being more commonly used than the third.

1. Testosterone propionate in a dosage of 100 mg intramuscularly twice or three times a week. If response is obtained a dosage of 3500 – 4000 mg should be obtained over about four months, with a subsequent dose reduction. Nandralone decanoate (Deca-durabolin), a less virilizing alternative administered i.m. weekly or fortnightly is as effective, more convenient and generally a preferred alternative.
2. Oral therapy – Methyl testosterone 50 – 100 mg per day, dissolved sublingually avoids the necessity for frequent patient attendance but is more expensive.
3. Implantation therapy is now rarely used. Pellets of 500 – 750 mg are implanted subcutaneously. If unpleasant side effects result it is not possible to interrupt therapy promptly.

Oestrogens

Between 30 and 40 per cent of post-menopausal patients respond but the majority for less than a year. The further past the menopause the greater the likelihood of benefit whilst local recurrence and a long DFI are favourable factors. As with androgens further relief may be obtained on cessation. Side effects include nausea, vomiting and uterine haemorrhage especially on discontinuation. Fluid retention may also occur.

Oestrogens are usually administered orally. The commonest and cheapest is diethyl stilboestrol 10–20 mg daily. Other preparations are dienoestrol, 10 mg daily; and ethinyl oestradiol 3 mg daily. Oestrogens can also be given parenterally.

Prednisone

Prednisone combined with thyroxine, appears to be of some value, though probably many remissions are subjective only due rather to the feeling of well-being engendered by the coricosteroids than to any effect on the tumour.

Prednisone depresses secretion of ACTH and thus adrenal oestrogen. However, there is an increase in gonadotrophins and so, if the ovaries are capable of responding, oestrogen secretion will be maintained. Thus, patients aged under 60 years require oophorectomy. As prednisone also interferes with thyroid function this hormone should also be administered. The suggested dosage is prednisone 30 mg three times daily and thyroxine 0·1 mg three times daily. With this dose, complications can occur and careful supervision is required.

Progestogens

There seems little to choose between the various preparations and norethisterone acetate (SH420) is probably as good as any. As with most hormones it is without benefit in younger women, in visceral disease and in the presence of a short disease-free interval. Accordingly it is of maximum benefit in older women with a longer disease-free interval and predominantly local recurrence of disease. An overall 30 per cent response rate is common, the figure depending upon the predictive factors ranging from zero where all are unfavourable to 80 per cent where the converse exists.

Anti-oestrogens

Now possibly the most widely used compound, tamoxifen (Nolvadex) is simple to administer and devoid of unpleasant side effects. About 40 per cent of patients respond to a dose of 10 mg four times daily, favourable factors being much as for norethisterone acetate. A recent prospective study comparing oestrogens with Nolvadex suggested the latter to be less upsetting and perhaps more effective, so it would seem preferable. It is of value in patients who have either failed to respond to chemotherapy or having responded subsequently relapsed. Remission rates encountered in this situation are similar to those obtained when the agent is used as first line treatment.

Aminoglutethimide

6-Aminoglutethimide, an interesting agent, is attracting increasing attention (Koelmeyer et al. [99]). Originally developed as an anti-convulsant, shortly thereafter it was noted to have certain undesirable endocrinological side effects which led to its withdrawal from general use. The drug inhibits the first step in the secretion of the whole range of adrenal steroids and has been likened to a medical adrenalectomy. This action can to some degree be overridden by a compensatory rise in ACTH secretion which can be suppressed by cortisone. There is also an inhibition of the conversion of androgens to oestrogens in the peripheral tissues.

Hall [76], possibly the first to use this drug in the treatment of advanced breast cancer, obtained a 33 per cent response rate amongst nine patients whilst Griffiths et al. [73] and Harvey et al. [80] also obtained useful results. More recently Smith [156] indicated that 37 per cent of patients showed evidence of objective response and that as with a surgical adrenalectomy a higher proportion, in this case 53 per cent of patients with bony deposits experienced rapid and marked subjective relief.

Koelmeyer et al. amongst 55 patients all of whom were progressive after prior chemo- or endocrine therapy obtained similar results. In this series adrenal suppression was confirmed by evaluation of the 9 am serum cortisol level and maintaining it below 100 nmol per litre. This necessitated individual dosage adjustment to achieve such a level. They concluded that it is of value in selecting patients for surgical adrenalectomy. It is however unclear whether a surgical adrenalectomy would produce better results and certainly the morbidity is greater, so aminoglutethimide may well have a role as an end in itself.

Recommended dosage is 250 mg orally four times daily and cortisone 25 mg twice daily with fluorocortisone 0·1 mg twice daily if electrolyte imbalance is noted. Principal side effects are drowsiness especially in older women which requires short term dose reduction and also a self-limiting skin rash.

Oophorectomy

This benefits about 25 per cent of pre- and menopausal patients for 6–9 months. Radiation is probably inferior to surgery which is relatively trivial and removes ovarian function swiftly.

Adrenalectomy

Usually combined with oophorectomy this produces regression in perhaps 40 per cent of patients and is of particular value in bony metastases. The patient and her doctor must be warned that there must never be any interruption of cortisone maintenance disease and that infection or stress require a prompt dose increase or serious catastrophe, if not death, may result.

Hypophysectomy

This operation has the advantage of eliminating ACTH which acts both on normal and ectopic adrenal tissue as well as prolactin and growth hormone.

It appears that bony metastases, a long DFI and relative youth combine to provide the best outcome. The procedure has been attempted by introducing radioactive seeds by the nasal route but blindness, rhinorrhoea, meningitis and haemorrhage from the cavernous sinus are encountered whilst pituitary tissue may persist and maintain function. The combination of surgery and intracellular radiation with Yttrium 90 in wax seems to overcome this problem. Beta rays are rapidly absorbed and radiation dosage at distances greater than 0·75 cm from the source is well within tolerance. Response rates are comparable with adrenalectomy. Possibly results obtained by adrenalectomy and hypophysectomy will be matched by aminoglutethimide and this may render both operations unnecessary.

CHEMOTHERAPY

The first reports on cytotoxic agents published about 1960, were concerned with single agents administered on a continuous basis. Cyclophosphamide, methotrexate and 5-fluorouracil were initially used, followed by the vinca alkaloids and more recently adriamycin. Generally objective response rates obtained were of a similar order to endocrine therapy namely, around 25–30 per cent, though adriamycin appears more effective with up to 50 per cent being claimed. Over the next decade the advantages of drug combinations at regular intervals became appreciated, and consequently this gradually predominated over single agent therapy. First reports (Greenspan, [72]) with a combination of cytotoxic and endocrine therapy claimed an 81 per cent response rate. This was followed by Cooper [44] who with cyclophosphamide, methotrexate, fluorouracil and vincristine and prednisone claimed a 90 per cent complete remission rate amongst 60 patients. Hannon [77] utilizing a 5-day regimen with the same four cytotoxic agents obtaining a response rate of 100 per cent from 14 patients, a figure never since equalled. A more representative estimate of results with these drugs would be a response rate between 50 and 60 per cent. Recently several randomized prospective studies comparing single agents with combinations have been performed. These show convincingly that combinations produce superior response rates of somewhat better duration. In consequence if chemotherapy is to be used it is best as a combination. Indeed preliminary use of single agents may prejudice its results.

It became clear that combination chemotherapy was superior in inducing response to endocrine therapy, though the price paid was greater in terms of toxicity and inconvenience, and demands upon hospital facilities were considerable. As a result the 5-day regimen failed to gain general acceptance, certainly in the UK. For this reason, amongst others the British Multicentre Collaborative Breast Chemotherapy Group was established in 1973. The underlying objectives of this group were to design chemotherapy regimens more compatible with the patient's requirements. In other words treatment must be convenient to administer, tolerable in terms of toxicity and therapeutically effective. Convenience implies that the patients should not spend more than one night in the hospital or better still not be admitted at all. This is an important consideration as hospitalization interferes considerably with the woman's domestic and social life and possible business commitments. It must be remembered that whilst percentage tumour regression produced by a regimen is often the yardstick of its effectiveness, as far as the patient is concerned life quality is supreme and the ability to maintain normal activity most relevant. Also a central issue is treatment toxicity. Adherence to the therapeutic principles discussed above goes a considerable way towards reducing unpleasant side effects, but a number remain commonplace. Thus whilst mucositis, marrow depression sufficient to cause symptoms, neuropathy and cardiac complications should not occur, nausea, vomiting and hair loss are commonplace as may be a general non-specific debility and mental depression, which whilst less defined can be most troublesome. This is in part drug-induced, and probably psychological factors play a significant part. Chemotherapy therefore should maintain the maximum therapeutic efficiency compatible with the minimum subjective disturbance. Supportive measures designed to overcome the inevitable consequence of treatment should always be used and improvement continually pursued. Commencing with the premise that no treatment could be more convenient than that administered by one intravenous injection, the Group designed such a regimen with the four drugs mentioned and a three-weekly cycle. This was significantly less toxic, but of less therapeutic benefit. Thus 5-day chemotherapy produced 59 per cent responses at 3 months, falling to 44 per cent by the 12 month period whilst the figures for the 1-day were 49 per cent and 17 per cent. A 2-day system was then devised with the same drugs administered on days 1 and 8 of a four weekly cycle. This produced objective results comparable to the 5-day regimen but with greater convenience and less toxicity. Epilation in particular was reduced by half. The problem still remained that at 12 months the initial remission rates had dropped by more than half to under 30 per cent.

The next step was to attempt to further raise and also to prolong the remission rates. Adriamycin was incorporated in the 2-day regimen and a study of 2-day chemotherapy with and without adriamycin was undertaken. The 2-day chemotherapy produced an objective remission rate of 60 per cent whilst adriamycin raised this to 78 per cent, though the overall duration of response remained the same, the median benefit obtained being under 12 months. At this stage following reports by Price and Goldie [136] that good remission rates were produced by a regimen administered over a period of about 24 hours, the group decided to re-evaluate 1-day treatment. To obviate hospital admission the regimen devised consisted of an intravenous bolus of adriamycin, vincristine and 5-fluorouracil followed by oral leukeran and methotrexate over 24 hours. This was compared with the 2-day adriamycin containing regimen, and has produced an initial objective remission rate of 80 per cent, not dissimilar from other reports of adriamycin in combination regimens. Unsuccessful efforts were also made to prolong the duration of remission by utilizing oral maintenance therapy. A situation has now been reached where initial remission figures are excellent, but maintenance remains a problem. A number of methods are being explored, thus the Multicentre Group are currently evaluating the alternating use of two non-cross-resistant combinations of three drugs, whilst an interesting but preliminary report (Edelstyn et al. [56]) suggests that ICRF 159 (Razoxane) appears capable on its own of maintaining complete remission once achieved by intensive therapy as described.

COMBINED CYTOTOXIC AND HORMONE THERAPY

There have been a number of reports concerning simultaneous administration of chemotherapy and hormones. A prospective randomized study (Rubens et al. [148]) compared two groups of patients both of whom received combination chemotherapy and one additionally norethisterone acetate. No advantage could be attributed to progestogen in terms of response rate or duration, though interestingly they did seem to demonstrate better marrow tolerance and less nausea and vomiting. Prednisone added to chemotherapy has been studied by American groups, no advantage being demonstrated. Decadurabolin was similarly evaluated (Edelstyn et al. [56]) the suggestion being that patients who received this hormone had a somewhat higher incidence of response which was of greater duration. Interestingly as in the progestogen study, bone-marrow depression was less marked. Alternatively Ahmann et al. [2] claims that in pre-menopausal women treated by oophorectomy followed by immediate chemotherapy objective response rates were significantly superior to a group in whom chemotherapy was delayed until the disease recurrence. It is worth observing that as cytotoxic agents are effective against cyclic cells concomitant use of hormones in a setting where they might inhibit tumour activity is unlikely to be of value. On the other hand were the growth to be possibly stimulated as by the use of oestrogens in the pre- or peri-menopausal setting then possibly a better therapeutic effect might be achieved. Such a study presents obvious problems.

Estracyte

This agent, in a sense in a class of its own, combines an alkylating agent and an oestrogenic sterol which may act as an anti-oestrogen. Whilst its therapeutic potential is presently uncertain there is evidence to suggest that it will have an important role. Thus, in a series of 44 post-menopausal women with advanced breast cancer, most of whom had relapsed following chemotherapy (Alexander [4]), 38 per cent had a definite objective response.

MANAGEMENT OF THE PATIENT WITH ADVANCED BREAST CANCER AND PROGRESS AFTER CHEMOTHERAPY

Patients with predominantly bony metastases and in reasonable general conditions may benefit from 6-aminoglutethimide. No major series has been reported but limited personal experience suggests the procedure to be worthwhile. In addition tamoxifen is of value. Amongst just under 100 such patients tamoxifen 10 mg four times daily produces good quality control in 40 per cent of instances. This figure, comparable with that obtained when the agent is used as primary therapy does not support the contention that systemic agents used as second line therapy tend to produce poorer results than when used *ab initio.* Responses in this series occurred predominantly in older women with local disease, and were somewhat less amongst those patients who originally had not responded to chemotherapy when compared with those who had.

Alternative Chemotherapeutic Regimens

Following failure of the initial chemotherapy, worthwhile response to alternative regimens is uncommon and if it does occur is of short duration. Such salvage chemotherapy is probably unjustified provided the primary treatment was one generally recognized as effective in its own right.

CHEMOTHERAPY INDUCED PROBLEMS

Without doubt chemotherapy can be associated with toxicities ranging from a mere transient subjective discomfort to an overwhelming rapidly fatal situation. It is however fair comment that these toxicities are attributable in greater part to the therapist than to the therapy. In selecting a patient for cytotoxic chemotherapy, a number of factors have to be considered, and if these are given due weight, then treatment should be compatible with the recipient enjoying good quality worthwhile life, the objective of any therapy.

Age

Older patients do not tolerate treatment well. Thus in general it is unwise to administer chemotherapy to women over 75 years and perhaps 70 years of age should be the upper limit. However, treatment has been successfully and uneventfully given to older women, and a decision should be reached on the biological rather than strictly chronological age.

General Condition

Advanced malignant disease carries a progressive debility and cachexia, and this must adversely effect the capacity to tolerate therapy. Rather than constituting an absolute bar to chemotherapy, treatment should be modified with dosage reduction of perhaps one-third in the early courses, levels being increased should the patient improve.

Specific Ailments

Cardiac Disease

Whilst a number of drugs possess a potential cardio-toxic effect, adriamycin is paramount, and a cumulative dose of 550 mg/m^2 surface area should not be exceeded. In view of the cardiotoxicity of this agent it is probably wise to omit it unless there are strong contrary reasons.

Liver Disease

Pre-existing non malignant or extensive metastatic liver disease, especially if liver biochemistry is impaired. Adriamycin is largely metabolized in the liver and in such circumstances this may be impeded with increased toxicity. Doses should be modified, though as good responses can be obtained in hepatic metastatic disease they may be increased later. Methotrexate should also be administered cautiously in this situation.

Renal Function

Considerably increased methotrexate toxicity may be experience in the presence of renal disease, and it is necessary to obtain preliminary blood urea levels and preferable creatinine clearance figures.

Effusions

Accumulation of fluid in body cavities can have serious implications for methotrexate. The drug tends to accumulate in such fluid being released slowly and this increases toxicity. Such effusions should first be drained or if this is impracticable or undesirable then methotrexate should be withheld or alternatively a prolonged folinic acid rescue instituted, preferably with monitoring of serum methotrexate levels.

Pancytopenia resultant upon Marrow Replacement

This is not a total contraindication to chemotherapy. Marrow function can be improved by drugs such as vincristine, bleomycin and indeed prednisone, combined perhaps with cautious utilization of anti-metabolites. Despite the above precautions toxicities will be encountered in a minority of patients and on an occasional basis. The management of severe bone-marrow depression, or mucositis will not be discussed here but a few points can be made.

Epilation

A distressing experience for some women, but more readily accepted if its possibility is explained before chemotherapy is commenced. A head band inflated to just above systolic pressure may help in some instances, but is painful and many find it difficult to accept. An alternative method is scalp cooling. This employs a number of bags containing a fluid which can be cooled in an ordinary domestic refrigerator to below 0 °C and yet not freeze. These are applied to the scalp some quarter of an hour before chemotherapy commences and kept in place for half an hour subsequently. Whilst not affording complete protection certainly the incidence of total and severe epilation is significantly reduced with little subjective discomfort. This may be time-consuming but is worthwhile.

Anorexia, Nausea and Vomiting

Certainly the commonest and probably the most unpleasant side effects. In certain instances, they can be so severe as to cloud the entire quality of life and even prevent the woman continuing with therapy. Whilst undoubtedly drug induced, psychological factors play a part; thus not a few patients feel nauseated and indeed vomit prior to drugs administration. One approach is to give the patient a tranquilizing agent which she should commence taking 24 hours prior to chemotherapy. When the chemotherapy intravenous giving system is established, the first agent should be an anti-emetic such as metoclopramide 10 mg which should then be taken orally at 6-hourly intervals for the succeeding 24–48 hours depending on the subjective state. If vomiting persists it may be preferable to use an alternative anti-emetic which should be given intramuscularly at home. There is anecdotal evidence that hydrocortisone 100 mg intravenously immediately followed by 10 mg oral administration combined with maxolon has additional benefit. The patient should have an experienced counsellor available before treatment commences and regularly thereafter. Staff administering chemotherapy should be aware of the various problems which can arise and it is their responsibility to make sure that further counselling is given when and as necessary. Without doubt psychological factors play a part in many of the problems encountered and that competent counselling can reduce these.

Placement of Cannula

Meticulous attention must be paid to the accurate placement of the intravenous cannula. In view of the need to change syringes frequently a 'butterfly' arrangement should be utilized as this is more secure. Drug extravasation particularly of vinca alkaloids and adriamycin can cause excruciating pain which persists for months and a deep full thickness skin ulcer may result which ultimately requires excision and grafting. Apart from possible medicolegal consequences, serious extravasation can do much to negate the effects of otherwise successful treatment.

PSYCHOLOGICAL FACTORS

To save a woman by surgical intervention and then deny her the emotional support necessary to form a different lifestyle and accept an altered body image is a contradiction in terms.

Any therapist involved in the total care of a woman with breast cancer is faced with an enormous professional challenge. Initially, and not least, he must help his patient to accept the presence of a serious, potentially fatal disease. From being a 'well' woman with a lump, the patient is changed, often overnight, into a 'sick' woman, needing hospitalization and extensive treatment. This sudden change of status can be confusing and disorientating. Patients regularly complain that they felt well until they came for treatment, and find it difficult to grasp the severity of their situation.

Cancer is still an emotive word in our community, conjuring up visions of doom and despair [92, 107, 113, 132, 168, 169]. Such generally held attitudes may reflect and even exaggerate the threat implied by the disease. Women with breast cancer must cope with these existing phantasies concerning the illness [104]. In addition, many fear diagnosis of malignancy. Such fears often pre-empt the illness, but crystalize with detection of the lump [78]. Whilst most women have sufficient personality integration to face such fears and come for diagnosis, some with markedly depressive or defeatist personalities may defer coming for biopsy because of their inherent sense of hopelessness [115]. Such hopelessness may arise either from existant, but often erroneous, myths concerning the illness, or from the woman's own deep rooted defeatism. Many women are afraid of surgery, and waiting for the biopsy, or its results can be distressing [78]. Maguire [116] noted anxiety and depression in 31 per cent of his patients prior to biopsy, and several writers have stressed the need for pre-operative counselling [50, 79, 104, 118]. Little is known about the psychological effects of mastectomy, although it has been argued that the breast has no essential function and that a woman confronted with cancer should accept its removal as a relatively small sacrifice to make for the sake of her health. On the other hand, in our society, the breasts have assumed an especial sexual and maternal significance [7, 141], and the loss of a breast might be equated with loss of femininity.

Mastectomy, simple or radical, is one way of reducing the total tumour burden, but there is no guarantee of cure. On the contrary it faces the woman with a major operation, itself traumatic, and undoubted permanent mutilation. Disfigurement may prove a real threat to the woman's self-image, and to her general psychological adjustment, and suicide may occur or be contemplated. Perhaps for this reason, given a simple but full explanation concerning alternative surgical procedures, it is probable most women would opt for lumpectomy alone. Where more extensive surgical intervention has occurred it is not surprising to find evidence of emotional upset following the event.

Several recent surveys have noted the presence of anxiety, depression or embarrassment following mastectomy. Roberts et al. [143] reported anxiety and depression in 51 per cent of the women they studied. Buls et al. [29] noted that a third of their patients were anxious or embarrassed because of their breast loss, and this showed no signs of diminution with time. Maguire et al. [116] found that a third of their patients had sexual problems following mastectomy, although none had consulted a general practitioner on the matter. Witkin [172] emphasized the mastectomee's concern over sexual desirability, her fear of rejection, and/or pity and the danger facing her marriage. She noted feelings of worthlessness, changed self-image, shame, mourning for breast loss, and insomnia, and emphasized the need for postoperative counselling of both patients and their sexual partners. Similarly Klein [104], Asken [7] and Dietz [50] emphasize that a husband may be more afraid of hurting his wife's feelings than of a scar, and may need help in knowing how best to help her. Klein states that unless support can be given to such men many, full of uncertainty and conflicting emotions, may express their concerns by withdrawing and retreating from the situation: the wife may interpret this behaviour as rejection, thereby compounding the problem. Both husband and wife may become depressed and disparate, affecting the emotional life of all family members, including children. Younger children may feel deserted by a hospitalized and convalescent mother, and older children may become a prey to fantasies centring on mutilation or mortality. Asken notes that children may develop school problems as a response to their mother's inexplicable depression. Women who have sustained major surgical intervention may have to endure the added discomfort of a stiff shoulder or painful chest wall. Buls et al. found that 32 per cent of the women they studied had subsequent chest wall problems, whilst 26 per cent reported shoulder difficulty. Forty four per cent of their sample had lymphoedema. Healey [82] noted that the psychological distress caused by lymphoedema centred on self-consciousness of the enlarged arm in the presence of others, difficulty in fitting clothes, and changes in life style reflecting embarrassment in social situations.

Treatment for breast cancer is rarely confined solely to surgery. As mentioned elsewhere radiotherapy and/or chemotherapy are commonly used in all but the earliest cases. Neither is without its distressing side effects. Maguire has emphasized the depressing nature of radiotherapy; patients are frequently left exhausted, and, without proper understanding of the treatment, believe that such feelings must argue for a worse prognosis. Kardinal and Cupper [96] and Burton [31] both emphasize the distressing side effects produced by chemotherapy particularly in advanced disease. Mouth ulceration is painful and may reduce appetite, and stimulate additional fears concerning reactivation of disease. Hair loss may contribute to feelings of ugliness and unacceptibility. Weight gain, increasing musculature, and the development of additional superficial hair due to androgen therapy may additionally confuse the patient, disturbing her sense of sexual identity. Probably most distressing of all are the nausea and vomiting produced by some chemotherapeutic regimens. Commencing during therapy, and often lasting for several days afterwards, sickness can so erode feelings of well-being that the patient may question whether it is really worth continuing with the therapy. In extreme cases patients become so afraid of the experience that they vomit on the way to hospital, even before the drugs are given.

Generally, from the patient's standpoint, any treatment will be tolerated best if it produces a sense of well-being. If the patient comes for treatment feeling ill, and goes away feeling better, he will accept the intervening therapy in reasonably good part. Unfortunately, as Burton emphasized, with many of the treatments presently used to combat breast cancer, the reverse is true. Following therapy some women feel worse than they did before. Many confide that before therapy began they felt well and were coping adequately, following it they feel tired, depressed, achey and sick. Many patients are perplexed by such feelings, and incorrectly attribute them to an acceleration of the disease. Because secondary spread is sited within the body, where they cannot assess its progress or regression, they monitor the success of their therapy by their own sense of physical well-being, and when faced with distressing treatment related side effects fear the disease is extending.

Most women appreciate the risk of recurrence in breast cancer and understandably many fear death. Several studies [10, 116, 139, 141, 142] have noted the distress such fears can produce. Younger patients may become angry and bitter [78, 96] yet desist from voicing such feelings because of their fears of rejection. Older patients may perceive the illness as a confirmation of the debilitating effects of old age [7] and become demoralized because they cannot see the value of struggling against it. McIntosh [113] has stated the damaging effects of uncertainty on patient's morale, and several studies have argued for the honest interchange of information between the doctor and the cancer patient [3, 70, 97]. Erwin [61] argues for a blend of hope and honesty and advocates involvement of the husband wherever possible. Other disease related fears may include that of contagion (Kennedy et al. [98]) or the fear that the disease was somehow caused by, or was a punishment for, the individual's misdeeds. Kardinal and Cupper [96] comment: 'It does seem surprising that in the twentieth century so many patients would feel that their cancers are a punishment for evil doing. Some patients seem to feel that nothing as terrible as cancer should happen to anyone unless it be retribution.' Other patients regularly harbour more realistic fears, for example, fears for the future may preclude realistic life planning. Kennedy has emphasized that patients may fear they will lose their jobs, and Weismann [171] noted their apprehensions concerning diminishing self-reliance.

Whatever the specific fears or worries most patients do seem to show a phasic response to their disease. At first they are confused, shocked or disorientated, wondering how they could possibly have 'caught' cancer. Some deny the gravity of their situation warding off the full implications of the diagnosis by maintaining that their illness is not the real thing, but rather some pre-malignant condition caught in good time. Later, when treatment makes denial impossible many patients become depressed, and some may dwell on the possibility of recurrence or death. At this stage, patients need optimistic updating of information, and constant reminders of the most hopeful aspects of their situation. Kennedy et al. [98] have stressed the need for a positive attitude on the patient's part in terms of combating the disease. Patients do best who have a positive determination to fight the disease, and Kennedy emphasizes that patients 'cured of advanced cancer' often become stronger people: 'Psychologic strength is often gained from having faced the stress of primary cancer and survived. There is elation, increased zest for life, and a greater appreciation of the commonplace. With each check-up visit concern of recurrence decreases, confidence increases, and fear diminishes, though it never disappears. Residual concern even after years without evidence of disease is common.' Similarly, Witkin [172] found that where a positive attempt is made by a husband to share his wife's experience, and support her through them, the marriage not only survives, but is often strengthened by the experience.

Several writers, for example Bronner-Huszar [26] Laxenaire et al. [110], and Shonfield [154] have noted the importance of an early return to work and normal activity as a means of effectively dealing with the high levels of anxiety produced. They also emphasize the importance of mobilizing family support. Weisman [171] and Burton [31] have both found that patients without family support show evidence of greater anxiety, and experience more difficulty in accepting treatment than those who are fully supported. Weismann comments: 'Every patient, regardless of coping competence or overall vulnerability has moments of distress in which problems pyramid. These may be transient, quickly abating like an abrupt fall in temperature. But they may persist or recur, like a smouldering low grade fever with an occasional 'spike' .... When patients were asked to rate themselves according to the most important or urgent problems at peak moments of psychological distress, non-medical problems predominate.' Thus, the quality of a patient's previous life is a predicative factor in determining his ability to combat and overcome the illness.

Even well supported patients do not escape practical problems however. After treatment many women find the scar tissue tender and sore to touch. Poorly fitting clothes, especially an ill-fitting bra or prosthesis, can be uncomfortable. Radiation may cause burning, and the whole area becomes inflamed, making difficulties even at night when bed clothes may rub. Even when a good prosthesis has been fitted, and there are no physical complications, some women feel asymmetrical, and find their remaining breast of questionable significance, either fearing that it also may be invaded by the disease, or feeling unwilling to display it as a sexual symbol next to the scar. Many women worry about straightforward practical problems such as how soon they may bathe or sunbathe the area, or how much use they may make of the adjacent arm in terms of housework or child care. Counselling concerning such practical problems is clearly imperative.

Beeby and Broeg [16] suggest a programme of practical and emotional intervention to support to woman with breast cancer. First he advocates the need to improve the woman's physical well-being. Exercises should be devised to obtain and maintain the complete range of shoulder and arm motion. An attempt should be made to correct any postural deformities, and to combat possible ill effects of lymphoedema. Such exercises could be introduced preoperatively to prevent postoperative pneumonia, muscle degeneration pooling of lymph in extremities, and postural deformities. Postoperative exercises should aid the woman's rehabilitation at home. Beeby's second objective is the restoration of the woman's previous physical appearance. He argues for breast reconstruction and describes the considerable psychological improvement obtained by silicone implants. Harwell [79] and Buls et al. [29] reinforce this point. Buls confirms that the knowledge and use of the prosthesis is not universal. Many mastectomees do not know of the existence of a prosthesis, let alone of the range and variety of prostheses available. One-third of the woman Buls studied said they had never been counselled in such matters. Beeby's final objective in rehabilitating the breast cancer patient is concerned with re-establishing her emotional stability. She should be helped to accept the loss of her breast, assisted to see her new self as an object worthy of love, and encouraged to lead a normal and full life. Beeby sees pre- and postoperative counselling as a mandatory part of this process. In this he agrees with Klein, Markel, Harrell, Dietz, Witkin, and Weismann. Indeed, Witkin goes further in believing that the husband should also be counselled, and Renneker and Cutler [142] even advocate in-depth psychotherapy. Weismann has devised a series of exercises to improve coping strategies, and believes that effective psycho-social intervention can have a beneficial effect on the patient's emotional well-being.

Ideally, the breast cancer patient should be given opportunities to express her fears and apprehensions at each stage in the disease's progress and treatment. Opportunities should be given for her to ask practical questions and to receive advice and support. Information concerning the illness should be constantly updated, and husband should be counselled regarding their wife's situation wherever possible.

FACTORS RELEVANT TO CANCER BEHAVIOUR

Formulation of a rational treatment policy for breast cancer requires an understanding of the relationships between certain clinico-pathological features of the cancer and its likely behaviour. Some points which are appropriate to this matter will now be discussed.

Histology

This has been well reviewed by Fisher [64] who concludes that much of the evidence relating various histology features to prognosis is retrospective and as might be expected there are considerable disagreements between findings. However it seems that certain cell types, namely medullary, mucinous tubular and adenocystic do pursue a more favourable course. Fisher's findings are that the infiltrating duct carcinoma is the commonest cancer (50 per cent). Compared with other cancers it is more likely to be histologic Grade III and to demonstrate lymphatic invasion and a clinically positive axilla. Combinations of infiltrating duct cancers with other tumour types constitute the second commonest tumour type and it is interesting that these show less lymphatic invasion, few clinically positive axillae, a lower malignant histological grade and fewer non-invasive multicentric growths, although there is a higher association with invasive multicentre growths. The clinical significance of pure and mixed tumour cell populations remains uncertain.

Lobar Carcinoma

First described as an *in situ* growth an unknown proportion develop into, or become associated with the invasive variety. The prognosis is relatively poor.

Histological Grading of Malignancy

There is a definite relationship between histological malignancy and prognosis which is further strengthened when pathological staging is also taken into account.

Cell Reaction

It has been suggested that a lymphoid reaction at the tumour periphery and within the growth itself is a favourable finding. Evidence however is by no means clear. Fisher concludes that the reaction indicates the degree of tumour malignancy rather than a host immunological response.

Circumscription

There is a tendency for the growth to assume either a circumscribed or relatively more infiltrative form. In Fisher's series 40 per cent of tumours were grossly circumscribed but the figure fell to 17 per cent on microscopic examination. Lack of circumscription is associated with more treatment failures, certainly in the short term, though longer term results are not yet available.

Blood Vessel, Lymphatic and Peri-neural Invasion

These findings are all more likely to be associated with nodal involvement, and therefore with a poorer prognosis.

Lymph Node Involvement

This has been reviewed by Hughes and Forbes [88] who conclude there is no truth in the suggestion [46] that lymph nodes possess a beneficial influence and their removal might be harmful. It is unlikely that immunity plays a significant role once the tumour has reached a diameter in excess of one millimetre and, whilst admitting host resistance has some ill-defined role, such considerations cannot at present play a part in clinical management. They find no evidence to support the observation [59] that 75 per cent of lymph nodes palpable prior to local mastectomy, disappeared subsequently, concluding that malignant lymph nodes show a steady growth progression consistent with the original primary tumour. Tumour deposits in lymph nodes indicates the probability of systemic disease. There is a significant but not absolute relationship between node status and tumour behaviour. Where nodes are clear the five year recurrence figure is 20 per cent. With any nodal involvement it is 66 per cent rising to 81 per cent with four or more nodes involved. With a median time from recurrence to death of seven months, mortality figures do not lag far behind. The significance of microscopic axillary involvement has been looked at by Fisher [64]. In a group of patients in whom initial pathological examination of the axilla was negative, subsequent intensive re-examination revealed occult tumour in 24 per cent. Apart from indicating the fallibility of standard pathological techniques, the finding seemed of little clinical significance, there being no correlation with survival. This is in agreement with the findings of Huvos who demonstrated that survival with either micrometastases (<2 mm) or no metastases was similar, both being superior to macrometastases (>2 mm), although treatment failure rates seemed similar between micro- and macrometastases. However the subgroup of micrometastatic nodes, less than 1·3 mm had a similar outcome to node negative patients both in terms of treatment failure and survival. Other conclusions were that the number rather than the size of involved nodes was of paramount significance and that extranodal extension of disease constituted a grave omen.

Relationship between Primary Tumour Dimensions and Prognosis

Langlands and Kerr [108], reporting on almost 4000 patients with primary breast cancer treated by local mastectomy and radiotherapy came to the following conclusions.

1. Primary tumour size in the absence of clinical node disease
   Tumours less than 2 cm have a 5-year crude survival rate of 80·5 per cent falling to 62 per cent at 10 years. From 2–5 cm the respective figures are 67 and 44 per cent. The median survival for patients with 1·0 cm tumours is 16·6 years and for tumours larger than 5 cm 2·7 years. Extrapolation indicated the median survival for a half-centimetre tumour at about 21 years.
2. Primary tumour size in the presence of clinical node disease.
   For a tumour less than 2 cm, 5-year survival is 75·6 per cent, the 10 year figure being 51 per cent. For larger growths the figures are 54·6 per cent and 34 per cent.

In conclusion, the median survival for tumour less than 2 cm without nodes is 14·5 years whilst for the larger ones the figure is 8·2 years. With nodes the respective figures were 13 and 6·5 years, so primary tumour size is apparently of great prognostic consequence, smaller stage II possessing a better prognosis than larger stage I tumours. It must be noted that these figures are without histological verification of node status.

Tumour Fixation

By itself tumour fixation does not appear to influence prognosis. Hughes and Forbes [88] consider that tumour size is more significant than attachment to nearby tissues. If a tumour is small but attached to skin or muscle this may mean that it originated close to such a structure, and the finding is simply a 'geographic accident'. A larger but mobile tumour situated deeply within the breast substance may indicate that the tumour has to extend further before fixity can develop. They suggest that if the extent of fixity is greater than the tumour diameter or other skin findings are present the tumour is excessively aggressive.

Multifocality and Bilaterality

Between 7 and 10 per cent of patients will develop carcinoma of the second breast, a figure 4–7 times greater than that amongst the general population. Nevertheless this is less than would be expected, for more than 50 per cent of women with lobular *in situ* carcinoma may demonstrate bilaterality whilst Urban [163] claims that amongst women who have the opposite breast biopsied 20 per cent had bilateral tumours and 54 per cent *in situ* lobular cancer. These figures are greater than the cancers which subsequently develop so clearly cancers do not necessarily progress, they may even regress, otherwise bilateral mastectomy would have commended itself to the many and not, fortunately, remained the practice of a diminishing number of extremist practitioners.

The observation also has implications for the management of the primary cancer. It is traditional and probably appropriate to advocate some form of mastectomy on the grounds of multifocality in that breast. However it does seem reasonable to assume that both breasts form a single pathophysiological 'organ' whose existance in two halves is an attractive but incidental finding. Unless it is assumed that breast cancer has a local explanation such as trauma, then the influences controlling cancer behaviour must be systemic, so the whole organ must be exposed to these in similar fashion, e.g. what happens in one half must happen in the other. Thus if tumours known to be present in the remaining half do not manifest themselves after removal of the other half, might they not perhaps have behaved similarily in the half removed by surgery had they been given the chance. The microscope and pathologist's mounted specimen see events in one moment of time – certainly there is strong evidence that even invasive breast cancer is not necessarily an inexorably progressive situation such considerations are not simply academic – they may have eventually considerable practical implications too.

Influence of Age

The traditional view that breast cancer is a more aggressive disease in younger women has recently been questioned by Mueller and Ames [122] who carried out a detailed study of age as a prognostic factor, basing figures on more than 3500 patients. Amongst women under 50 years of age half of all the deaths occurred within 11·5 years, in the age group 51–70 years this period shortened to 7·2 years, and in the 71 or older group it was 4 years. However these results are based on deaths from all causes and other factors must assume greater significance in older women. Nevertheless a life table analysis of patients dying from breast cancer only did support their findings. The situation is not entirely clear, but their conclusions seem reasonable, i.e. that whilst most women who develop breast cancer will eventually die from their disease, the rate at which this occurs is slower in younger women, the disease being more aggressive in the older age groups.

REFERENCES

1. Adair F., Berg J., Lourdes J. et al. (1974) Long term followings of breast cancer patients: the 30 year report. *Cancer* **33**, 1145–1150.
2. Ahmann D. L., O'Connell M. J., Hahn R. G. et al. (1977) An evaluation of early or delayed adjuvant chemotherapy in pre-menopausal patients with advanced breast cancer undergoing oophorectomy. *N. Engl. J. Med.* **297**, 356–60.
3. Aitken Swan J. and Easson E. C. (1959) Reactions of cancer patients on being told their diagnosis. *Brit. Med. J.* **1**, 779–781.
4. Alexander L. L. (1979)
5. Allegra J. L., Lippman M. E., Thompson E. B. et al. (1978) An association between steroid hormone receptors and response to cytotoxic chemotherapy in patients with metastatic breast cancer. *Cancer Res.* **38**, 4299–304.
6. Anderson J. M., Stimson W. H. and Kelly F. (1976) Preclinical warning of necrudescent mammary cancer by pregnancy-associated alpha-macroglobulins. *Brit. J. Surg.* **63**, 819–822.
7. Asken M. J. (1975) Psychoemotional aspects of mastectomy: a review of the literature. *Am. J. Psychiatry* **132**, 56–60.
8. Atkins H., Hayward J. L., Klugman D. J. et al. (1972) Treatment of early breast cancer: a report after 10 years of a clinical trial. *Br. Med. J.* **2**, 423.
9. Baldwin R. W. (1975) *In vitro* assays of cell medicated immunity to human solid tumour: problems of quantitation, specificity and interpretation. *J. Natl. Cancer Inst.* **55**, 745.
10. Bard M. and Sutherland A. M. (1955) Psychological impact of cancer and its treatment: IV Adoption to radical mastectomy. *Cancer* **8**, 656–659.
11. Barnes B. A. (1977) Cost benefit analysis of surgery: current accomplishments and limitations. *Am. J. Surgery* **133**, 438–46.
12. Bataini J. P., Picco C., Martin M. et al. (1978) Relation between time-dose and local control of operable breast cancer treated by tumourectomy and radiotherapy or by radical radiotherapy alone. *Cancer* **42**, 2059–65.
13. Bauer H. W. and Ax W. (1977) Detection of sensitized human blood lymphocytes by agglutination with basic peptides: a possible test for malignant disease. *Brit. J. Cancer* **36**, 708–12.

14. Baum M. (1976) The curability of breast cancer. *Brit. Med. J.* **1**, 439–442.
15. Beatson G. T. (1896) *Lancet* **2**, 104–107.
16. Beeby J. and Broeg P. E. (1970) Treatment of patients with radical mastectomies. *Phys. Ther.* **50**, 40–3.
17. Bennett A., McDonald A. M., Simson J. S. et al. (1975) Breast cancer. *Prostaglandins* **9**, 377–84.
18. Bhattacharya M., Chatterjee S. K. and Barlow J. J. (1976) Uridine 5'diphosphatase-galactose: Glycoprotein galactosyltransferase activity and sialic acid content in rats with metastasizing mammary tumours. *Science* **195**, 577–579.
19. Bond W. H. (1968) *Treatment of Carcinoma of Breast.* Amsterdam, Excerpta Medica.
20. Bonadonna G. (1976) Combination chemotherapy as an adjuvant treatment in operable breast cancer. *N. Engl. J. Med.* **294**, 405–416.
21. Borthwick N. M., Wilson D. W. and Bell P. A. (1977) Carcinoembryonic antigen (CEA) in patients with breast cancer. *Eur. J. Cancer* **13**, 171–176.
22. Brinkley D. and Haybittle J. L. (1971) Treatment of Stage 2 carcinoma of female breast. *Lancet* **2**, 1086–1089.
23. Brinkley D. and Baybittle J. L. (1975) The curability of breast cancer. *Lancet* **2**, 95–7.
24. British Breast Group 1970.
25. British Multicentre Collaborative Breast Chemotherapy Group 1973.
26. Bronner-Huszar (1971).
27. Bruce H. A. and Forrest A. P. (1971) The surgeon and cancer research. Bruce Memorial Lecture. *Can. J. Surg.* **14**, 19–30.
28. Buffkin D. C., Webber M. M., Davidson W. D. et al. (1978) Ornithine as a possible marker of cancer. *Cancer Res.* **38**, 3225–9.
29. Buls J. C., Jones I. H. and Bennett R. C. (1976) Women's attitudes to mastectomy for breast cancer. *Med. J. Aust.* **2**, 336–8.
30. Burker.
31. Burton J. (1978) Attitudes towards death and of scientific authorities on death. *Psychoanal. Rev.* **65**, 415–32.
32. Bussolati G., Ghiringhello B. and DiCarlo F. (1977) Lactalbumin synthesis in breast-cancer tissue. *Lancet* **2**, 352.
33. Byar D. P., Simon R. M. and Friedewald W. T. (1976) Randomised clinical trials. Perspectives on some recent ideas. *New Engl. J. Med.* **295**, 74–80.
34. Caceres E. (1977) Actinomycin D in the treatment of metastatic osteogenic sarcoma. *Cancer Treat. Rep.* **61**, 498–9.
35. Cadeau B. J., Blockstein M. E. and Malkin A. (1974) Increased incidence of placenta-like alkaline phosphatase activity in breast and genito-urinary cancer. *Cancer Res.* **34**, 729.
36. Calle R., Pilleron J. P., Schlienger P. et al. (1978) Conservative management of operable breast cancer: ten years' experience at the Foundation Clinic. *Cancer* **42**, 2045–53.
37. Cercek L. and Cercek B. (1974) Involvement of cyclic-AMP in changes of the structuredness of cytoplasmic matrix (SCM). *Radiat. Environ. Biophys.* **11**, 209–212.
38. Chu T. M., and Nemoto T. (1973) Evaluation of carcinoembryonic antigen in human mammary carcinoma. *J. Natl. Cancer Inst.* **51**, 1119.
39. Cole M. P. (1964) The place of radiotherapy in the management of early breast cancer. *Brit. J. Surg.* **51**, 216–220.
40. Cole M. P. (1970) Deca-durabolin compared with cyclophosphamide. In: Joslin C. A. F. and Gleave E. N. (ed.), *Clinical Management of Advanced Breast Cancer.* Cardiff, Alpha Omega Press.
41. Coombes R. C., Hillyard C. J., Greenberg P. B. et al. (1900) Plasma-immunoreactive calcitonin in patients with non-thyroid tumours. *Lancet* **1**, 1080–108.

42. Coombes R. C., Powles T. J. and Gazet J. C. (1977) A biochemical approach to the staging of human breast cancer. *Cancer* **40,** 937–44.

43. Coombes R. C., Powles T. J. and Neville A. M. (1977a) Evaluation of biochemical markers in breast cancer. *Proc. R. Soc. Med.* **70,** 843–5.

44. Cooper . . (1969) Combination chemotherapy in hormone resistance breast cancer. *Proc. Am.*

45. Cowen A. E., Korman M. G., Hoffman E. F. et al. (1978) Radioimmunoassay of sulfated lithocholates. *J. Lipid Res.* **18,** 693–703.

46. Crile G. Jr (1965) Rationale for cutting thick skin flaps in operation for cancer of the breast. *Cancer* **18,** 795.

47. Cuschieri A. (1975) Urinary hydroxyproline excretions and survival in cancer of the breast. *Clin. Oncol.* **1,** 127.

48. Cuschieri A., Jarvie R., Taylor W. H. et al. (1978) Three centre study on urinary hydroxyproline excretion in cancer of the breast. *Br. J. Cancer* **37,** 1002–1005.

49. Dickinson J. P. and Caspary E. A. (1973) The chemical nature of cancer basic protein. *Br. J. Cancer* **28,** Suppl. 1. 224–228.

50. Dietz J. H. (1969) Rehabilitation of the cancer patient. *Med. Clin. North Am.* **53,** 607.

51. Dowsett M., Easty G. C., Powles T. J. et al. (1976) Human breast tumour-induced osteolysis and prostaglandins. *Prostaglandins* **11,** 447.

52. Duffy M. J. and Duffy G. J. (1977a) Multiple steroid receptors in male breast carcinoma. *Clin. Chim. Acta* **85,** 211–214.

53. Duffy M. J. and Duffy G. J. (1977b) Peroxidose activity as a possible marker for a functional oestradiol receptor in human breast tumours (proceedings). *Biochem. Soc. Trans.* **5,** 1738–9.

54. Easson E. C. (1976) Postoperative radiotherapy in breast cancer. In: Forrest A. P. M., and Kunkler P. B. (ed.) *Prognostic Factors in Breast Cancer.* London, Livingstone.

55. Edelstyn G. J. A., Gillepsie P. T. and Greball F. S. (1967) The radiological demonstration of osseous metastases. *Clin. Radiol.* **18,** 158–62.

56. Edelstyn G. A., MacRae and MacDonald F. M. (1979) Improvement of life quality in cancer patient undergoing chemotherapy. *Clin. Oncol.* **5,** 43–49.

57. Editorial (1979) Age and death in breast cancer. *Br. Med. J.* **1,** 211.

58. Editorial (1979) Tumour marker in breast cancer. *Br. Med. J.* **1,** 1036.

59. Edwards M. H., Baum M. and Magarey C. J. (1972) Regression of axillary lymph nodes in cancer of the breast. *Br. J. Surgery* **59,** 776–9.

60. Ege G. B. (1978) Internal mammary lymphoscintigraphy: a rational adjuvant to the staging and management of breast carcinoma. *Clin. Radio.* **29,** 453–6.

61. Erwin

62. Field E. J. and Caspary E. A. (1970) Lymphocyte sensitization: an *in vitro* test for cancer. *Lancet* **2,** 1337.

63. Fisher B. et al. (1977) L-phenylalamine mustard (LPAM) in the management of primary breast cancer. *N. Engl. J. Med.* **292,** 117.

64. Fisher E. R. (1978) The pathologist's role in the diagnosis and treatment of invasive breast cancer. *Surg. Clin. North Am.* **58,** 705–21.

65. Forrest A. P. M. (1970) Workshop discussion In: Joslin C. A. F. and Gleave E. N. (eds.), *The Clinical Management of Advanced Breast Cancer.* Cardiff, Alpha Omega Press.

66. Freed E. J. and Caspary E. A. (1970) Lymphocyte sensitisation: an *in vitro* test for cancer. *Lancet* **2,** 1337–1341.

67. Frenning et al. (1978).

68. Galasko C. S. B. (1969) The detection of skeletal metastases from mammary cancer by gamma camera scintography. *Br. J. Surg.* **56,** 757.

69. Gielen F., Dequeker J. and Drochmans A. (1976) Relevance of hydroproline excretion to bone metastasis in breast cancer. *Br. J. Cancer* **34**, 279–85.
70. Gilbertsen V. A. and Wangensteen O. H. (1962) Should the doctor tell the patient that the disease is cancer. *CA* **12**, 82–6.
71. Gold P. and Freedman S. O. (1965) Demonstration of tumor-specific antigens in human colonic carcinomata by immunological tolerance and absorption techniques. *J. Excerpta Med.* **121**, 439–62.
72. Greenspan E. (1963) Response of advanced breast cancer to the conservation of the anti-metabolite, methotrexate and alkylating agent thiotepa. *J. Mt. Sinai Hosp. N.Y.* **30**, 246.
73. Griffiths C. T., Hall T. C., Saba Z. et al. (1973) Preliminary trial of 6-aminoglutethimide in breast cancer. *Cancer* **32**, 31–7.
74. Grosser N. and Thompson D. M. (1975) Cell-mediated antitumour immunity in breast cancer patients evaluated by antigen-induced leukocyte adherence inhibition in test tubes. *Cancer Res.* **35**, 2571–9.
75. Guzzo C. E., Pachas W. N., Pinals R. S. et al. (1969) Urinary hydroxyproline excretion in patients with cancer. *Cancer* **24**, 382.
76. Hall T. C. (1969) Endocrinologic factors in the design of more selective antitumour agents. *Cancer Res.* **29**, 2412.
77. Hannon (1971)
78. Harker (1972)
79. Harrel H. (1972) To lose a breast. *Am. J. Nursing* **72**, 676.
80. Harvey S. R., Girota A. and Nemoto T. (1976) Immunochemical studies on carcino-embryonic antigen reactive glycoproteins from carcinomas of the colon and breast separated by concanavalin. Affinity chromatography. *Cancer Res.* **36**, 3486–94.
81. Harvey S. R., Van Dusen L. and Howell J. (1976b) Immunochemical studies on the onco-fetal properties of carcinoembyonic antigen. In: Fishman W. H. and Sall S. (ed.), *Onco-developmental Gene Expression.* New York, Academic Press.
82. Healey J. E. (1971) Role of rehabilitation medicine in the care of the patient with breast cancer. *Cancer* **28**, 1666–1668.
83. Henderson M. and Kessell D. (1977) Alterations in plasma sialytransferase levels in patient with neoplastic disease. *Cancer* **39**, 1129–34.
84. Hendriek J. C. and Franchimont P. (1974) Radio-immunoassay of caesein in the serum of normal subjects and of patients with various malignancies. *Eur. J. Cancer* **10**, 725–730.
85. Hoch S. O., Longmuire R. L. and Hoch J. A. (1975) Unique DNA binding protein in the serum of patients with various neoplasms. *Nature* **255**, 560–2.
86. Hollinshead A. C., Jaffurs W. T., Alpert L. K. et al. (1974) Isolation and identification of soluble skin-reactive membrane antigens of malignant and normal breast cells. *Cancer Res.* **34**, 2961–8.
87. Horwitz K. B., Costlow M. E. and McGuire W. L. (1975) MCF-7. A human breast cancer cell line with estrogen and progesterone and glucocorticoid receptors. *Steroids* **26**, 785–795.
88. Hughes L. E. and Forbes J. F. (1978) Early breast cancer: II Management. *Brit. J. Surg.* **65**, 764–72.
89. Ip C. and Dao T. L. (1978) Alterations in serum glycosyltransferases and 5-nucleostidase in breast cancer patients. *Cancer Res.* **38**, 723–8.
90. Jacobs A., Slater A., Whittaker J. A. et al. (1976) Serum ferritin concentration in untreated Hodgkin's disease. *Brit. J. Cancer* **34**, 162–166.
91. Jacoby B. and Bagshaw K. D. (1972) A radioimmunoassay for placental-type alkaline phosphatase. *Cancer Res.* **32**, 2413.
92. James J. R. (1970) Sexual activity and cancer. *Lancet* **1**, 776.

93. Jonat W. and Maass H. (1978) Some comments on the necessity of receptor determination in human breast cancer. *Cancer Res.* **38,** 4305–6.
94. Kaae S. and Johansen H. (1967) Single versus radical mastectomy in primary breast cancer. In: Forrest A. P. M., and Kunkler P. B. (eds.), *Prognostic Factors in Breast Cancer.* London, Livingstone.
95. Kardinal C. G. and Carolla R. L. (1977) Recent advances in the management of cancer of the breast. *J. Am. Osteopath. Assoc.* **76,** 259–63.
96. Kardinal C. G. and Cupper H. T. (1977) Reaction of patients with advanced breast cancer to their diagnosis and treatment. *Milit. Med.* **142,** 374–6.
97. Kelly W. D. and Friesen S. R. (1950) Do cancer patients want to be told? *Surgery* **27,** 822.
98. Kennedy B. J., Tellegen A. and Kennedy S. (1976) Psychological responses of patients cured of advanced cancer. *Cancer* **38,** 184–91.
99. Keoleyer T. D., Stephens E. J. W. and Wood H. F. (1978) Experience with 6-amonoglutethimide in the treatment of metastatic breast cancer. *Clin. Oncol.* **4,** 323–327.
100. Kessell D. and Allen J. (1975) Elevated plasma sialytransferase in the cancer patient. *Cancer Res.* **35,** 670–2.
101. Kessell D., Samson M. K. and Shah P. (1976) Alterations in plasma sialytransferase associated with successful chemotherapy of a differentiated tumour. Case report. *Cancer* **38,** 2132–4.
102. Kiang D. T. and Kennedy B. J., (1978) Factors affecting estrogen receptors in breast cancer. *Cancer* **40,** 1571–6.
103. Kirkman S. and Henk J. M. (1979) The value of bone scanning in the study of breast cancer. *Clin. Radio.* **30,** 11–14.
104. Klein R. (1971) A crisis to grow on. *Cancer* **28,** 1660–1667.
105. Kleinberg D. L. (1975) Human alpha-lactalbumin: measurements in serum and in breast organ cultures by radioimmunoassay. *Science* **190,** 276–8.
106. Knight W. A., Livingston R. B., Gregory E. J. et al. (1977) Estrogen receptor as an independent prognostic factor for early recurrence in breast cancer. *Cancer Res.* **37,** 4669–71.
107. Knoph A. (1976) Changes in women's opinions about cancer. *Soc. Sci. Med.* **10,** 191–5.
108. Langlands A. O. and Kerr G. R. (1978) Prognosis in breast cancer, the relevance of clinical staging. *Clin. Radiol.* **29,** 599–606.
109. Laurence D. J. R. and Neville A. M. (1972) Foetal antigens and their role in the diagnosis and clinical management of human neoplasms: a review. *Brit. J. Cancer.* **26,** 335–355.
110. Laxenaire M., Chardot C. and Bentz L. (1971) Quelques aspects psychologiques du malade cancereux. A propos de 80 observations. *Presse Med.* **79,** 2497–500.
111. McGuire W. L., Zava D. T., Horwitz K. B. et al. (1978) Hormone Receptors and Breast Cancer. In: Griffiths K., Neville A. M. (eds.), *Tumour Markers.*
112. McGuire W. L. (1975) Current status of oestrogen receptors in human breast cancer. *Cancer* **36,** 638.
113. McIntosh J. (1974) Processes of communication information seeking and control associated with cancer: a selective review of the literature. *Soc. Sci. Med.* **8,** 167.
114. MacKay E. N. and Sellars A. H. (1965) *Breast Cancer at the Ontario Cancer Clinics 1938–1956.* A statistical review. Ontario Medical Statistics Branch. Ontario Department of Health.
115. Magarey C. J. and Todd P. B. (1976) Breast loss and delay in breast cancer diagnosis, behavioural science in surgical research. *Aus. N.Z. Surg.* **46,** 1–3.
116. Maguire C. P., Lee E. G., Bevington D. J. (1978) Psychiatric problems in the first year after mastectomy. *Brit. Med. J.* **1,** 963.

117. Marcus D. M. and Zinberg N. J. (1975) Measurement of serum ferritin by radioimmunoassay: results in normal individuals and patients with breast cancer. *J. Natl. Cancer Inst.* **55,** 791–5.
118. Markel W. M. (1971) The American Cancer Society's program for the rehabilitation of the breast cancer patient. *Cancer* **28,** 1676–78.
119. Meakin J. W., Allt W. E. and Beale F. W. (1977) Ovarian irradiation and prednisone following surgery for carcinoma of the breast. In: Salmon F. E. and Jones S. E. (ed.), *Adjuvant Therapy or Cancer.* Amsterdam, North-Holland.
120. Meyer J. S. and Facher R. (1977) Thymidine labelling index of human breast carcinoma. Enhancement in vitro labelling by 5-fluorouracil and 5-fluoro-2'-deoxyuridine. *Cancer* **39,** 2524–32.
121. Monacco M. E., Bronzert D. A., Tormey D. C. et al. (1977) Casein production by human breast cancer. *Cancer Res.* **37,** 749–753.
122. Mueller C. B. and Ames F. (1978) Bilateral carcinoma of breast, frequency and mobility. *Can. J. Surg.* **21,** 459–65.
123. Nevill A. M. and Cooper E. H. (1976) Biochemical monitoring of cancer: a review. *Ann. Clin. Biochem.* **13,** 283–305.
124. Nevill A. M., MacKay A. M., Westwood et al. (1975) Human tumour-associated and tumour specific antigens. Some concepts in relation to clinical oncology. *J. Clin. Pathol.* **28,** Suppl. 6, 102.
125. Nevinny H. B. (1969) Prophylactic oophorectomy in breast cancer therapy. *Am. J. Surg.* **117,** 531–6.
126. Nissen–Meyer (1968) Of ovarian function in primary carcinoma of the breast. In: Forrest A. P. M. and Kunkler P. B. eds., *Prognostic Factors in Breast Cancer.* Edinburgh, Livingstone.
127. Nissen–Meyer R., Kjellgren K., Malmo K. et al (1978) Surgical adjuvant chemotherapy. *Cancer* **41,** 2088–98.
128. Nordenskjoid (1978)
129. Norton L. and Simon R. (1977) Tumour size, sensitivity to therapy and design of treatment schedules. *Cancer Treat. Rep.* **61,** 1307.
130. Parsons R. G., Hoch J. A., and Longmine R. L. (1978) A correlation of serum C3DP levels with chemotherapeutic management of cancer patients. *Cancer* **41,** 2099–106.
131. Parsons R. G., Langmine R. L. and Hoch S. O. (1977) A clinical evaluation of serum C3DP levels in individuals with malignant disease. *Cancer Res.* **37,** 692–5.
132. Paterson R. and Aitken Swan J. (1954) Public opinion on cancer: a survey among women in the Manchester area. *Lancet* **2,** 857–61.
133. Powles T. J., Clark S. A., Easty D. M. et al. (1973) The inhibition by aspirin and indomethacin of osteolytic tumour deposits and hypercalcaemia in rats with Walker tumour and its possible application to human breast cancer. *Brit. J. Cancer* **28,** 316–321.
134. Powles T. J., Coombes R. C., Nevill A. M. et al. (1977) 15 keto –13, 14 dihydro-prostaglandin E2 concentrations in the serum of patients with breast cancer. *Lancet* **2,** 138.
135. Powles T. J., Leese C. L. and Bondy P. K. (1975) Hydroxyproline excretion in patients with breast cancer and response to treatment. *Brit. Med. J.* **2,** 164.
136. Price L. A. and Goldie J. H. (1971) Multiple drug therapy for disseminated malignant tumour. *Brit. Med. J.* **4,** 336.
137. Price, Hill and their colleagues.
138. Priestman T. J. (1978) Recent advances in cytotoxic therapy for gastrointestinal carcinoma. A review. *Proc. R. Soc. Med.* **71,** 195–8.
139. Quint J. (1963) The impact of mastectomy. *Am. J.* **63,** 88–92.

140. Ravdin R. G., Lewison E. F. and Slaek N. H. (1970) Results of a clinical trial concerning the worth of prophylactic oophorectomy for breast carcinoma. *Surg. Gynecol. Obstet.* **131,** 1055–64.
141. Ray C. (1977) Psychological implication of mastectomy. *Brit. J. Soc. Clin. Psychol.* **16,** 373–7.
142. Renneker R. C. and Cutler M. (1952) Psychological problems of adjustment to cancer of the breast. *J. Am. Med. Ass.* **148,** 833–835.
143. Roberts M. M., Furnival S. G. and Forrest A. P. M. (1972) The morbidity of mastectomy. *Brit. J. Surg.* **59,** 301.
144. Rosato F. E. (1967) Serum glycoproteins in the evaluation of breast cancer. *Surg. Gynecol. Obstet.* **124,** 1291–4.
145. Rosato F. E. and Seltzer M. H. (1969) Serum protein bound fucose and carcinoma of the female breast. *Am. J. Surg.* **118,** 61–4.
146. Rosato F. E., Seltzer M. H., Mullen J. et al. (1971) Serum fucose in the diagnosis of breast cancer. *Cancer* **28,** 1575–9.
147. Rosenblum M. G., Duire B. G., Salmon S. E. et al. (1978) Metabolism of (14C) spermidine and (14C) putnescine in normal volunteers and in cancer patients. *Cancer Res.* **38,** 3161–3.
148. Rubens R. D., Begent R. H., Knight R. K. et al. (1978) Combined cytotoxic and progestogen therapy for advanced breast cancer. *Cancer* **42,** 1680–6.
149. Russell D. H., Gullino P. M., Marton L. J. et al. (1975) Polyamine depletion of the MTW9 mammary tumour and subsequent elevation of spermidine in the sera of tumour-bearing rats as a biochemical marker of tumour regression. *Cancer Res.* **34,** 2378–81.
150. Russell D. H. and Russell S. D. (1975) Relative usefulness of measuring polyamines in serum, plasma and urine as biochemical markers of cancer. *Clin. Chem.* **21,** 860–3.
151. Sabolovic D., Sabolovic N. and Moutte A. (1975) Agglutination of peripheral blood lymphocytes from cancer patients and not from healthy controls with the F2A1 histone fraction. *Brit. J. Cancer* **32,** 28–33.
152. Syeberth H. W., Segre G. V. and Morgan J. L. (1975) Prostaglandins as mediators of hypercalcaemia associated with certain types of cancer. *N. Engl. J. Med.* **293,** 1278–83.
153. Shinzinger
154. Shonfield J. (1972) Psychological factors related to delayed return to an earlier life-style in successfully treated cancer patients. *J. Psychosom. Res.* **16,** 41–44.
155. Skipper H. E., Schabel F. M. and Wilcox W. S. (19) Experimental evaluation of potential anticancer agents. *Cancer Chemother. Rep.* **35,** 1–111.
156. Smith (1978)
157. Steward A. M., Nixon D. and Zamcheck N. (1974) Carcinoembryonic antigen in breast cancer patients: Serum levels and disease progress. *Cancer* **33,** 1246–52.
158. Stimson W. H. (1971) Studies on the changes in the concentration and total mass of individual serum proteins during late pregnancy. *Clin. Biochem.* **5,** 3–12.
159. Thomas J. M. (1978) Failure to detect ultra-abdominal metastases from breast cancer: a case for staging laparotomy. *Brit. Med. J.* **2,** 157–159.
160. Tormey D. C., Waalkes T. P., Ahmann D. et al. (1975) Biological markers in breast carcinoma. 1. Incidence of abnormalities of CEA, HCG, three polyamines and three minor nucleosides. *Cancer* **35,** 1095.
161. Tormey D. C., Waalkes T. P., Snyder J. J. et al. (1977) Biological markers in breast carcinoma. III Clinical correlations with carcinoembryonic antigen. *Cancer* 39, 2397–404.

162. Turnbull A. R., Turner D. T., Chant A. D. et al. (1978) Treatment of early breast cancer. *Lancet* **2,** 7–9.
163. Urban J. A. (1978) Management of operable breast cancer: the surgeon's view. *Cancer* **42,** 2066–77.
164. Veronesi U. (1977) Surgical treatment of primary breast cancer according to disease extent. *Clin. Biol. Res.* **12,** 347–57.
165. Waalkes T. P., Gehrke C. M., Zumwalt R. W. et al. (1975) The urinary excretion of nucleosides of ribonucleic acid by patients with advanced cancer. *Cancer* **36,** 390–398.
166. Waalkes
167. Wagner R. K. and Jungblut P. W. (1976) Oestradiol and dihydrotestosterone receptors in normal and neoplastic human mammary tissue. *Acta Endocrinol. (Kbh)* **82,** 105–20.
168. Wakefield J. (1962) The organization of public education about cancer. *Monthly Bull. Ministry Health (London)* **21,** 82–8.
169. Wakefield J. (1970) The social implication of cancer. *Radiography* **36,** 93–5.
170. Wang D. Y., Bulbrook R. D., Hayward J. L. et al. (1975) Relationship between plasma carcinoembryonic antigen and prognosis in women with breast cancer. *Eur. J. Cancer* **11,** 615.
171. Weismann A. D. (1977) Coping behaviour and suicide in cancer. In: Cullen J. W. (ed.) *Cancer: The Behavioural Dimensions.* New York, Raven Press.
172. Witkin M. H. (1975) Sex therapy and mastectomy. *J. Sex Marital Ther.* **1,** 290–293.
173. Woo K. B., Waalkes T. P., Ahmann D. L. (1978) A quantitative approach to determining disease response during therapy using multiple biologic markers: application to carcinoma of the breast. *Cancer* **41,** 1685–703.
174. Woods
175. Woods K. L. and Heath D. A. (1977) The radioimmunoassay of human lactalbumin. *Clin. Chim. Acta* **78,** 129–33.
176. Zangerle P. F., Hendrick J. C., Thirion A. et al. (1976) In: Franchimont P. (ed.) *Cancer Related Antigens.* Amsterdam, Elsevier.

The task of compiling the list of references for this chapter has been difficult and I have failed to locate them all. Rather than delay publication I have left some references incomplete.

Editor.

James G. Pearson

4 Management of Cancer of the Oesophagus

Oesophageal cancer is a disease likely to yield to early diagnosis and treatment. However, in most communites it is still characterized by late diagnosis, with tumour spread beyond cure by loco-regional treatment, and management complicated by starvation, and sometimes cardiovascular disease, emphysema and the effects of overuse of alcohol. In the UK and North America only five per cent of patients survive five years after diagnosis and good palliation is not easy to accomplish. Nevertheless, during the last 40 years there have been important improvements in both diagnosis and in radiation and surgical treatment, and further improvement is expected. So far there is no systemic treatment effective enough for general use.

In this chapter, emphasis is placed on the improvements which have taken place in radiotherapy in the context of the other important developments.

PRESENTATION AND INVESTIGATION OF OESOPHAGEAL CANCER

In reported series all but one per cent of oesophageal cancers are carcinomas. The infrequent non-carcinomatous malignancies are sarcoma, pseudosarcoma, carcinosarcoma, malignant melanoma, carcinoid, granular cell myoblastoma, and verrucous squamous cell carcinoma, for all of which surgical treatment is preferable; and Hodgkin's disease and non-Hodgkin's lymphomas, for which radiotherapy either alone or combined with chemotherapy is the optimum treatment. Direct invasion of the oesophagus by bronchial carcinoma and gastric carcinoma is common, and also occurs from thyroid carcinoma. There are rare instances of blood-borne metastases to the oesophagus from other sites. Patterns of incidence, histology, spread, the extent of the tumour, its site in the oesophagus, the patient's sex, the presence of other diseases and the nature of the treatment facilities available all influence the management of the disease.

INCIDENCE AND AETIOLOGY

Case [25] explained the need for contemporary arrays of age specific death rates over many decades, by sex, and for each community studied, with analysis of the data by cohorts, if moderate differences in mortality are to be correctly related to the biological impact of environmental factors. Oesophageal cancer mortality can vary as much as one hundredfold between communities and significant epidemiological observations are possible even from only moderately precisely gathered data. In most communities the disease is so highly lethal that mortality is within five per cent of the incidence. Greater errors arise from imprecise death certification and incomplete recording of incidence. Few communities have adequate data about occupation, location of habitation and dietary practices throughout each individual's lifetime. Another factor of interest which is incompletely recorded is the site of the tumour in the oesophagus.

Age

In most communities the age specific incidence of oesophageal cancer is low until the fifth decade, thereafter rising with increasing rapidity with advancing age. This tendency is exaggerated in a community experiencing a decreasing incidence in successive cohorts. In some communities the incidence has increased so rapidly in successive cohorts that the more usual pattern of increasing incidence with age has been overwhelmed for a few decades during which the middle aged showed a higher incidence than the elderly. These features are well demonstrated by cohort analysis [25].

Sex

In most communities oesophageal cancer is more common in males than in females. In North-West Brittany and Normandy there is a very high incidence in males, related to alcohol and tobacco use, with a 25 : 1 male : female ratio. The alcohol and tobacco related high incidence in Durban and Johannesburg is mainly in domestically disrupted urban male blacks [20]. There are well defined communities in the Transkei in Africa and in a belt from Iran to North China where the incidence is high in both men and women. The sharp geographic gradients in incidence are often more marked in females [36]. In Finland, north Sweden, Scotland and the Welsh population of Wales there is a moderately high incidence, the male : female ratio is approximately one, relatively more of the cases in females are in the cervical oesophagus, there is no evidence of an important alcohol-tobacco factor in the females, and there is an association between the now uncommon Paterson-Kelly (Plummer-Vinson) syndrome and upper oesophageal cancer in women [78]. In Canada, the incidence is low and the male : female ratio is 2·5 : 1. In the USA, with a higher incidence in blacks, the male : female ratio is 4·5 : 1 for blacks and 3·6 : 1 for whites [59].

Site

Incidence by site is less well documented. Cancer registry and death certification data lack subclassification by the level of the tumour in the oesophagus. Studies often reflect patterns of referral rather than whole community experience. Radiotherapists usually see more cervical and upper and mid thoracic tumours, while surgeons see more lower third tumours. In northern Europe, post-cricoid carcinoma is confined to women, but in parts of Egypt, Iraq and Thailand it occurs more often in men [47]. In the high incidence communities of the Caspian littoral of Iran, mid and lower oesophageal cancers predominate. Whole population reporting of epidermoid carcinoma of the oesophagus in south-east Scotland has been attempted from 1931 to 1969, and this goal had been approached closely in the last decade of that period. Nine hundred and fifty-eight female patients had tumours almost evenly distributed throughout the oesophagus. One thousand and seventy-four males showed a markedly increasing incidence from few in the neck to a majority in the lower oesophagus [111].

Geography

Day [36] and Haas and Schottenfeld [59] describe the epidemiology of oesophageal cancer. In a belt extending from Iran to northern China there are areas of very high incidence. Diet and culture vary widely among those areas and highly restricted diets which may be deficient are common, but there is no suggestion that alcohol and tobacco are significant factors. In the Taihang mountains in the north-west of the Chinese province of Honan, oesophageal cancer is very common, with an age standardized incidence of 130/100 000 population per year, which is fifty times more frequent than in most European countries, North America or other parts of China [30]. The Kazakhs, Turkomen and Uzbeks (former central Asian nomads), the Islamic peoples of Gonbad and Gorgan regions of northern Iran, the Bantu of the Transkei and the blacks of Natal in South Africa experience more cancer in the oesophagus than at any other site. There is a patchy distribution of very high incidence in many East and South African communities, but in West Africa the disease is a rarity. In the Caribbean, incidence is high in Puerto Rico, Jamaica and Curaçao and in South America it is high in the north of Chile. In Europe and North America the highest incidence in males is in the north-west of Brittany and Normandy, possibly associated with the consumption of apple cider distillates and tobacco usage [36, 139, 141]. In France as a whole (especially in males), in Switzerland, and in Finland (males and females) incidence is high at about 7/100 000 per year. In the UK it is 5·5/100 000 per year. In Denmark, Germany and in USA blacks it is 3·5/100 000 per year. In USA whites, Canada, Italy, Netherlands the incidence is low at less than 3/100 000 per year. The incidence is 4·1 in New Zealand, 3·4 in Japan, 2·8 in Australia, and 2·4 /100 000 per year in Israel [25, 40, 59].

Secular Trends

In parts of the Transkei, the high incidence of oesophageal cancer has been observed to develop as an epidemic since about 1945 [22], and similarly in Durban [19]. Over the same period in the USA the incidence has been increasing in blacks and remains stable in whites [123]. Since about 1945 there has been a decreasing incidence of upper oseophageal carcinoma associated with the Paterson-Kelly (Plummer-Vinson) syndrome in undernourished, iron-deficient women in parts of Britain and Scandinavia – a decrease probably associated with improved nutrition [69]. In England and Wales the mortality from oesophageal cancer for successive cohorts decreased over a thirty year period: males aged 50–54 years born around 1901 experienced only 27 per cent of the mortality of 50–54 year-old males born around 1871 [25], but in the last decade an increasing incidence has been observed for both sexes in the Birmingham area [147].

Associated Factors

Steiner [132] found that only about five per cent of oesophageal cancers arise in association with a pre-existing organic lesion. Such lesions are achalasia [45, 130, 143], Chagas' disease [43], Paterson-Kelly syndrome [2, 3, 78, 120], lye strictures [17, 73], ionizing radiation [53, 107], head and neck cancer with which there is a ten-fold increased risk of oesophageal cancer [51], previous gastric surgery [125], malabsorption syndrome [155] and tylosis [26, 127].

There are commonly occurring and often cross-related associated factors of less easily determined aetiological significance, such as heavy use of alcohol and tobacco [12, 13, 139, 140, 152], and malnutrition and specific dietary factors [30, 41, 59, 65, 68, 86, 133]. The swallowing of tobacco pipe tar (injonga) in the Transkei, and opium pipe dross (sukhteh) in north-east Iran are possible factors, since both substances are strongly mutagenic [62].

Most authors suspect a complex multifactorial aetiology with much variation in the dominant factors among different communities. For some the dominant factors are alcohol and tobacco, while for others the factors are various nutritional deficiences or the presence of specific elements in the diet [36, 41, 59].

Implications

The treatment of oesophageal cancer is more successful with a small localized tumour, in a young patient, in a female, in the absence of any other disease which makes radiotherapy or surgery more difficult, and in a community in which the disease is common enough for the team of radiotherapist and surgeon to acquire great skill. Surgery is most successful for tumours in the lower third while radiotherapy is most successful in the upper two-thirds. Where many of the patients are male, especially alcoholic derelict, heavy smoking males, coexistent liver damage, lung damage, heart damage, or mental impairment militate against successful irradiation or resection. The above factors influence management and prognosis and they vary widely among communities.

Logan and LeRoux [84], who have extensive experience of the surgical management of oesophageal cancer both in Edinburgh, Scotland and Durban, South Africa, state that the presentation and response to treatment of oesophageal cancer in high incidence groups of South Africans is so unfavourable compared with the Edinburgh experience that it seems to be a different disease.

In very high incidence areas of Honan province in North China, where oesophageal cancer is much the commonest cancer, mass screening by oesophageal cytology is practicable (using a net covered balloon catheter to obtain specimens). Thirteen per cent of those screened had mild dysplasia, 1·2 per cent had severe dysplasia and 0·9 per cent had carcinoma. Some dysplasias were reversed following dietary adjustment. Others were followed closely until carcinoma developed, the carcinoma usually being diagnosed early, thus raising the resection rate to 82 per cent, lowering the operative mortality to 4 per cent, and raising the 5-year survival rate to 29 per cent. Until 1971, the overall mortality rates remained close to the incidence rates. Amongst the patients treated surgically were some with in situ carcinoma and others with tumours of less than 1 cm [23].

In the Edinburgh area, where oesophageal cancer constitutes only 2 per cent of all cancer, no cases were found by screening. The smallest tumour was 2 cm in diameter but the mean tumour size in patients planned for radical treatment was greater than 6 cm. Half of the patients were females, and few were impoverished derelicts. Between 1949 and 1967, when radical treatment was surgery for 432 patients and radiotherapy for 288, the 5-year survival of these 720 radically treated patients was 13·3 per cent (*see Fig. 4.3*).

Few 1-year survivors and no 5-year survivors have been reported following treatment in some series comprising mainly male patients, many of whom were impoverished, undernourished, alcoholic smokers. Alcoholism militates against early diagnosis. Alcoholism and heavy smoking militate against successful treatment by either radiotherapy or surgery, because of cardiac and respiratory impairment.

Adenocarcinoma in the oesophagus and any cancer developing following a lye stricture or previous heavy irradiation should be treated surgically. For carcinomas in the upper two-thirds of the oesophagus and for those developing in aged patients irradiation will generally be the treatment of choice.

Accordingly, the best management of oesophageal cancer is highly dependent on many parameters which vary widely among communities.

PATHOLOGY

Squamous Cell Carcinoma

The oesophagus is normally lined by stratified squamous epithelium and 95 per cent of its cancers are squamous carcinoma.

Adenocarcinoma

Adenocarcinoma arising in the stomach and invading the lower oesophagus causes dysphagia. Whether it is more, or less, common than squamous oesophageal carcinoma as a cause of dysphagia depends on the relative incidence of gastric and oesophageal cancer in the community. The cardia usually resists the spread of squamous oesophageal carcinoma into the stomach but gastric adenocarcinoma freely invades the oesophagus.

Primary oesophageal adenocarcinoma is rare [119]. The described incidence varies: 9 per cent [14]; 8 per cent [129]; 2·6 per cent [85]; 2·3 per cent [138]; 0·8 per cent [9]. It may occur at any level in either sex. Adenocarcinoma bleeds more, is more commonly associated with distant blood-borne and widespread lymph node metastases, and responds less well to radiotherapy than squamous carcinoma [35].

There are also carcinomas so undifferentiated as not to be recognizably squamous or glandular. Even rarer are mixed squamous and adenocarcinomas, muco-epidermoid carcinoma, adenoid cystic carcinoma and, at the cardia, collision carcinoma [39].

Grading

Oesophageal squamous carcinoma is usually undifferentiated and usually Broder's Grade III or IV [21]. Using a three grade classification, Marcial et al. [89] found 83 per cent of 211 patients to be Grade II. Vaeth [142] stresses the desirability of relating grade to clinical stage and response to treatment but Gowing [54] describes great variation in grade within the same tumour. Grading on the basis of a small endoscopic biopsy may be misleading. Nakayama [97] documents the relationship between the 5-year survival rate and the degree of malignancy determined on microscopy of 370 operative specimens. Each was studied in respect to cellular morphology, pathological alignment, and the grade of infiltration. He found a close correlation between prognosis and each of these parameters.

Site

Carcinoma may occur at any level in the oesophagus but its incidence at the different levels varies widely among communities, between the sexes, and over periods of time – presumably due to the different impact of various aetiological factors.

Appelqvist [9] found oesophageal carcinoma to be more localized and more curable when situated on the left lateral wall rather than on the right lateral, anterior or posterior walls.

Size

With the exception of the Chinese experience with the screening programme in the very high incidence area in Honan, oesophageal cancer is diagnosed late. In the report by Appelqvist [9] of 623 patients in Helsinki, at the time of radiographic diagnosis 12 per cent of men and 22 per cent of women had a tumour less than 4 cm long, and in 49 per cent of men and 38 per cent of women the primary tumour was more than 8 cm long. Tumour length was greater in the lower oesophagus. Beyond a 4-cm length of tumour the severity of dysphagia does not accurately reflect tumour size.

Macroscopic Appearance

The early stages of the disease are symptomless and rarely observed in the absence of a screening programme. On radiography and endoscopy the tumour presents as an ulcerating mass, an ulcer with everted margins, an excavating ulcer, an ulcerated stricture, or a pedunculated mass. Not uncommonly there is a narrowed segment lined by apparently intact mucosa which is only moderately irregular because infiltration by carcinoma has provoked a fibrous reaction which is the main cause of the stenosis.

Direct Spread

The greatest direct spread occurs in the submucosa. Preferential spread in this layer tends to be more extensive proximally than distally [16] and commonly extends more than 1 cm and frequently more than 5 cm beyond the gross margin of the tumour. The submucosal spread may be massive but is frequently detectable only on microscopy. Pallor of the overlying mucosa may be the only sign. Satellite nodules may be present. Local cure is jeopardized unless treatment encompasses a 5-cm margin beyond the gross margins of the tumour. Miller [92] analysed surgical experience of persistent or recurrent carcinoma at the proximal line of resection of the oesophagus and he concluded that a margin of 12 cm proximal to the gross tumour is necessary to reduce anastomotic recurrence to a really low level. The submucosal layer extends proximally into the pharynx and distally into the stomach, and so may the oesophageal cancer. However, massive gastric invasion by squamous carcinoma is uncommon.

By the time of diagnosis, both the circumferential and longitudinal muscle layers have usually been penetrated although the muscle is less readily invaded than the submucosa. Initially the muscle layers are invaded along the pathways of the blood and lymphatic vessels.

The oesophagus has no serosa. After penetrating the muscularis the tumour spreads through the loose peri-oesophageal adventitia to surrounding organs. Most commonly invaded are the trachea and bronchi into which a fistula may develop, the hili and pulmonary ligaments, the aortic adventitia, and also the pleura, pericardium, large veins, thyroid, recurrent laryngeal nerves, diaphragm, and left lobe of the liver, depending on the level of the tumour [80]. The elastic media of the aorta and the aponeuroses overlying the vertebral bodies offer, for a time, more effective barriers. Appelqvist [9] found extraoesophageal spread grossly evident at operation in 46 of 154 patients. He found tumour still localized to the oesophagus more frequently in women than men, especially in the upper oesophagus. He also observed evidence of more extensive spread in longer tumours and in anaplastic tumours. However, 13 per cent of tumours over 8 cm long were still free from grossly visible spread.

Lymphatic Metastases

Lymphatic spread occurs early in these usually poorly differentiated tumours, first into the rich submucosal plexus, then through the muscularis to the paraoesophageal lymph nodes at the level of the tumour, and thereafter to more remote lymph nodes, sometimes skipping intermediate nodes. From the upper third of the oesophagus, paraoesophageal, retropharyngeal, lower deep cervical and supraclavicular nodes may be invaded. From the middle third, after invasion of local paraoesophageal nodes, there is frequently invasion of quite remote nodes superiorly in the neck, or inferiorly around the cardia and along the left gastric artery. Tracheobronchial nodes extending into the hili of the lungs may also be invaded. From the lower third, beyond the local nodes, spread is commonly to below the diaphragm to the paracardial, left gastric, and coeliac axis nodes and less commonly to nodes along the upper border of the pancreas, in the splenic hilum, or upwards to the middle third drainage area. Appelqvist [9] reported that in 70 per cent of surgically treated patients with lower and middle third tumours who had lymphatic metastases there was involvement of subdiaphragmatic nodes – especially along the left gastric artery. Of 26 patients who had surgery for upper third tumours, five had lymphatic metastases and half of these were subdiaphragmatic.

Appelqvist found no metastases in biopsied scalene nodes in patients with primary oesophageal cancers less than 4 cm long, 8 per cent if the primary was 4–8 cm and 21 per cent if the primary was more than 8 cm. Scalene node metastases were more frequently on the right side from upper and middle third tumours and more frequently on the left side from lower third tumours.

LeRoux [80] found histologically proved cervical node metastases to be the contraindication to operative treatment in 26 out of 102 inoperable patients. Histological confirmation of lymph node metastases in the mediastinum or abdomen was obtained in 145 (61 per cent) of 236 patients submitted to resection for squamous carcinoma. Forty-nine of the 145 patients with proved lymph node metastases had other evidence of spread beyond the oesophagus but only 4 had other spread without lymph node metastases.

Gunnlaugsson and his collaborators [58] found positive nodes in 78 of 162 patients submitted to curative resection for squamous oesophageal cancer and in 174 of 245 patients submitted to curative resection for adenocarcinoma of the cardia. The higher the tumour in the oesophagus, the lower was the incidence of lymph node metastases.

Blood-borne Metastases

The plexus of thin-walled veins in the oesophageal submucosa, the perioesophageal venous plexus, and the connections between lymphatics and veins are routes by which tumour emboli are likely to enter the bloodstream. However, one third of the patients die from the local complications of the tumour without readily detectable blood-borne metastases at autopsy. The recorded incidence of metastases depends on their visibility, on whether the observation is clinical, radiographic, by scanning, at operation, or at autopsy, and on the thoroughness of selection of material for microscopy. The commonest clinical evidence of blood-borne metastases is gross nodular hepatomegaly. Less massive liver metastases may be suspected or confirmed after biochemical tests, radionuclide scans, CT scans, ultrasonography, or laparoscopy, laparotomy or autopsy. The radiographic detection of metastases is most common in the lung, and much less common in bone. Of 280 patients subjected to thoraco-laparotomy for squamous oesophageal cancer LeRoux [80] found that 15 had liver metastases and 1 had a renal metastasis revealed only at operation. In a study of deaths occurring during the first six years following treatment by radical irradiation, of 208 patients with squamous oesophageal cancer, Pearson [108] attributed one half of the deaths mainly to locally recurrent tumour, one quarter mainly to blood-borne metastases which were most frequently in the liver and lungs, and one quarter mainly to non-malignant diseases. Goodner and Turnbull [52] found bone metastases during the last three months of life in 5 per cent of 1909 patients with oesophageal cancer. In a collected series of 824 autopsies on patients who died from oesophageal cancer, Dormanns (1939) reported metastases to the liver in 32 per cent, lungs and pleura in 21 per cent, bone in 8 per cent, kidneys in 7 per cent, and adrenals in 3 per cent. In a series of 154 autopsies on patients dying from carcinoma of the oesophagus or cardia, Appelqvist [10] found metastases in the liver associated with 35 per cent of the cardia cancers, 25 per cent of the lower third cancers, 15 per cent of the middle third cancers and 9 per cent of the upper third cancers. The other common sites for blood-borne metastases were lungs 12 per cent, adrenals 7 per cent, kidneys 5 per cent, bones 5 per cent, and the pancreas 5 per cent.

Implications

Full histological appraisal may be difficult if based only on material secured at endoscopy. Nevertheless the distinction between squamous carcinoma and adenocarcinoma is important to the choice between radiotherapy and surgery. If radiotherapy is intended, it is important to determine, as accurately as is possible on the basis of endoscopic biopsies, the degree of differentiation of the carcinoma. The more undifferentiated the carcinoma, the greater is the margin to be allowed around the demonstrable tumour in defining the volume to be irradiated and the lower is the appropriate radiation dose.

The level of the carcinoma in the oesophagus, and even which side of the oesophagus it lies on, for any one size of primary, influence the probability of local lymphatic or blood-borne spread, the prognosis, the technical feasibility of successful surgery, the choice between radiotherapy and surgery, and the definition of the volume to be irradiated.

Tumour size is a vital factor but large size alone does not rule out all hope of cure. Even when the demonstrable tumour is 8 cm long cure may still be worth attempting provided there are no other contraindications to radical treatment.

It is vital to estimate as precisely as possible the limits of direct infiltration by the tumour, the extent of regional lymphatic metastases, and whether viable blood-borne metastases have been established. This information is needed to make the best choice between radiotherapy and surgery, to avoid a pointless and possibly life threatening attempt to cure by radiation or resection when only palliation is possible, and to plan the optimal margins for the irradiated volume.

DIAGNOSTIC PROCEDURES

History of Symptoms

At first the cancer causes no symptoms.

The early recognition of the significance of the first symptom is the most important process which may lead to confirmation of the diagnosis and treatment whilst cure is still possible, Edwards [44]. The patient may notice vague discomfort, a slight foreign body sensation, or slight pain on swallowing. Painless, intermittent, obstructive dysphagia, first for solids, is the first symptom for 65 per cent of the patients and pain on swallowing for 13 per cent [9]. Less frequently the first symptom is chest, back or abdominal pain, dyspepsia, anorexia, weight loss, haematemesis, melaena, cough, or hoarseness. The cancer may remain symptomless until about two thirds of the circumference has been stiffened by tumour. Later, the dysphagia is for liquids as well as solids and is unremitting. The patient adapts, first by cutting his food smaller, then by taking only creamy soft food, and finally only liquids. So poorly is the public educated that patients will tolerate dysphagia for an average of four months before they seek medical advice. In some communities delay approaches eight months, by which time dysphagia is total and survival thereafter is measured in days rather than in months.

In a patient with achalasia, lye stricture, or Paterson-Kelly syndrome, a change in the character of longstanding dysphagia may not be recognized to be due to cancer until too late. In achalasia, the oesophageal lumen is wide and the tumour can grow to a large size before causing noticeable obstruction. For these reasons a carcinoma which complicates cardiospasm is rarely operable or curable by radiotherapy.

Clinical Signs

On examination, if the cancer is still curable there will be no abnormality or merely weight loss. Occasionally, even a curable patient may be very emaciated. The commonest clinical evidence of spread beyond the oesophagus is an enlarged, hard, lower deep cervical lymph node, or an enlarged nodular liver [80]. Ten per cent of patients present with a haemoglobin below 10 g/100 ml.

Radiology

In many series half of the patients referred to hospital with dysphagia have oesophageal cancer. If treatment is to be worthwhile the correct diagnosis must be made without delay. The principles of the radiographic diagnosis of early oesophageal cancer using air-contrast technique as well as an oesophagus well filled with barium, using cineradiography or videotape as well as static views, using both recumbent and vertical postitions, and using tangential views around the whole circumference, are described by many authors [34, 51, 74, 93, 135, 153, 156]. Yamada, Suzuki and their collaborators at Tokyo Womens' Medical College have detected nine oesophageal cancers less than 2·5 cm in extent by using these techniques to investigate patients with minimal symptoms.

The radiological examination, whether positive or negative, must be followed by oesophagoscopy. A normal oesophagogram is not a reason for not undertaking oesophagoscopy. Small tumours, even though symptomatic, may not be easily demonstrable radiographically. Oesophagoscopy without a radiological examination is equally inappropriate. If the cause of dysphagia cannot be found and the symptoms persist it is essential to avoid false reassurance. The patient must be re-investigated at least once a month or until dysphagia is no longer present.

Unfortunately, the common presentation, after many months of symptoms, is with a large tumour, easy to diagnose and impossible to cure, impassable by the oesophagoscope and with a lower limit and whole intraluminal extent better demonstrated by radiography than oesophagoscopy. For most such patients the cancer is so advanced that no amount of sophisticated investigation will result in benefit. The life at stake is that of the patient with less impressive symptoms and a small, elusive or barely detectible cancer, a patient for whom a negative examination followed by false reassurance may be a great tragedy.

Appelqvist [9] documents a false negative diagnosis resulting from 25 per cent of the first and 4 per cent of the second barium examinations of the tumour area with rather more errors in males than females, for lower oesophageal tumours, and for small tumours. At the lower end the main problem is to distinguish between carcinoma and peptic ulcer with stricture. Carcinoma usually causes more distortion but the two lesions may be undistinguishable and, indeed, may co-exist.

In the neck and to a lesser degree in the upper thorax, anterior displacement and distortion of the trachea by the mass of oesophageal tumour is well demonstrated by a lateral soft tissue X-ray. Computerized axial tomography demonstrates any massive extension beyond the oesophageal wall and is particularly helpful for radiotherapy planning [77, 142].

A chest X-ray which must include a lateral view and ideally whole lung tomography or computerized tomography, is part of the search for metastases. A thickened posterior tracheal stripe seen in the lateral chest X-ray has enabled Putman et al. [117] to identify mid-oesophageal carcinoma in three patients who were asymptomatic at the time. A huge soft tissue mass, air in an oesophagus stiffened by infiltrating tumour, a fluid level above severe obstruction [81], or pneumonitis or lung abscess due to aspiration or oesophagotracheal fistula, are usually evidence of extensive and incurable cancer. However a relatively small, severely stenosing but still curable tumour may be associated with a fluid level above the obstruction and aspiration pneumonitis.

To achieve better definition of tumour extent pneumomediastinography has been suggested by Holub and Simecek [64] and azygos venography by Crummy et al. [33], Humeau et al. [66], and Carlyle et al. [24].

The ^{32}P uptake test is used by Nakayama [96, 97], Nelson and Lanza [101], and Suzuki et al. [135] to localize a symptomatic oesophageal cancer which has evaded detection by both radiography and endoscopy. Suzuki and his collaborators now use a 0·5 cm diameter beta detector introduced through the biopsy channel of the fibreoptic oesophagoscope, 6–12 hours after an intramuscular injection of 8 μCi/kg body weight of ^{32}P.

A radionuclide bone scan, skeletal X-rays, and a liver scan are carried out in the search for distant metastases.

Endoscopy, Biopsy and Cytology

Oesophagoscopy, bronchoscopy, mediastinoscopy, laparotomy and thoracotomy all have a place. Even when rigid instruments had to be used, oesophagoscopy was contraindicated only if excessively dangerous due to rigidity of the spine, the presence of large anterior spinal osteophytes which make perforation of the posterior wall of the cervical oesophagus a grave risk, or a large aortic aneurysm [128]. With the flexible fibreoptic scope oesophagoscopy is performed in almost all patients in whom an oesophageal carcinoma is suspected, unless disease advanced beyond useful treatment has already been demonstrated by simpler means. However, fixity of the tumour is more readily appreciated using the old-fashioned rigid oesophagoscope (the fibreoptic scope can now be stiffened for this purpose). The purpose of oesophagoscopy is to visualize the tumour; to record the level of its proximal limit and, if possible, its distal limit, both measured in centimetres from the upper alveolus; to judge its fixity by gently pressing the beak of the instrument to one side; to take brushings and washings for cytology, and to take biopsies for histology. The vocal cords should be examined for paralysis due to tumour interrupting one or other recurrent laryngeal nerve. Separate tumour nodules may be detected above or below the main tumour due to submucosal lymphatic spread. Submucosal spread may produce a funnel-like narrowing impeding advance of the oesophagoscope so that no tumour is seen and biopsy through the overlying normal mucosa fails to reach the tumour. The more distal narrowed lumen may then be gently explored with a bougie, followed by angled biopsy forceps with which it may be possible to feel a nodule or ulcer from which a specimen may be taken. Simple ulcers and fibrous tissue are difficult to grasp, normal mucosa tends to tear and tumour is much easier to bite. To take too deep a bite from normal oesophagus or from the depths of an ulcer crater invites perforation [136]. Progressive dilatation of the narrowed segment with bougies over several days may permit the tumour to be seen and biopsied. Brushings and washings from beyond the stricture will lead to positive cytology in cases where a satisfactory biopsy is not possible. Energetic dilatation as a method of treatment of carcinoma is pointless because any benefit is transitory, and dangerous because the likelihood of perforation makes the procedure more risky than oesophagectomy [112]. Tanner [136] states: 'It is a stimulus to the endoscopist in his search, to remember that when a patient first begins to complain of dysphagia over the age of 40, there is over a 90 per cent chance that the cause is a malignant lesion affecting the oesophagus.' Therefore, if no abnormality is found, but the symptoms persist, the examination should be repeated.

Appelqvist [9] describes the difficulty of early diagnosis and the prevalence of medical delay: in 315 (45 per cent) of 701 patients with carcinoma of the oesophagus or cardia the first visit to a physician did not lead to further examination or therapy, resulting in the loss of approximately 19 weeks per patient before a successful consultation.

In expert hands, cytology is one of the most highly productive methods of diagnosis, giving correct answers in 95 per cent of cases and sometimes giving the diagnosis of an early, curable cancer in the presence of apparently normal radiology, endoscopic examination and biopsy [18, 28, 63, 115, 116, 136, 144, 151, 154]. The Chinese oseophageal cancer study group in Honan province has used specimens collected for cytology by the abrasive balloon technique in mass screening surveys in high incidence areas to detect both pre-malignant changes and early oesophageal cancer [30].

In a patient without other certain evidence of incurability, a palpable cervical lymph node should be excised for histological examination. In the absence of a palpable lymph node, a blind scalene node biopsy is not indicated because the yield of positive findings is so small.

Akovbiantz et al. [5] performed mediastinoscopy on patients with oesophageal cancer and retrieved histologically positive lymph nodes in 6 of 12 patients with middle third lesions and in 1 out of 4 patients with lower third tumours. The mortality of the procedure is less than 0·1 per cent [11] and the morbidity is low [94]. Baskind [15] found a pick up rate of only 5 per cent of 100 mediastinoscopies in oesophageal cancer. Marchand [88], a proponent of mediastinoscopy in lung cancer, has ceased to use it in oesophageal cancer.

Laparotomy permits biopsies of paracardial, left gastric and the coeliac lymph nodes [57, 94, 98]. Rubin [122] discusses the value of this procedure.

Nordenström [103] describes fine needle exploration and aspiration biopsy of the oesophagus and mediastinum by a paravertebral approach.

There may still remain the occasional patient, especially with a small carcinoma in the presence of fibrosis at the cardia, for whom the diagnosis will only be made at thoraco-laparotomy.

A biochemical screen may provide a lead to the diagnosis of liver metastases.

Alexander et al. [6] find that even in squamous carcinoma of the oesophagus advancing cancer is probable if the carcinoembryonic antigen levels are rising rapidly.

Implications

The seriousness of dysphagia is emphasized [99]. There is need for earlier recognition of the significance of the rather unimpressive, intermittent pre-dysphagic symptoms; yet the patient is often a heavy user of alcohol and tobacco with impaired perception; and in a low incidence area the physician may see only one patient with oesophageal cancer in a working lifetime.

The next need is for rapid referral to a diagnostic team capable of detecting a superficial, half-centimetre carcinoma causing only slight localized rigidity or slight mottling of rugae, without actual stenosis.

Hardly surprisingly these needs are met only in high incidence areas where there has been appropriate education. Ackerman et al. [1] describe the work of the Institute for Cancer Research, Chinese Academy of Medical Sciences, Peking, in Linhsien County in Honan where the incidence of oesophageal cancer is probably the highest in the world. An effective screening programme has been mounted and many symptomless, small, invasive oesophageal cancers, cancer in situ, and premalignant conditions are discovered and successfully treated. So far the diet which probably causes these cancers remains little changed.

In low incidence areas high risk patients such as those previously successfully treated for buccal, pharyngeal and laryngeal cancer could benefit from screening [8, 51].

Cytology is an excellent diagnostic tool.

In spite of the unfavourable outlook for most patients with large tumours causing severe obstruction, full work-up with a view to cure is still necessary as long as tumour spread far beyond the oesophagus has not been demonstrated. A patient with a tumour up to about 8 cm long, even when obstruction is complete and emaciation severe, may still, occasionally, be curable.

Mediastinoscopy and laparotomy are valuable diagnostic measures, giving a high yield of information, in particular about lymphatic and liver metastases. However, as a preliminary to radiotherapy, especially when the patient is frail and old, these more aggressive investigations are not so frequently justified because the irradiated volume will in any event include nearby lymph nodes, and probably cannot be enlarged to include more remote nodes without the need to lower the radiation dose to an ineffective level. For the patient with occult, remote lymphatic or blood-borne metastases, radiotherapy given with the intent to cure will still palliate, although with higher treatment morbidity than would be risked were it known from the outset that only palliation was possible. Such radiation morbidity may be less than the morbidity of laparotomy or mediastinoscopy.

PROGNOSTIC FACTORS

The most important measurable factors influencing prognosis are tumour extent, treatment, sex, site, histology, age and general condition, and the community in which the patient lives [110]. They are complexly interrelated.

Tumour Extent

Given present diagnostic methods, in the individual patient there is always conjecture about the true extent of the cancer. In most sites a metastasis of one hundred million cells (half a centimetre in diameter) goes undetected. Only limited samples can be examined under the microscope. Nevertheless, the extent of demonstrable tumour remains the best guide to prognosis.

The UICC TNM Classification (8) and related national systems of staging (e.g. American, 1973) are being used increasingly. The clinical and pathological classification of the Japanese Society for Esophageal Diseases [70] is especially detailed.

In the oesophagus as in other sites early cancer is highly curable. In Linhsien County Hospital, Honan, 58 (86 per cent) of 69 patients with stage 0 oesophageal cancer are alive 5 years after surgical treatment, and 133 (52 per cent) of 255 stage 1 and 11 patients survived for 5 years [1].

In 701 patients with carcinoma of the oesophagus and cardia treated by radiotherapy or surgery, Appelqvist [9] reports 5-year survival rates in patients with tumours less than 4, 4–8, and more than 8 cm of 21, 9, and 1 per cent respectively. In the Edinburgh series there was a similar experience with patients treated by irradiation. On the occasions when the locoregional eradication of an oesophageal cancer more than 8 cm long is achieved the patient usually dies later from distant metastases.

Although a patient's untreated cancer always increases in extent with time the length of the history by itself is not a useful guide to prognosis [9]. Some slow growing tumours with a long history are still at an early stage, and some aggressive, rapidly growing tumours present at a late stage after a short history.

Lymph node invasion often indicates incurable disease but when confined to nodes lying close to the primary, long survival is still possible following loco-regional treatment by radiation or surgery [58].

Treatment

Oesophageal cancer untreated by radiation or surgery usually kills the patient within a year of onset of symtoms; the mean survival is seven and a half months [106, 126]. Yet even the short remaining life of a frail old patient or one with extensive disease may be further shortened by a major surgical procedure or radiotherapy to too high a dose or too great a volume. It is essential to match the aggressiveness of the investigation and treatment to the fortitude of the patient. Radiotherapy, surgery, and nutritional support applied with skill and wide experience of the disease will shorten the life of few, improve the quality of remaining life for many, and restore to a few the expectation of a life normal in both length and quality. There are various therapeutic or palliative procedures discussed later which may lengthen or unintentionally shorten a patient's life by a month or two but in general they should be applied only when there is a real prospect of the remaining life being enjoyable.

Sex

Female patients have a better prognosis than males whether they are young or old, treated by radiation or surgery, and whether their tumours are in the upper or lower half of the oesophagus [110]. The better prognosis of females has been observed by many [9, 79, 92, 95, 97, 134, 145, 158].

Site

In a centre where both radiotherapy and surgery are available and collaboration between the disciplines is close, prognosis may not vary greatly with the site of the tumour in the oesophagus [9]. However, many series show a worse prognosis for tumours in the upper thorax linked with the early invasion of trachea, bronchi and aorta which occurs at that level. This is likely to be an even greater limitation for surgery than for radiotherapy.

Histology

Patients with well differentiated squamous carcinoma have the best prognosis. Adenocarcinoma is worse because it is commonly associated with a larger primary tumour and a higher incidence of distant metastases [9, 32, 46, 58, 80, 92]. Resection, if possible, is superior to radiation as treatment for adenocarcinoma because adenocarcinoma is marginally less radiosensitive than squamous carcinoma and because irradiation below the diaphragm is complicated by reduced tolerance of the normal tissues.

Undifferentiated carcinoma has the worst prognosis [9, 80]. The local response of undifferentiated carcinoma to radiotherapy is excellent, with rapid relief of symptoms and eradication of tumour within the irradiated volume but the patient usually dies from distant metastases within a few months. A similar outcome awaits those who survive resection of an undifferentiated carcinoma.

Younghusband and Aluwihare [158] report a series of 77 patients treated by oesophagectomy amongst whom those with histological evidence of an immune response in the tumour and lymph nodes have a reduced incidence of tumour extension beyond the oesophagus, fewer lymph node metastases, and longer survival.

Age and General Condition

Advanced age, cardiovascular and respiratory disease, smoking, heavy alcohol consumption, and prolonged starvation militate against successful irradiation, and may also contraindicate surgical treatment. However, it must not be overlooked that a patient, even an aged patient, may be in very poor condition solely due to starvation caused by relatively small, metastasis-free, curable oesophageal cancer.

The Community where the Patient Lives

In affluent communities in which large resources are devoted to alcohol, tobacco, education, and medical facilities, patients with oesophageal cancer usually present with late disease. Between 2 and 9 per cent are alive 5 years later.

In some less affluent communites – even in some of the communities in Africa in which the disease is epidemic and the oesophagus is the commonest site of cancer – late presentation, too late for it to be possible to modify the course of the disease, is so general that 5-year survival is unknown [114].

In another less affluent community (Linhsien County) where the disease is epidemic and radiotherapy is primitive, education of the populace and the medical profession together with a screening campaign result in early diagnosis, high operability and a high resection rate, low operative mortality, and 507 (43 per cent) of 1308 patients alive 5 years later [1].

THE TREATMENT OF OESOPHAGEAL CANCER: RADIOTHERAPY FOR CURE

Technique

Clinical lore, developed by the analysis of experience with thousands of 'anecdotal cases', guides everday practice until it can be replaced by more scientifically determined facts. The following observations are based largely on experience of practice in Edinburgh, Scotland, from 1951 to 1969, a review of Edinburgh records from 1931 to 1950, and Edmonton, Canada, practice from 1970 to 1979.

Curative radiotherapy of carcinoma of the oesophagus is worth attempting if:

1. The histology is squamous or undifferentiated carcinoma.
2. There are no detectable distant metastases.
3. The demonstrable length of the primary tumour and any detectable lymph node metastases extends over no more than 9 cm (less for a frail old patient).
4. There is no invasion of trachea, bronchi, thyroid, stomach or vertebrae (the commonly present bulging of the posterior tracheal wall without demonstrable invasion is not a contraindication).
5. The patient's general condition is good enough for him to tolerate the course of radiotherapy (dehydration and emaciation do not rule out an attempt at cure if the demonstrable tumour is small enough).

The greater the magnitude of unfavourable factors such as great age and emaciation or advanced circulatory, respiratory or metabolic disease, the smaller must be the demonstrable tumour for cure to be attempted. Werner and his associates [148, 150] lucidly describe the indications and contraindications for various categories of treatment.

It is highly desirable, but impossible, to have complete information about the true extent of the tumour in order to plan the target volume for irradiation (metastases of less than 10^8 cells (0·5 cm) are rarely detected). The normal practice is complete non-invasive investigation which includes optimum photon and radionuclide imaging, haematology, and a biochemical profile. Also normally essential are oesophagoscopy, biopsies, brushings and washings. Bronchoscopy is necessary unless the tumour is remote from the trachea. More invasive investigations such as mediastinoscopy, laparotomy and thoracotomy are not usual preliminaries to irradiation [15]. The target volume chosen for irradiation without the evidence from these more aggressive investigations will usually cover all the tumour if it is indeed curable. A tumour which can only be encompassed by a much larger volume will usually not be controlled by the lower radiation dose which must be prescribed for a larger volume.

The average patient planned for radical treatment is not unacquainted with alcohol and tobacco, chronic bronchitis and emphysema, and has a demonstrable length of moderately undifferentiated squamous carcinoma of 6 cm. The correction of starvation, dehydration, anaemia, and infection are commenced, and without delay radiotherapy is given using 20 equal fractions, 1 fraction per day, 5 times a week to a total dose which ranges between 4800 and 5300 rad throughout a 15 cm long by 6·5 cm diameter (somewhat rounded off) cylindrical volume. A 4, 6 or 8 MeV linear accelerator is used. If unusually low tolerance is expected a reduction in volume rather than in dose, is indicated. Only for the larger very undifferentiated carcinomas is a dose of 200–300 rad less given to a volume rarely exceeding an 18 × 7·5 cm cylinder. Rarely is the volume less than a 12 × 6 cm cylinder, even for the small tumours. The irradiated volumes vary over a smaller range than the estimated tumour volumes. Patients with smaller volumes are given the benefit of a slightly wider margin and, if they are not too old and frail, an extra 250 rad of dose. For patients with larger tumours the margin is less and the risk of geographic miss greater but the dose is kept up. Even for the same dose the larger tumours are more likely to recur locally. Because most of the larger tumours are associated with occult distant spread, a higher treatment morbidity is not inflicted for the sake of the rare cure which would be at the expense of optimum palliation for the large majority.

A lower local failure rate awaits earlier diagnosis, improved definition of the extent of tumour, and an improved therapeutic ratio, whether it be achieved by improved fractionation, hypoxic cell sensitizers, HPO_2, neutrons, pions, heavy ions, or super-additive combinations with hyperthermia or cytotoxic drugs – or whatever improvements lie in the future.

For the radical irradiation of oesophageal cancer it is suggested that antero-posterior opposed fields should never be used. Even that 'moderate radical dose' which locally eradicates only 50 per cent of oesophageal cancer is too great a threat to the functional integrity of the spinal cord. There are numerous published reports of paraplegia resulting from the treatment of oesophageal cancer using techniques which irradiate the spinal cord to the same dose as the oesophagus, and radiation pneumonitis has been a frequently reported complication. Not one of the 401 patients radically irradiated in Edinburgh from 1949 to 1969 (*see Fig. 4.2*) was treated with an antero-posterior opposed pair, and over 180 lived more than a year, but only one developed partial, transient transverse myelitis, and only one (who had scleroderma) suffered significantly from irradiation pneumonitis.

Since 1955 radical irradiation of the thoracic oesophagus has usually been by three symmetrically arranged fields at 120° to each other, the anterior field applied with the patient supine, and the two postero-lateral fields applied with the patient prone. Orthogonal planning films were prepared separately for the supine and prone positions and the two plans were integrated using the centre of the target volume, placed at the isocentre, as the common reference point. In every case the planning was three dimensional in that the relationship of the spinal cord to the target volume was determined 1 cm within the rostral and caudal ends of the target volume as well as in the central transverse plane. In the central plane a more detailed calculation was performed. The long axis of the target volume was usually orientated at an angle to the horizontal and sometimes at an angle to the sagittal plane, so as best to fit the volume suspect of invasion by tumour without encroaching on the spinal cord.

In recent years, using a more modern linear accelerator which can swing below the couch, the patient remains supine throughout treatment (*see* 8MeV, *Fig. 4.1*) and either an anterior and two postero-lateral fields or a vertically upwards posterior and two antero-laterals may be used. Supine is the most relaxed, precisely reproducible treatment position and for this reason is almost invariably preferred. With a modern machine the oblique fields can readily be shaped by blocks so that the treated volume becomes a gently curved sausage shape, fitting the curve of the spine, thus affording greater security to the spinal cord without loss of tumour coverage [48].

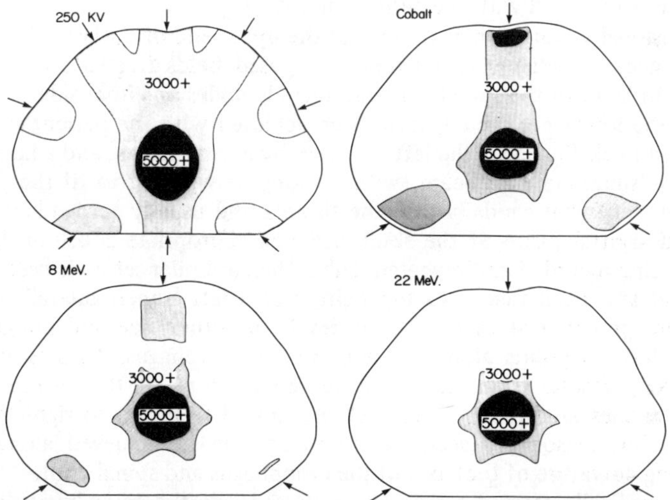

Fig. 4.1 Four dose distributions for the mid tumour cross section of the same patient. The higher the energy the better the localization of the absorbed radiation in the target volume. (Reproduced from Pearson [117] by courtesy of 'Cancer'.)

Prager [113] and Lewinsky [82] have studied the attractions of the prone position to increase the separation between oesophagus and spinal cord.

In the Edinburgh practice since 1955 the shape of the lung has been reconstructed on the main plane plan from the orthogonal planning films and anatomical knowledge, and the decreased absorption in lung has been calculated separately for each field. For the more complexly varying tissue depths and lung thicknesses between the neck and the upper thorax a different technique was introduced in 1957 to treat a volume angled to fit snugly in front of the spinal cord, if necessary from cricoid to main carina, using two antero-lateral fields, again with the patient supine. Two planning films were prepared with a diagnostic beam perpendicular to the intended treatment beam, barium in the oesophagus, and the appropriate body surface contour outlined by soft wire. Then contours were prepared, the lung shape drawn in, and planning done in the main plane and in planes 1 cm within either end of the target volume. Compensation was achieved rather crudely by wedging for an appropriate number of fractions across the long axis and then across the short axis of each field. Deeley and Francois [37] solved this problem with a combination of a stepped field in the long axis and wedge filtration across the short axis of each of the antero-lateral fields. In the early 1950s in Liverpool a standard brass block wedged diagonally across each rectangular antero-lateral field was used to make this correction (Garrett, 1971). Now these needs are more elegantly and precisely met using CT scans at appropriate levels, simulator fluoroscopy and planning films with barium, and a perspex shell and compensators – still with the patient supine [77].

Occasionally, for a small tumour at the upper end of the oesophagus in a long necked patient, two laterally opposed fields treat a satisfactory volume in front of the spinal cord and include nodes on either side.

For the lower neck, cures have been achieved with the patient supine, head and neck flexed to the left, steadied by a head clamp, and a horizontal right 'supero-lateral' beam, with its long axis angled to fit the spine, directed somewhat caudally into the thorax, and usually perpendicular to the mid sagittal plane of the skull, using an appropriate couch angle, all angles being recorded and repeated daily. Then a similar set-up is used with the head and neck flexed to the right, and a left 'supero-lateral' beam. Plans are prepared at each of three levels on either side and integrated using reference points along the axis of the oesophagus. An inescapable complexity results from the changing relationships of the surrounding normal tissues as the head and neck are moved from left to right lateral flexion, but reasonably accurate dosimetry can be achieved along the (changing curvature of the) axis of the oesophagus and spinal cord.

Most radically treated patients have started radiotherapy while still able to swallow liquids or soft solids. Many have been treated as out-patients. They have received advice on the preparation of a rich liquid diet. Usually the tumour starts to shrink and swallowing improves towards the end of the second week of treatment, and the patient then improves rapidly. The symptoms of irradiation oesophagitis also commence during the second week of treatment and are a great burden to the few patients whose dysphagia was insignificant at the start of treatment, but cause little additional suffering to the more typical patient who starts treatment with severe dysphagia. Irradiation oesophagitis reaches a maximum during the fourth and final week of treatment, continues unabated for the first week after treatment, and takes another two weeks (sometimes longer) to settle down. Medication has little useful effect on the pathology but antacid mucilage with a mild mucosal analgesic may give comfort. The main supportive measure is a copious, very bland, nutritionally rich liquid diet flavoured and timed to the patient's taste.

An intelligent, spirited patient may feel cheated if not forbidden alcohol and tobacco, cheated of a discipline which aids him to another purpose in life – to instruct young friends and relatives to forego self-destructive practices. This phenomenon has been observed in some northern Indian and Eskimo patients but rarely is the urban patient so paternalistic.

Radical radiotherapy is occasionally still indicated in a dehydrated patient with complete or almost complete dysphagia. For such patients intravenous hydration and feeding have been preferred to either intubation or enterostomy. Intravenous management is usually very successful for the two or three weeks required before the tumour shrinks. Marcial [89] has also had this experience. It avoids any further delay before commencing irradiation and also avoids the hazard of intubation in the face of complete obstruction. For the patient who can still swallow liquids and whose tumour is soon to regress, intubation contributes nothing but an unnecessary hazard. The presence of a tube through the tumour adds further trauma at the site of an infected ulcer and adds to the fibrosis which attends healing as the tumour regresses. This may cause a stricture at the site of healing which without intubation may be less severe or avoided [109].

There is considerable variation in the rate of shrinkage of the tumour following radiotherapy. The average tumour will shrink to half its pre-treatment bulk by the end of treatment and 2 months later mucosal healing is complete. Healing may occur with minimal fibrosis and complete relief of dysphagia, or the tumour may be replaced by a fibrous stricture. If this residual stricture seriously impairs nutrition, gentle bouginage should be attempted. Of the 5-year survivors, half never require bouginage, a quarter need one dilatation, and the remaining quarter need repeated bouginage, in some cases for over a year. Bouginage is hazardous, must not be started until two or more months after irradiation, and *must* be very gentle. Several such patients, cancer free at autopsy, have died as a consequence of rupture of the oesophagus by a bougie.

If the philosophy of the treatment team is to administer moderate radical dose radiotherapy such as 20 fractions of 250 rad in 4 weeks (or 28 fractions of 200 rad in 5½ weeks) to a 15 × 7 centimetre cylindrical volume, half the 5 cm-long tumours will be eradicated (more than half of the smaller tumours and less than half of the larger tumours), and for the majority of the patients so treated who are not cured because of local failure or occult spread beyond the target volume, such a moderate radical dose and volume achieves good palliation, with a low radiation morbidity.

When local failure occurs, the cancer can be detected, with or without distant metastases, usually between 6 and 12 months, but occasionally as much as 30 months later [112]. Potentially operable patients, those who are not too frail and who remain free from detectable distant metastases, must be followed closely with a view to salvage by surgical resection should a local recurrence develop. Such surgery is technically more difficult than oesophageal resection in the unirradiated patient but may occasionally be very successful [109]. The majority of the patients who suffer local failure of radiotherapy are not suitable for surgery, some because distant metastases have appeared since irradiation, and some because of various criteria of inoperability present before the initial decision to irradiate. As dysphagia worsens a strictly liquid but rich diet is advised. When nutrition is no longer adequate with this regimen, the oesophageal lumen can be kept open a little longer by means of intubation.

Morbidity of Radical Radiotherapy

Using the above technique the worst complication is local recurrence of the oesophageal cancer. Otherwise, morbidity is low. Treatment mortality is less than 1 per cent. Radiation oesophagitis occurs in all patients. Less than 1 per cent suffer symptoms from lung or skin reactions. A faint paramediastinal lung opacity can be detected on the chest X-ray in nearly all cases. Radiation osteitis of the spine occurs after three years in 10 per cent of the long term survivors (especially if there is already senile osteoporosis), but the symptoms are minimal [79, 112]. Radiation myelitis does not occur with good radiotherapy technique unless there is some unusual extra hazard such as the need to attempt cure in a patient who has had previous radiotherapy but refuses alternative surgical treatment. One of the 401 patients treated in this series developed a partial cord lesion, which recovered completely after 5 months. Oesophagotracheal fistula has not been a complication of the technique described above. Patients with detectable tumour invasion through to the tracheal mucosa have not been irradiated for cure but have been treated with lower dose palliative irradiation. High dose irradiation of such a patient might well cause a fistula. Patients with established oesophagotracheal fistula have rarely been treated with irradiation. In these cases, irradiation would be expected to enlarge the fistula as the tumour shrinks. Oesophagotracheal fistula commonly results from the advance of untreated oesophageal cancer. In a report of 111 patients with oesophago-respiratory fistula Martini et al. (1970) found no evidence that radiotherapy was a significant cause. In fact they reported one patient whose fistula was healed by irradiation.

Half of the long term survivors require dilatation of a stricture. This is not a radiation stricture. When a tumour which has destroyed the whole thickness of the oesophageal wall around its whole circumference is eradicated by radiotherapy healing occurs by fibrosis and causes a stricture. If the cancer destroys both muscle layers around only half the circumference healing following radiation cure will produce a fibrous scar which merely kinks the oesophageal wall, may be asymptomatic and will not require bouginage. If the cancer infiltrates without destroying the muscle, radiation cure leaves a normal functioning, stricture-free oesophagus which is also radiographically normal.

Results of Radiotherapy for Cure

The most important benefit is restoration of months or years of enjoyable life that would otherwise be lost. Of the patients radically irradiated in Edinburgh from 1949 to 1967 41 per cent survived 1 year and 17 per cent 5 years (*see Fig. 4.4*). For those whose cancer is not eradicated the main concern is for the quality of their remaining life. Most live more than six months. If local recurrence occurs, the outlook is indeed gloomy but even these patients have usually had restoration of normal or improved swallowing for a period of months up to a year or two. For radiation failure, surgical salvage is occasionally possible but always difficult. Many are treated merely by intubation which usually makes maintenance on a liquid diet possible for a few weeks, or occasionally months, but is not without mortality. Once cure is recognized to be no longer possible, enterostomy is avoided. Of those dying within 5 years from causes other than local recurrence half die from distant metastases and half die from causes other than cancer. After the first 3 years most of the deaths are due to other causes [108].

Forty-eight of the patients irradiated between 1949 and 1967 (*see Fig 4.3*) lived more than 5 years and each had a normal voice and a normal stomach and had regained normal or excessive weight. Those under retiring age were working and nearly all were taking a normal diet.

RADIOTHERAPY FOR PALLIATION

To palliate is to improve the quality of the patient's remaining life. When cure is seen to be impossible, there is rarely occasion for a major procedure which itself induces symptoms. To prolong a life of suffering is not good palliation. In the Edinburgh series 35 per cent of the patients were demonstrably incurable and for another 10 per cent the chance of cure was remote (*see Fig. 4.2*). Those with very advanced disease received 'no treatment' which means excellent nursing with anxiety and pain-relieving medication, but no direct attack on the tumour. Of the 35 per cent judged incurable about half received palliative irradiation of the primary tumour: 4500–4800 rad in 20 fractions in 4 weeks to a restricted volume, allowing a smaller margin around the detectable tumour than is used for radical treatment, or appropriately modified doses given in 5 or 10 fractions. Significantly smaller doses than the above risk prolonging rather than relieving distressing dysphagia. The results were similar to those of other authors who have observed that 75 per cent of patients experience worthwhile relief of dysphagia following radiotherapy, some remaining euphagic until they die from distant metastases [76, 79, 89]. If a patient is going to die from his cancer within one year, as do 95 per cent of those not selected for radical treatment, and relief of dysphagia is indicated, palliative irradiation is usually the preferred initial treatment. It is less of a burden to the patient than intubation or a bypass operation. If relief of dysphagia is inadequate or if, after a few months of improved swallowing, a local recurrence develops, a decision as to palliative intubation or no further treatment is made.

For patients with pain or discomfort from metastases remote from the primary tumour, satisfactory short term palliation frequently results from simple single fraction or 5 fraction radiation treatment.

SURGERY FOR CURE

The surgical treatment of early oesophageal cancer in the hands of an experienced team is attended by good results. A person born in Linhsien County (population 720 000) near the Taihang Mountains in the Anyang Administrative Region of Honan Province, has at least a 10 per cent chance of getting carcinoma of the oesophagus. The disease has been recognized there for about 2000 years. Their screening programme brings to light many early cases and the staff of Linhsien County Hospital is very experienced in managing the disease. Of 324 patients of stages 0, I, and II treated surgically since 1964 and followed more than 5 years, 191 (59 per cent) survive for 5 years. The resection rate is 95 per cent and the operative mortality is 5 per cent [1]. No other team has reported such good results. In most reports in which the extent of disease at the time of diagnosis is analyzed in detail about 80 per cent of patients already have evidence of spread of the cancer beyond the oesophagus [9, 80, 92, 102, 111].

There are now several surgeons or surgical teams reporting more than 20 patients living 5 or more years after surgical treatment of carcinoma of the oesophagus or carcinoma of the oesophagus and cardia. Amongst these are [1, 4, 9, 23, 29, 46, 58, 80, 83, 92, 97]. With the exception of Linhsien County where the diagnosis is made early and a high order of surgical skill has been acquired, there is no community where it has been shown that as many as 10 per cent of the patients developing oesophageal cancer are alive 5 years later as a consequence of surgical treatment. There are reports of elite teams of patients, surgeons and nursing staff, characterized by fortitude and less than hopelessly advanced cancers at a site in the oesophagus suited to the well-practised techniques of the highly skilled surgeons, achieving 5-year survival rates of 20 per cent or more. Before this expertise developed in the 1940s the long term survival of a patient with carcinoma of the thoracic oesophagus was a rarity (*see Fig. 4.2*). However, those patients who have died from a surgical procedure for oesophageal cancer greatly outnumber the 5-year survivors from such procedures and may well outnumber the 1-year survivors. The more successful experiences are the most widely published. It is salutory to peruse cancer registry reports. Of patients who developed oesophageal cancer in the USA from 1965 to 1969, only 3 per cent of males and 6 per cent of females survived 5 years.

SURGERY FOR PALLIATION

Progressive dysphagia is a distressing symptom which finally leads to death. For a patient without hope of cure, it is necessary to find some palliative procedure to relieve dysphagia without inflicting unwarranted additional suffering. All except the most agressive surgeons will conclude that a palliative oesophagogastrectomy or a bypass operation with stomach or colon is too large a procedure to inflict on an incurable patient who is going to die within a few months to a year. Dysphagia can probably be relieved by palliative radiotherapy. If this fails, or if dysphagia recurs several months later, intubation is then indicated. Ammann and Collis [7] report better results with a specially modified Souttar tube than with the pull-through Mousseau-Barbin type. Hegarty et al. [60, 61] also prefer the pulsion to the traction technique because of the lower mortality, lower morbidity and shorter hospitalization. In their report of 181 intubations over a 15-month period in the Oesophageal Cancer Unit at the University of Natal in Durban, their preference for the Proctor-Livingstone tube is recorded. Following intubation, 16·6 per cent of patients failed to leave hospital alive, which is a not unreasonable mortality at this advanced stage of the disease when set against the benefit to the survivors of restoration of ability to swallow liquids which may last several months, and occasionally more than a year.

Oesophagotracheal or oesophagobronchial fistula due to carcinoma of the oesophagus is most satisfactorily treated by intubation. In their report of 62 intubations for malignant oesophago-respiratory fistula Hegarty et al. found the best technique to be the insertion of a Proctor-Livingstone tube by the pulsion technique. Seventy-five per cent of patients so treated returned home swallowing satisfactorily and relieved of respiratory distress. Ong and Kwong [104] advocate a more aggressive approach. Eighteen patients with a malignant oesophago-respiratory fistula were treated by resection or bypass of the lesion. Nine (50 per cent) died within a month. Five (28 per cent) died between 1 and 6 months, four of them having experienced benefit. Three achieved good palliation and died later between 6 and 12 months. One was still living at the time of the report, 2 months after bypass.

Gastrostomy or jejunostomy as definitive treatment are mentioned only to be condemned. Dysphagia is not relieved and a miserable existence aspirating and continually spitting out saliva may be cruelly prolonged.

COMBINATIONS OF RADIOTHERAPY AND SURGERY

Loco-regional or local treatment such as radiotherapy or surgery must fail to cure the 80 per cent of patients who already have more remote tumour spread [111]. However, some patients still free from remote spread die as a consequence of surgery, or primary recurrence within the irradiated volume, or recurrence at the margins of the irradiated or resected tissues. Many different combinations of irradiation and surgery have been tried in attempts to reduce these hazards. Robertson et al. [121] lucidly outline the reasons for expecting benefit from preoperative irradiation. Akakura et al. [4] and Yamashita et al. [157] found that, during a period when surgical technique altered little, the introduction of full preoperative irradiation to a dose of 5000 to 6000 rad in 4–6 weeks, followed 2–4 weeks later by resection, was associated with a striking improvement in resectability, reduction in the incidence of tumour at the margins of resection, and improvement in 5-year survival. Nakayama [97] reports that preoperative irradiation (500 rad × 4) and three stage oesophagectomy and reconstruction have decreased operative mortality and increased survival. Rambo et al. [118], Parker and Gregorie [105] and Marks et al. [90] have extensive experience of a preoperative dose of 4500 rad in 18 fractions in three and one half weeks and they conclude that preoperative irradiation offers a distinct advantage. Seymour and Petit [124] and Nègre et al. [100] favour preoperative irradiation. The group at the Fu Wai Hospital in Peking [49] and Doctor and Sirsat [38] have studied the effect of a range of doses used preoperatively. Werner et al. [148, 150] have developed an impressive overall plan for the management of clearly categorized stages of oesophageal cancer using preoperative methotrexate and irradiation; or methotrexate and radiotherapy without surgery. Their early results are exciting. Guernsey et al. [56] used doses of 6600 rad in seven weeks preoperatively and concluded such a dose is too high. After a trial of 800 rad × 3 preoperatively in 70 patients, Groves and Rodríguez-Antúnez have discontinued the practice.

Postoperative irradiation may be inferior to preoperative irradiation because the blood supply and oxygenation of the residual tumour, and therefore its radiosensitivity, are believed to be reduced after surgery. However, in 39 patients who underwent curative resection of oesophageal cancer and were found to have no lymph node metastases, Kasai et al. [71] observed increased survival in those given postoperative irradiation, but there was no benefit from postoperative irradiation if lymph node metastases were present.

Thus there are indications that radiotherapy and surgery can usefully be combined but due to lack of suitable controls none of the evidence constitutes incontrovertible proof.

COMPARISON OF RADIOTHERAPY AND SURGERY

Localized Treatment

Radiotherapy is a loco-regional method of treatment which can cure only if the cancer is localized. Surgical treatment is limited in a similar manner. There are minor differences which can be critical for some patients. The surgeon may resect the whole oesophagus but leave tumour behind on the trachea, aorta, pericardium or in lymph nodes. The radiotherapist will irradiate a larger volume circumferentially around the oesophagus than the surgeon can resect but the length of oesophagus irradiated will be less than the surgeon removes in a total oesophagectomy. An oesophagogastrectomy performed below the aortic arch may well remove a smaller margin of oesophagus above the tumour than would be irradiated.

Local Radiation Failure versus Operative Mortality

Radiotherapy frequently fails because the tumour recurs at the primary site. Such failures are less common in favourable patients with smaller tumours which are also associated with less occult distant spread. The treatment mortality for moderate dose radical radiotherapy is much less than the operative mortality for radical surgery. These disastrous features of the two methods of treatment tend to have a similar effect on long term survival but operative death kills a patient about six months earlier than a local recurrence following radiotherapy (*see Fig. 4.4*).

Level of the Tumour

It has been observed by many radiotherapists that radiotherapy tends to be rather more effective in the upper two-thirds of the oesophagus (*see Fig 4.3*). Most surgeons report fewer problems with the resection of lower third tumours. Evaluation of the significance of level in the Edinburgh material is complicated by the cross linkages with sex, age and method of treatment. Similar numbers have been irradiated in the upper, middle and lower oesophagus but 281 at the lower end compared with only 25 at the upper end have been treated surgically. However, at all three levels the survival rates are higher following radiotherapy. The differences are statistically significant at the upper end (25 per cent vs. 16 per cent), in the middle (16 per cent vs. 9 per cent) and overall (17 per cent vs. 11 per cent), but imperceptible in the lower oesophagus (12 per cent vs. 11 per cent). However, the comparability of the surgical and radiation groups is impossible to establish with precision in the absence of a properly randomized trial. The 103 patients with lower third tumours treated by radiotherapy include a distinctly higher proportion of older patients, but not a higher proportion of females, than the 281 surgically treated. There is no evidence that site, *per se*, is an important prognostic factor in this series, but because of the cross linkages between site, sex, age and method of treatment – because more patients with upper end tumours are female, younger and irradiated – upper end tumours are associated with a better prognosis.

Age

The older the patient the more hazardous is radical treatment by surgery or radiotherapy, but age is less a limitation for radiotherapy than surgery.

Survival

No carefully designed, prospective, randomized trial has ever been carried out to compare surgery and radiotherapy or combinations of the two in the management of any category of patient with oesophageal cancer.

There remains an element of conjecture in any provisional conclusions drawn on the basis of material so far available. The attraction of the Edinburgh material for this purpose is that it is the work of a team of radiotherapists and surgeons who together provide all the treatment for this disease for a well defined and stable population of 1·3 million people. In the later years of the study the patients include all those recorded in the regional cancer registry. The surgical component of the material constitutes a remarkable record as reported by LeRoux [80] and Logan [83]. The radiotherapy component has benefited greatly from the availability of a 4MeV linear accelerator since 1955. Radiotherapists have gained vital insight into the likely extent and anatomy of the tumour to be included in the target volume by working closely with their surgical colleagues in the clinic, the operating room and in the autopsy room. Neither the surgery nor the radiotherapy of oesophageal cancer will be optimal in the hands of occasional practitioners.

The Edinburgh experience is of disease apparently more extensive than at the Linhsien County Hospital but less extensive than in Durban, Port Elizabeth, Johannesburg or Cape Town. In the Edinburgh series there are as many females as males, which is a factor favouring longer survival not present to the same degree in most other series.

Figs. 4.2–4.4 should be examined together.

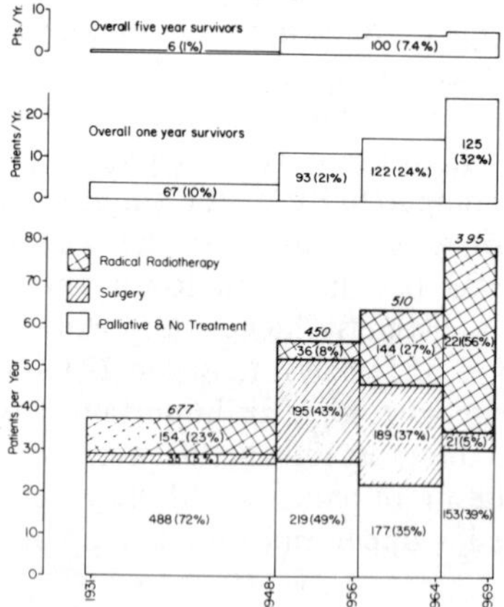

Fig. 4.2. Distribution of 2032 patients with squamous carcinoma of the oesophagus seen in hospitals in the Edinburgh area during four periods of 18, 8, 8, and 5 years between 1931 and 1969.

Fig. 4.2 shows the distribution of 2032 patients with squamous carcinoma of the oesophagus seen in hospitals in the Edinburgh area during four periods of 18, 8, 8, and 5 years between 1931 and 1969. The vertical scale shows the absolute numbers of patients per year. The trend towards

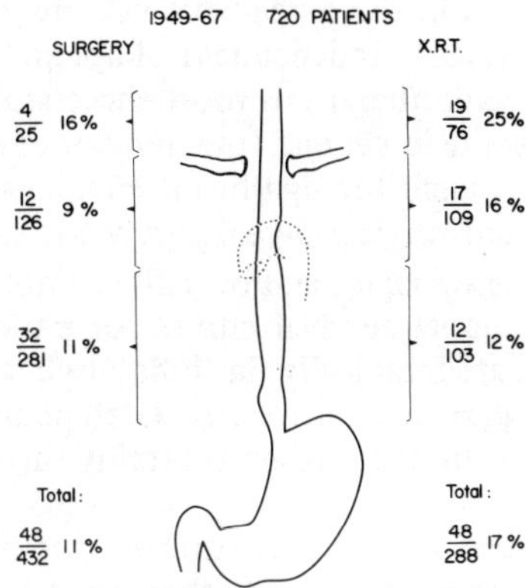

Fig. 4.3. The 5-year survival fractions and percentages are shown for 720 patients treated radically for squamous oesophageal cancer in Edinburgh from 1949 to 1967. (Reproduced from Pearson [111] by courtesy of 'Cancer.')

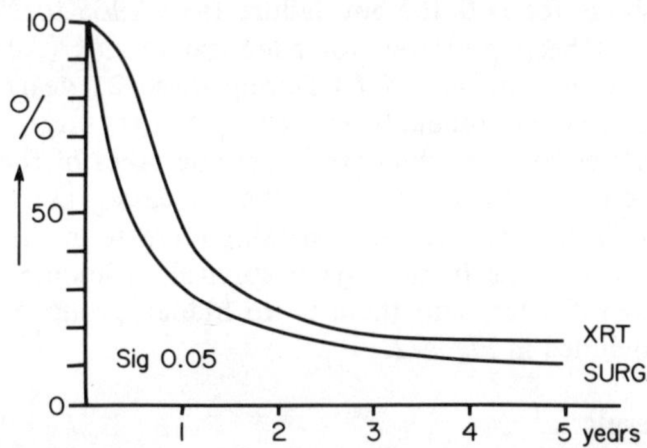

Fig. 4.4. The actuarial survival curves for patients with squamous oesophageal cancer treated radically in Edinburgh from 1949 to 1969.

more patients per year represents the increasing proportion referred rather than increasing incidence. The percentages are out of the total number of patients which occurs in each period. From 1949 to 1969 the trend towards the wider use of radiotherapy for the initial treatment is associated with an increase in 1-year survival rate, a maintained overall 5-year survival rate and an increasing absolute number of 1 and 5-year survivors occurring in the community.

In *Fig. 4.3* the 5-year survival fractions and percentages are shown for 720 patients treated radically for squamous oesophageal cancer in Edinburgh from 1949 to 1967. Four hundred and thirty-two patients were treated by surgery and 288 by radiotherapy. Ninety-six survived for 5 years. The site differences in the 5-year survivals are partly attributable to age and sex factors but in part, independent of age and sex, survival by site varies with treatment. Radiotherapy is most successful towards the upper end and surgery towards the lower end (the number of cervical oesophageal tumours resected is too small for significant comparison). The difference between radiotherapy and surgical 5-year survival is significant ($P<0{\cdot}05$) for the upper and mid oesophagus, and overall, but not for the lower third. *Fig. 4.4* shows the actuarial survival curves for patients with squamous oesophageal cancer treated radically in Edinburgh from 1949 to 1969 show a significantly higher survival for irradiated patients at 1 and 5 years ($p = 0{\cdot}05$), mainly due to the higher mortality in the first 2 months following surgery.

The practice has been to treat by surgery for thoracic oesophageal cancer (followed occasionally by radiotherapy salvage) and by radiotherapy for cervical oesophageal cancer from 1949 to 1956; surgery for lower half tumours and radiotherapy for upper half tumours (and for particularly old and frail patients with small tumours) from 1957 to 1964; and initial radiotherapy at all levels for squamous carcinoma and wider use of surgical salvage for radiotherapy failure from 1965 to 1969. Throughout, surgery has been preferred for adenocarcinoma. (Adenocarcinomas are excluded from *Figs. 4.2–4.4.*) During these 21 years the definitive treatment has been radiotherapy for 401 patients, surgery for 405, and palliative measures for 549. Whatever view one takes of the causes of the effects observed over these 21 years, the increasing use of megavoltage irradiation has been attended by a striking increase in the overall 1-year survival and no decrease in the 5-year survival. A hundred patients have lived more than 5 years and there is no hidden group of unfavourable patients not included in *Fig. 4.2*.

Functional Result

The long term survivors following radiotherapy constitute a particularly fortunate group from the functional point of view. Most are euphagic, regain normal weight, and retain a normal functioning larynx, normal lungs, and normal cardia, and a normal functioning stomach.

CHEMOTHERAPY

Chemotherapy benefits only a small minority of patients with oesophageal carcinoma and is curative in none. Therefore it is reserved for the patient beyond further help by radiotherapy or surgery (Cline, 1971) or for use in combination with radiotherapy and surgery.

For squamous carcinoma of the oesophagus the use of chemotherapy is limited by the toxicity of the drugs which are effective in bringing about tumour regression and the short duration of such regressions. Werner et al. [148, 150] have developed a successful overall plan of management which combines methotrexate with either radiotherapy or surgery or both.

Bleomycin, discovered by Umezawa and his associates in 1962 in Japan, concentrates in the skin and is sometimes effective in squamous carcinoma [67, 146] but can cause pneumonitis proceeding to fibrosis, which may be fatal. Elderly smoking drinkers are not good candidates for this drug. Kolarić et al. [75] describe the treatment of advanced oesophageal cancer with bleomycin, irradiation and a combination of bleomycin and irradiation, with reduction of selection factors between the three groups by using each regimen exclusively during each of three successive time periods. They observed a median duration of remission of 9 months in the combined therapy group as compared with 6 months when treatment was by radiotherapy alone and only 3 months when treatment was by bleomycin alone. Kelsen et al. [72] treated 47 patients with oesophageal carcinoma with a combination of cis-platinum and bleomycin and feel that the combination, although highly toxic, is worthy of further study. Soreide et al. [131] draw attention to the dangers of greatly increased toxicity when bleomycin and irradiation are combined. Werner [149], in the course of a very extensive experience of the management of oesophageal cancer, has studied both bleomycin and methotrexate in combination with radiotherapy and finds methotrexate preferrable.

For adenocarcinoma presenting in the oesophagus, chemotherapy follows the same pattern as for gastric cancer. 5-Fluorouracil may benefit 20 per cent of the patients beyond further help by surgery or radiotherapy. The benefit may be gained with little toxicity and may occasionally last six months or longer. A reasonable dose is 12·5 mg per kg body weight once weekly until toxicity develops or until it is clear that there is no benefit.

A large research programme continues the search for more effective drugs and combinations of drugs.

PROSPECTS FOR IMPROVEMENT

For most patients treatment fails because of the great extent of tumour by the time the diagnosis is made. The Chinese experience in Linhsien County proves that in a high incidence area a screening programme can be made to work and early diagnosis and treatment by an experienced team really does produce better results.

There are technical improvements in radiotherapy which will reduce the local failure rate and increase the volume of local and regional disease which can be irradiated radically.

1. Better definition of the optimum dose–time–fractionation factors.
2. A better therapeutic ratio within the irradiated volume using selective hypoxic radiosensitizers.
3. A better therapeutic ratio within the target volume and better localization of the absorption of radiation energy to the target volume using neutrons, heavy ions, or *pi*-mesons.

4. It may be possible to get a more than additive effect preferentially on the tumour cells, and therefore a better therapeutic ratio, by combining irradiation with hyperthermia or suitable cytotoxic drugs.

Surgical mortality has been dramatically reduced in the hands of the most experienced practitioners and these benefits are being extended more widely.

More advantageous combinations of surgery with radiotherapy or with radiotherapy and chemotherapy are likely to be developed in the way that has been possible for cancer in several other sites. (Werner et al. [148, 150].)

Surgical salvage following radiation failure may be more successful if a technique is developed to determine at an earlier date and with more precision in just which patients a local recurrence is developing. At present some patients die needlessly from an operation carried out on suspicion of local radiation failure when in fact the radiation has eradicated all tumour. Many more patients die because the fact of local failure of radiotherapy is not established until it is too late for salvage surgery to be practicable.

SUMMARY

There are large variations between communities in the pattern of oesophageal malignant disease.

During the last 30 years there have been great improvements in the local effectiveness of both the radiation and surgical treatment of oesophageal cancer, not matched by improved diagnosis. Few patients are treated before the size of the primary tumour and the extent of metastases make cure impossible. The screening programme in North China is an exceptional experience in a very high incidence community which has lead to the diagnosis of many very early cancers which have been successfully treated by surgery.

In communities where there are good and closely associated radiotherapy and surgical facilities the greatest number of enjoyable patient years of life is likely to be contributed if patients with squamous carcinoma of the middle and upper thirds of the oesophagus are treated initially by radiotherapy, with surgery held in reserve for local recurrences, and patients with squamous carcinoma of the lower third and all adenocarcinomas are treated surgically unless medically unfit.

Patients with more advanced disease can usually be helped by palliative radiotherapy, with intubation held in reserve until an adequate fluid diet can no longer be swallowed.

Prevention is conceivable and would be preferable.

REFERENCES

1. Ackerman L. V., Weinstein I. B. and Kaplan H. S. (1978) Cancer of the esophagus. In: Kaplan and Tsuchitani (eds.), *Cancer in China*, New York, Liss; pp. 111–136.

2. Ahlbom H. E. (1936) Simple achlorhydric anemia, Plummer-Vinson syndrome, and carcinoma of the mouth, pharynx and oesophagus in women; observations at Radiumhemmet, Stockholm. *Brit. Med. J.* **2,** 331–333.
3. Ahlbom H. E. (1937) Prädisponierende Faktoren für Plattenepithelkarzinom in Mund, Hals und Speiseröhre. Eine Statistische Untersuchung am Material des Radiumhemmets, Stockholm. *Acta Radiol.* **18,** 163–185.
4. Akakura I., Nakamura Y., Kakegawa T. et al. (1970) Surgery of carcinoma of the esophagus with preoperative radiation. *Chest* **57,** 47–57.
5. Akovbiantz A., Aeberhard P., Linder E. et al. (1965) Die bedeutung der mediastinoskpie für die Beurteilung der Operabilität des Oesophaguscarcinoms. *Langenbecks Arch. Chir.* **313,** 360–363.
6. Alexander J. C., Chretien P. B., Dellon A. L. et al. (1978) CEA levels in patients with carcinoma of the esophagus. *Cancer* **42,** 1492–1497.
7. Ammann J. F. and Collis J. L. (1971) Palliative intubation of the esophagus. *J. Thorac. Cardiovasc. Surg.* **61** (6), 863–869.
8. Andrieu-Guitrancourt J., Brossard-Legrand M., Happich J. L. et al. (1975) Endoscopie systématique de l'oesophage au cours des cancers buccaux, pharingés et laryngés. *Ann. Otolaryngol. Chir. Cervicofac.* **92,** (12) 659–666.
9. Appelqvist P. (1972) Carcinoma of the oesophagus and gastric cardia. *Acta Chir. Scand.* Suppl. **430,** 3–92.
10. Appelqvist P. (1975) Carcinoma of the oesophagus and gastric cardia at autopsy in Finland. *Ann. Clin. Res.* **7,** 334–340.
11. Ashbaugh D. G. (1970) Mediastinoscopy. *Arch. Surg.* **100,** 568–573.
12. Audigier J. C., Tuyns A. J. and Lambert R. (1975) Epidemiology of oesophageal cancer in France. *Digestion* **13,** 209–219.
13. Auerbach O., Stout A. P., Hammond E. C. et al. (1965) Histological changes in esophagus in relation to smoking habits. *Arch. Environ. Health* **11,** 4–15.
14. Azzopardi J. G. and Menzies T. (1962) Primary oesophageal adenocarcinoma: confirmation of its existence by the finding of mucous gland tumours. *Brit. J. Surg.* **49,** 497–506.
15. Baskind A. and Marchand P. E. (1978) Discussion of diagnosis in carcinoma of the oesophagus. In: Silber W. (ed.), *Carcinoma of the Oesophagus.* Cape Town, Rotterdam; A. A. Balkema. pp. 211–216.
16. Bergman F. (1959) Cancer of the oesophagus: histological study of development and local spread of 10 cases of squamous cell carcinoma in the lower third of oesophagus. *Acta Chir. Scand.* **117,** 356–365.
17. Bigger I. A. and Vinson P. P. (1950) Carcinoma secondary to burn of the esophagus from ingestion of lye: report of a case. *Surgery* **28,** 887–889.
18. Bishop D., Lushpihan A. and Louis C. (1977) The cytology of carcinoma in situ and early invasive carcinoma of the esophagus. *Acta Cytol.* (*Baltimore*) **21** (2), 298–300.
19. Bradshaw E. and Schonland M. (1969) Oesophageal and lung cancers in Natal African males in relation to certain socio-economic factors: an analysis of 484 interviews. *Brit. J. Cancer* **23,** 275–284.
20. Bradshaw E. and Schonland M. (1974) Smoking, drinking and oesophageal cancer in African males of Johannesburg, South Africa. *Brit. J. Cancer* **30,** 157–163.
21. Burgess H. M., Baggenstoss A. H., Moersch H. J. et al. (1951) Carcinoma of the esophagus; a clinicopathologic study. *Surg. Clin. North Am.* **31,** 965–976.
22. Burrell R. J. W. (1969) Distribution maps of esophageal cancer among Bantu in the Transkei. *J. Natl. Cancer Inst.* **43,** 877–889.
23. Cancer Institute, Chinese Academy of Medical Sciences, Peking; (1975) Surgical treatment of carcinoma of esophagus and gastric cardia. An analysis of 1432 cases. *Chinese Med. J.* **1,** 60–63.
24. Carlyle D. R., Goldstein H. M., Wallace S. et al. (1976) Azygography in the pretreatment evaluation of oesophageal carcinoma. *Brit. J. Radiol.* **49,** 670–677.

25. Case R. A. M. (1961) Mortality from cancer of the oesophagus in England and Wales. In: Tanner N. C. and Smithers D. W. (eds.), *Neoplastic Disease at Various Sites. IV Tumours of the Oesophagus.* Edinburgh, London; Livingstone, pp. 11–25.
26. Clarke C. A., Howel-Evans A. W. and McConnell R. B. (1957) Carcinoma of oesophagus associated with tylosis. *Brit. Med. J.* **1**, 945.
27. Cline M. S. (1971) *Cancer Chemotherapy; Major Problems in Internal Medicine. I.* Philadelphia, London, Toronto; Saunders.
28. Cohen N. N. and Flowers W. (1969) Diagnosis of stenosing lesions of the esophagus using brush cytology. *Gastrointest. Endosc.* **15**, 213–224.
29. Collis J. L. (1971) Surgical treatment of carcinoma of the oesophagus and cardia. *Brit. J. Surg.* **58**, 801–804.
30. Coordinating Group for Research on Etiology of Esophageal Cancer in North China (1975) The epidemiology and etiology of esophageal cancer in North China. *Chin. Med. J.* **1**, 167–183.
31. Coordinating Groups for the Research of Esophageal Carcinoma, Honan Province and Chinese Academy of Medical Sciences (1975) Studies on relationship between epithelial dysplasia and carcinoma of the esophagus. *Chin. Med. J.* **1**, 110–116.
32. Cox R. (1957) The management of dysphagia due to malignant disease of the thoracic and abdominal oesophagus. *Ann. R. Coll. Surg. Engl.* **21**, 133–176.
33. Crummy A. B., Wegner G. P., Flaherty T. T. et al. (1968) Azygos venography. *Ann. Thorac. Surg.* **6**, 522–527.
34. Cummack D. H. (1969) Gastrointestinal X-ray diagnosis; a descriptive at last. Edinburgh, London; Livingstone.
35. Danoff B., Cooper J. and Klein M. (1978) Primary adenocarcinoma of the upper oesophagus. *Clin. Radiol.* **29**, 519–522.
36. Day N. E. (1975) Some aspects of the epidemiology of esophageal cancer. *Cancer Res.* **35**, 3304–3307.
37. Deeley T. J. and Francois P. E. (1958) A technique for the irradiation of the upper oesophagus in megavoltage therapy. *Brit. J. Radiol.* **3**, 395–396.
38. Doctor V. M. and Sirsat M. V. (1967) A histopathological study of pre-operative radiated carcinoma of the esophagus. *Clin. Radiol.* **18**, 422–427.
39. Dodge O. G. (1961) The surgical pathology of gastro-oesophageal carcinoma. *Brit. J. Surg.* **49**, 121–125.
40. Doll R. (1969) The geographical distribution of cancer. *Brit. J. Cancer* **23**, 1–8.
41. Doll R. (1977) The prevention of cancer. *J. R. Coll. Physns. Lond.* **11**, 125–140.
42. Dormanns E. (1939) Das oesophaguscarcinom: Ergebnisse der unter Mitarbeit von 39 pathologischen Instituten Deutschlands durchgeführten Erhebung über das oesophaguscarcinom (1925–1933). *Z. Krebsforsch* **49**, 86–108.
43. Earlam R. J. (1972) Gastrointestinal aspects of Chagas' disease. *Am. J. Dig. Dis.* **17**, 559–571.
44. Edwards D. A. W. (1974) Carcinoma of the oesophagus and fundus. *Postgrad. Med. J.* **50**, 223–226.
45. Ellis F. G. (1960) The natural history of achalasia of the cardia. *Proc R. Soc. Med.* **53**, 663–666.
46. Ellis F. H. Jr., Jackson R. C., Kreuger J. T. et al. (1959) Carcinoma of the esophagus and cardia. Results of treatment. 1946–1956. *N. Engl. J. Med.* **260**, 351–358.
47. Elsebai I. (1971) Cancer of the hypopharynx. UICC Bulletin. *Cancer* **9**, 1–2.
48. Flores A. (1978) Personal Communication.
49. Fu Wai Hospital and Institute for Oncology, Chinese Academy of Medical Sciences, Peking (1967) Combined preoperative irradiation and surgery for carcinoma of the esophagus. *China's Med.* **6**, 473–478.

50. Garrett M. J. (1971) Megavoltage technique for treatment of carcinoma of the post cricoid region. *Clin. Radiol.* **22,** 136–138.
51. Goldstein H. M. and Zornoza J. (1978) Association of squamous cell carcinoma of the head and neck with cancer of the esophagus. *Am. J. Roentgenol. Radium Ther. Nucl. Med.* **131,** 791–794.
52. Goodner J. T. and Turnbull A. D. M. (1971) Bone metastases in cancer of the esophagus. *Am. J. Roentgenol. Radium Ther. Nucl. Med.* **111,** 365–367.
53. Goolden A. W. G. (1957) Radiation cancer. A review with special reference to radiation tumours in the pharynx, larynx and thyroid. *Brit. J. Radiol.* **30,** 626–640.
54. Gowing N. F. C. (1961) The pathology of oesophageal tumours. In: Tanner N. C. and Smithers D. W. (eds.), *Tumours of the Oesophagus.* Edinburgh, London; Livingstone, pp. 91–135.
55. Groves L. K. and Rodríguez-Antúnez A. (1973) Treatment of carcinoma of the esophagus and gastric cardia with concentrated preoperative radiation followed by early operation. *Ann. Thorac. Surg.* **15,** 333–338.
56. Guernsey J. M., Dogget R. L. S., Mason G. R. et al. (1969) Combined treatment of cancer of the esophagus. *Am. J. Surg.* **117,** 157–161.
57. Guernsey J. M. and Knudsen D. F. (1970) Abdominal exploration in the evaluation of patients with carcinoma of the thoracic esophagus. *J. Thorac. Cardiovasc. Surg.* **59,** 62–66.
58. Gunnlaugsson G. H., Wychulis A. R., Roland C. et al. (1970) Analysis of the records of 1657 patients with carcinoma of the esophagus and cardia of the stomach. *Surg. Gynecol. Obstet.* **130,** 997–1005.
59. Haas J. F. and Schottenfeld D. (1978) Epidemiology of esophageal cancer. In: Lipkin M. and Good R. (eds.), *Gastrointestinal Tract Cancer;* pp. 145–172.
60. Hegarty M. M., Angorn I. B., Bryer J. V. et al. (1977a) Pulsion intubation for palliation of carcinoma of the esophagus. *Brit. J. Surg.* **64,** 160–165.
61. Hegarty M. M., Angorn I. B., Bryer J. V. et al. (1977b) Palliation of malignant oesophago-respiratory fistulae by permanent indwelling prosthetic tube. *Ann. Surg.* **185,** 88–91.
62. Hewer T., Rose E., Ghadirian P. et al. (1978) Ingested mutagens from opium and tobacco pyrolysis products and cancer of the oesophagus. *Lancet* **2,** 494–496.
63. Hishon S., Smithies A., Lovell D. et al. (1976) Cytology in the diagnosis of oesophageal cancer. *Lancet* **1,** 296–297.
64. Holub E. and Simecek C. (1968) Pneumomediastinography in carcinoma of the esophagus. *Thorax* **23,** 77–82.
65. Hormozdiari H., Day N. E., Aramesh B. et al. (1975) Dietary factors and esophageal cancer in the Caspian Littoral of Iran. *Cancer Res.* **35,** 3493–3498.
66. Humeau F., Gignoux M., Plombin P. et al. (1975) L'azygographie dans l'étude radiologique des tumeurs malignes de l'oesophage. *J. Radiol. Electrol. Med. Nucl.* **56** (3), 227–234.
67. Ichikawa T. (1969) The clinical effect of bleomycin against squamous cell carcinoma and further developments. Progress of antimicrobial and anticancer chemotherapy. *Proc. 6th Internat. Congr. of Chemotherapy* 1–3.
68. Iran – International Agency for Research on Cancer Study Group (1977) Esophageal cancer studies in the Caspian Littoral of Iran: Results of population studies – a Prodrome. *J. Natl. Cancer Inst.* **59,** 1127–1138.
69. Jacobsson F. (1961) The Paterson-Kelly (Plummer-Vinson) syndrome and carcinoma of the cervical oesophagus. In: Tanner N. C. and Smithers D. W. (eds.), *Neoplastic Disease at Various Sites. IV Tumours of the Oesophagus,* Edinburgh, London; Livingstone, pp. 53–60.
70. Japanese Society for Esophageal Diseases (1976) Guidelines for the clinical and pathological studies on carcinoma of the esophagus. *Jpn. J. Surg.* **6,** 69–86.

71. Kasai M., Mori S. and Watanabe T. (1978) Follow-up results after resection of thoracic esophageal carcinoma. *World J. Surg.* **2,** 543–551.
72. Kelsen D. P., Cvitkovic E., Bains M. et al. (1978) *cis*-Dichlorodiammineplatinum (II) and bleomycin in the treatment of esophageal carcinoma. *Cancer Treat. Rep.* **62,** 1041–1046.
73. Kivirantá U.K. (1952) Corrosion carcinoma of the esophagus: 381 cases of corrosion and nine cases of corrosion carcinoma. *Acta Otolaryngol. (Stockh.)* **42,** 89–95.
74. Koehler R. E., Moss A. A. and Margulis A. R. (1976) Early radiographic manifestations of carcinoma of the esophagus. *Radiology* **119,** 1–5.
75. Kolarić K., Maricic Z., Dujmovic I. et al. (1976) Therapy of advanced esophageal cancer with bleomycin, irradiation and combination of bleomycin with irradiation. *Tumori* **62,** 255–262.
76. Lachapèle A. P., Lagarde C. and Touchard J. (1964) Bilan de sept ans d'expérience de cycloroentgenthérapie du cancer de l'oesophage. *J. Radiol. Electrol. Med. Nucl.* **45,** 732–735.
77. Lane F. W. (1976) The case of irradiation – symposium on cancer of the esophagus. *Hosp. Pract.* October 68–73.
78. Larsson L-G., Sandström A. and Westling P. (1975) Relationship of Plummer-Vinson disease to cancer of the upper alimentary tract in Sweden. *Cancer Res.* **35,** 3308–3316.
79. Leborgne R., Leborgne F. Jr. and Barlocci L. (1963) Cancer of the oesophagus: results of radiotherapy. *Brit. J. Radiol.* **36,** 806–811.
80. LeRoux B. T. (1961) An analysis of seven hundred cases of carcinoma of the hypopharynx, the oesophagus and the proximal stomach. *Thorax* **16,** 226–255.
81. Levy J. I. (1966) The diagnosis of carcinoma of the oesophagus in the plain chest radiograph. *S. Afr. J. Radiol.* **4,** 1–5.
82. Lewinsky B. S., Annes G. P., Mann S. G. (1975) Carcinoma of the esophagus. *Radiol. Clin.* **44,** 192–204.
83. Logan A. (1963) The surgical treatment of carcinoma of the oesophagus and cardia. *J. Thorac. Cardiovasc. Surg.* **46,** 150–161.
84. Logan A. and LeRoux B. T. (1977) Personal communication.
85. Lortat-Jacob J. L., Maillard J. N., Richard C. A. et al. (1968) Primary esophageal adenocarcinoma: Report of 16 cases. *Surgery* **64,** 535–543.
86. McGlashan N. D. (1969) Oesophageal cancer and alcoholic spirits in central Africa. *Gut* **10,** 643–650.
87. McPeak E. and Warren S. (1948) Histologic features of carcinoma of the cardio-esophageal junction and cardia. *Am. J. Pathol.* **24,** 971–999.
88. Marchand P. E. (1978) Diagnosis in carcinoma of the oesophagus. In: Silber W. (ed.), *Carcinoma of the Oesophagus.* Cape Town, Rotterdam; Balkema, pp. 211–216.
89. Marcial V. A., Tomé J. M., Ubiñas J. et al. (1966) Role of radiation therapy in esophageal cancer. *Radiology* **87,** 231–239.
90. Marks R. D., Scruggs H. J. and Wallace K. M. (1976) Preoperative radiation therapy for carcinoma of the esophagus. *Cancer* **38,** 84–89.
91. Martini N., Goodner J. T., D'Angio G. J. et al. (1970) Tracheoesophageal fistula due to cancer. *J. Thorac. Cardiovasc. Surg.* **59,** 319–324.
92. Miller C. (1962) Carcinoma of the thoracic esophagus and cardia: a review of 405 cases. *Brit. J. Surg.* **49,** 507–522.
93. Moss A. A., Koehler R. E. and Margulis A. R. (1976) Initial accuracy of esophagograms in detection of small esophageal carcinoma. *Am. J. Roentgenol. Radium Ther. Nucl. Med.* **127,** 909–913.
94. Murray G. F., Wilcox B. R. and Starek J. K. (1977) The assessment of operability of esophageal carcinoma. *Ann. Thorac. Surg.* **23,** 393–399.

95. Mustard R. A. and Ibberson O. (1956) Carcinoma of the esophagus. A review of 381 cases admitted to Toronto General Hospital 1937–1953 inclusive. *Ann. Surg.* **144,** 927–940.
96. Nakayama K. (1956) Diagnosis of significance of radioactive isotopes in early cancer of alimentary tract, especially esophagus and cardia. *Surgery* **39,** 736.
97. Nakayama K. (1977) Experiences in the treatment of esophageal cancer of the upper and middle thoracic segment. *Surg. Annu.* **9,** 125–132.
98. Nakayama K. and Kinoshita Y. (1974) Surgical treatment combined with preoperative concentrated radiation: esophagus: treatment: cancer of the gastrointestinal tract. *JAMA* **227,** 178–181.
99. Nanson E. M. (1976) Dysphagia: caveat oesophagum. *NZ Med. J.* **83,** 109–111.
100. Nègre E., Pujol H., Gary-Bobo J. et al. (1976) L'irradiation pré-opératoire dans le traitement des cancers de l'oesophage thoracique. *J. Chir. (Paris)* **111,** 403–408.
101. Nelson R. S. and Lanza F. L. (1969) The clinical value of radioactive phosphorous (^{33}P) in the diagnosis of esophageal cancer. *Am. J. Dig. Dis.* **14,** 538–544.
102. Nicks R., Green D. and McClatchie G. (1973) A clinico-pathological study of some factors influencing survival in cancer of the oesophagus: a survey of ten years' experience. *Aust. NZ J. Surg.* **43,** 3–13.
103. Nordenström B. (1972) Paravertebral approach to the posterior mediastinum for mediastinography and needle biopsy. *Acta Radiol.* [*Diagn*] (*Stockh*) **12,** 298–304.
104. Ong G. B. and Kwong K. H. (1970) Management of malignant esophagobronchial fistula. *Surgery* **67,** 293–301.
105. Parker E. F. and Gregorie H. B. (1976) Carcinoma of the esophagus. Long term results. *JAMA* **235,** 1018–1020.
106. Parker E. F., Gregorie H. B., Arrants J. E. et al. (1970) Carcinoma of the esophagus. *Ann. Surg.* **171,** 746–751.
107. Pearson J. G. (1966) Radiotherapy of carcinoma of the oesophagus and postcricoid region in South East Scotland. *Clin. Radiol.* **17,** 242–257.
108. Pearson J. G. (1969) The value of radiotherapy in the management of esophageal cancer. *Am. J. Roentgenol. Radium Ther. Nucl. Med.* **105,** 500–513.
109. Pearson J. G. (1971) The value of radiotherapy in the management of squamous oesophageal cancer. *Brit. J. Surg.* **58,** 794–797.
110. Pearson J. G. (1974) Carcinoma of the oesophagus – operation or radiation. *Langenbecks Arch. Chir.* **337,** 739–743.
111. Pearson J. G. (1977) The present status and future potential of radiotherapy in the management of esophageal cancer. *Cancer* **39,** 882–890.
112. Pearson J. G. and LeRoux B. T. (1974) Malignant tumors of the esophagus. In: *Handbuch der inneren Medizin, Dritter Band/Erster Teil, Fünfte Auflage; Diseases of the Esophagus.* Berlin, Heidelberg, New York; Springer-Verlag, pp. 447–487.
113. Prager G. R. (1973) Vertebral fixation of the oesophagus. A symptom in the posterior mediastinum. *Radiol. Clin. Biol.* **42,** 174–175.
114. Procter D. S. C. (1968) Carcinoma of the oesophagus: a review of 523 cases. *S. Afr. J. Surg.* **6,** 137–169.
115. Prolla J. C. (1973) Histopathology and cytology in detection: esophagus: Cancer of the gastrointestinal tract. *JAMA* **226,** 1554–1556.
116. Prolla J. C., Taebel D. W. and Kirsner J. B. (1965) Current status of exfoliative cytology in diagnoses of malignant neoplasms of the esophagus. *Surg. Gynecol. Obstet.* **121,** 743–752.
117. Putman C. E., Curtis A. M., Westfried M. et al. (1976) Thickening of the posterior tracheal stripe: a sign of squamous cell carcinoma of the esophagus. *Radiology* **121,** 533–536.

118. Rambo V. B., O'Brien P. H., Miller M. C. III. et al. (1975) Carcinoma of the esophagus. *J. Surg. Oncol.* **7**, 355–365.
119. Raphael H. A., Ellis F. H. Jr. and Dockerty M. B. (1966) Primary adenocarcinoma of the esophagus: 18 years review and review of literature. *Ann. Surg.* **164**, 785–796.
120. Richards S. H., Kilby D. and Shaw J. D. (1971) Post-cricoid carcinoma and the Patterson-Kelly syndrome. *J. Laryngol. Otol.* **85**, 141–152.
121. Robertson R., Coy P. and Mokkhavesa S. (1967) The results of radical surgery compared with radical radiotherapy in the treatment of squamous carcinoma of the thoracic esophagus. The case for preoperative radiotherapy. *J. Thorac. Cardiovasc. Surg.* **53**, 430–440.
122. Rubin P. (1974) Comment: Pretreatment laparotomy: esophagus: treatment – localized and advanced: cancer of the gastrointestinal tract. *JAMA* **227**, 184–185.
123. Schoenberg B. S., Bailar III J. C. and Fraumeni J. F. (1971) Certain mortality patterns of esophageal cancer in the United States, 1930–67. *J. Natl. Cancer Inst.* **46**, 63–73.
124. Seymour E. Q. and Pettit H. S. (1973) An evaluation of long term survivors treated for cancer of the esophagus with preoperative X-ray therapy. *Radiology* **106**, 423.
125. Shearman D. J. C., Finlayson N. D. C., Arnott S. J. et al. (1970) Carcinoma of the oesophagus after gastric surgery. *Lancet* **1**, 581–582.
126. Shimkin M. B. (1951) Duration of life in untreated cancer. *Cancer* **4**, 1–8.
127. Shine I. and Allison P. R. (1966) Carcinoma of the oesophagus with tylosis. *Lancet* **1**, 951–953.
128. Smith C. C. K. and Tanner N. C. (1956) The complications of gastroscopy and oesophagoscopy. *Brit. J. Surg.* **43**, 396–403.
129. Smithers D. W. (1956) Adenocarcinoma of the oesophagus. *Thorax* **11**, 257–267.
130. Smithers D. W. (1961) Achalasia and tumours of the oesophagus. In: Tanner N. C. and Smithers D. W. (eds.), *Neoplastic Disease and Various Sites, IV. Tumours of the Oesophagus.* Edinburgh, London; Livingstone, pp. 61–67.
131. Söreide O., Janssen C. W., Kvam G. et al. (1976) Aorto-oesophageal fistula complicating carcinoma of the oesophagus. *Scand. J. Thor. Cardiovasc. Surg.* **10**, 79–84.
132. Steiner P. E. (1956) The etiology and histogenesis of carcinoma of the esophagus. *Cancer* **9**, 436–452.
133. Stephen S. J. and Uragoda C. G. (1970) Some observations of oesophageal carcinoma in Ceylon, including its relationship to betel chewing. *Brit. J. Cancer* **24**, 11–15.
134. Storey C. F. (1962) *Acquired Surgical Lesions of the Esophagus.* Springfield, Illinois; Thomas.
135. Suzuki H., Kobayashi S., Endo M. et al. (1972) Diagnosis of early esophageal cancer. *Surgery* **71**, 99–103.
136. Tanner N. C. (1961) Exfoliative cytological methods in the diagnosis of oesophageal tumours. In: Tanner N. C. and Smithers D. W. (eds.), *Neoplastic Disease at Various Sites. IV, Tumours of the Oesophagus.* Edinburgh, London; Livingstone, pp. 163–167.
137. Turnbull A. D. M. and Goodner J. T. (1970) Primary adenocarcinoma of the esophagus. *Cancer* **22**, 915–918.
138. Turnbull A. D., Rosen P., Goodner J. T. et al. (1973) Primary malignant tumors of the esophagus other than typical epidermoid carcinoma. *Ann. Thorac. Surg.* **15**, 463–473.
139. Tuyns A. J. (1970) Cancer of the oesophagus: further evidence of the relation to drinking habits in France. *Cancer* **5**, 152–156.

140. Tuyns A. J. and Audigier J. C. (1976) Double wave cohort increase for oesophageal and laryngeal cancer in France in relation to reduced alcohol consumption during the second world war. *Digestion* **14**, 197–208.
141. Tuyns A. J. and Massé G. (1975) Cancer of the oesophagus in Brittany: an incidence study in Ille-et-Vilaine. *Int. J. Epidemiol.* **4**, 55–59.
142. Vaeth J. M. (1978) Esophageal carcinoma. In: Gilbert and Kagan (eds.), *Modern Radiation Oncology*. Hagerstown, New York, San Francisco, London; Harper and Row, pp. 357–374.
143. VanTrappen G. and Hellemans J. (1974) Motility disturbances of the esophagus. In: *Handbuch der inneren Medizin Dritter Band/Erster Teil; Diseases of the Esophagus.* Berlin, Heidelberg, New York; Springer-Verlag, pp. 287–354.
144. Vilardell F. (1974) Exfoliative cytology of the esophagus. In: *Handbuch der inneren Medizin Dritter Band Erster Teil, Fünfte Auflage. Diseases of the Esophagus.* Berlin, Heidelberg, New York; Springer-Verlag, pp. 218–234.
145. Voutilainen A. and Koulumies M. (1965) Results of radiation therapy of cancer of the oesophagus. *Ann. Chir. Gynaecol. Fenn.* **54**, 40–51.
146. Wada T., Matsumoto Y. and Amano T. (1969) Chemotherapy of esophageal cancer with bleomycin. Progress in antimicrobial and anticancer chemotherapy. *Proc. 6th Internat. Congr. of Chemotherapy* 41–46.
147. Waterhouse J. A. H. (1974) Cancer handbook of epidemiology and prognosis. Edinburgh, Churchill Livingstone.
148. Werner I. D. (1978a) Pre and post-operative radical therapy for oesophageal carcinoma. In: Silber W. (ed.), *Carcinoma of the Oesophagus.* Cape Town, Rotterdam; A. A. Balkema, pp. 340–345.
149. Werner I. D. (1978b) The palliative management of squamous carcinoma of the intra-thoracic and intra-abdominal oesophagus. In: Silber W. (ed.), *Carcinoma of the Oesophagus.* Cape Town, Rotterdam; A. A. Balkema, 445–448.
150. Werner I. D. Silber W., Madden P. C. W. et al. (1975) Carcinoma of the thoraco-abdominal oesophagus. *S. Afr. Med. J.* **49**, 653–656.
151. Winawer S. J., Sherlock P., Belladonna J. A. et al. (1975) Endoscopic brush cytology in esophageal cancer. *JAMA* **232**, 1358.
152. Winder E. L. and Mabuchi K. (1973) Cancer of the gastrointestinal tract – esophagus: detection and diagnosis – etiological and environmental factors. *JAMA* **226**, 1546–1548.
153. Wiot J. F. and Felson B. (1973) Radiographic differential diagnosis – cancer of the gastrointestinal tract – esophagus. *JAMA* **226**, 1548–1552.
154. Witzel L., Halter F., Gretillat P. A. et al. (1976) Evaluation of specific value of endoscopic biopsies and brush cytology for malignancies of the oesophagus and stomach. *Gut* **17**, 375–377.
155. Wright J. T. and Richardson P. C. (1967) Squamous carcinoma of the thoracic oesophagus in malabsorption syndrome. *Brit. Med. J.* **1**, 540–542.
156. Yamada A., Kobayashi S., Kawai B. et al. (1972) Study on X-ray findings of early oesophageal cancer. *Australas. Radiol.* **16**, 238–246.
157. Yamashita H., Okura J., Yoshioka T. et al. (1972) Preoperative irradiation in treatment of carcinoma of the oesophagus. *Australas. Radiol.* **16**, 250–257.
158. Younghusband J. D. and Aluwihare A. P. R. (1970) Carcinoma of the oesophagus: factors influencing survival. *Brit. J. Surg.* **57**, 422–430.

E. M. Nordman and A. H. Rekonen

5 The Diagnosis of Brain Tumour Recurrences

INTRODUCTION

The diagnosis of recurrent brain tumours after surgical and/or radiation treatment causes difficulties in clinical work although there are several examination methods available: electroencephalography, angiography, pneumoencephalography, radioisotope scintigraphy and computerized tomography (CT). After surgery, for example, the cavity formed in the tumour area by operation affords space for the regrowing tumour [29] and the clinical symptoms remain dormant often for several months. On the other hand, for several weeks after radiotherapy the patient often presents the same cerebral symptoms as before treatment. Pneumoencephalography, too, may be misleading for a long time after operation in spite of regrowth of the tumour. The demonstration of a recurrent glioma by means of angiography is often delayed because the vascularity of the recurrence may be insignificant if compared with the primary tumour, as Winkelman and Deckar [29] pointed out. Nor is angiography suitable for regular follow-up. The clinical and neuroradiological diagnosis of recurrent brain tumour is cumbersome and the electroencephalographic findings are confusing because of the effects of the operation of the registered curves [3]. Radioisotope scintigraphy has been recommended for the follow-up of brain tumours after treatment [4, 25, 26]. The nuclear methods are less strenuous for the patient than the neuroradiological examinations.

In the diagnosis of both primary and metastatic brain tumours, Harper et al. [7] and Witcofski et al. [30] reported that brain scintigraphy has a definite position. Schneider et al. [24], using $^{99}Tc^{m}$-pertechnetate, reported that 80–90 per cent of brain tumours were visualized. However, the status of scintigraphy for recurrent tumours differs from the scanning of the untreated primary tumours. The treatment itself, radiotherapy or operation, causes a long-lasting effect in the area and the radionuclide uptake of the recurrent tumour may be weaker than in the untreated lesion.

In recent years computerized tomography has offered new possibilities in brain tumour diagnosis as well as in the early diagnosis of recurrences [20].

BRAIN SCINTIGRAPHY AFTER SURGERY

There are several factors which affect the uptake of a radionuclide after surgical treatment:

1. The blood/brain barrier after surgery is disturbed and a postoperative accumulation is seen in the operation area usually for about 2 months [19] but possibly up to 6 months [9] after operation.
2. The vascularity of the operation area is often increased immediately after the operation.
3. The defect in the skull caused by the operation diminishes the bony attenuation of radiation and increases the counts by about 13–16 per cent in the area of the defect [18].

BRAIN SCINTIGRAPHY AFTER RADIOTHERAPY

The accumulation of the isotope is affected by both surgical treatment and radiation treatment. Irradiation alone produces oedema in the irradiated area; this may be increased if there has been previous surgical intervention. Mallard [12] noted that 'after radiotherapy large areas of generally increased background were observed with ^{99}Tcm.' Wende [27] mentions that after radiotherapy some of the isotope remains in the brain.

In the series of Nordman and Holsti [15] 37 per cent of the patients with brain tumours treated by radiotherapy and 48 per cent of patients treated by a combination of surgery and irradiation survived for 2 years or more. The corresponding figures after 5 years were 24 per cent and 31 per cent. As the diagnosis of recurrent tumour in the brain leads to a new operation or in selected cases to a further course of radiation treatment [3] or chemotherapy given over a period of several months or years, the accurate diagnosis of a regrowth is important.

The prognosis of re-irradiated recurrent tumours in the brain is not unfavourable; 24 per cent of 25 patients were living for two years after treatment [15].

METHODS IN SCINTIGRAPHY

The formerly popular radiopharmaceuticals ^{203}Hg-Neohydrin and ^{131}I-serum-albumin have been out of use for many years. Technetium ^{99}Tcm, with its short half-life of 6 hours and optimal gamma-radiation energy of 140 keV for gamma camera imaging, is the isotope currently in routine use. It is given usually in the form of the pertechnetate and has a fairly high accuracy in brain tumour detection. The uptake of pertechnetate is based on its passive transport through the blood/brain barrier into the pathological lesion, but newer ^{99}Tcm radiopharmaceuticals seem to have an active take-up tendency. The most favourable results have been obtained with ^{99}Tcm-DTPA and ^{99}Tcm-glucoheptonate [11, 23]. With these agents a higher accuracy in scintigraphy of primary brain tumours and especially of cerebral metastases has been achieved. However, we have not seen any reports concerning the examination of recurrent brain tumours with DTPA or glucoheptonate.

The conventional brain scintigraphy is performed by taking pictures from 30 to 60 minutes after the injection of 10–20 mCi of ^{99}Tcm-pertechnetate, but a higher target to non-target ratio can be achieved if delayed pictures are taken 3–4 hours after the injection [22]. Nuclear angiography can also aid in the detection of recurrences and further vascular concepts can be studied with regional blood flow measurements.

In nearly all radionuclide centres a scintillation camera of the Anger type is in use. Its resolution is at present 4–6 mm and it is unlikely that there will be future major improvements in the images obtained from such apparatus. Computer-linked gamma camera systems make it possible to make quantitative measurements of the activity in the tumour and they may be of considerable use in follow-up studies, avoiding subjective estimations of the take-up pictures.

FOLLOW-UP STUDY OF PATIENTS WITH CEREBRAL TUMOUR

Thirty-one patients with brain tumours were examined with ^{99}Tcm-pertechnetate scintigraphy before and immediately after radiotherapy [17]. The results are shown in Table 5.1. In 12 cases a total or subtotal resection of the tumour was performed; in six inoperable cases a biopsy only was performed. Fifteen of the patients had a gliomatous tumour, two had other primary brain tumours, four had metastases of a histologically verified primary carcinoma, one a metastasis of unknown origin and nine had only a neuroradiological confirmation of the tumour. The radiotherapy was delivered with a ^{60}Co teletherapy unit to a dose of 5000–5500 rad in 6–8 weeks according to an individual treatment plan. Eighteen patients had further scintigraphy of the brain 3 months after the irradiation, 14 patients after 6 months, and 13 after 12 months. The examination was performed after an injection of 10 mCi ^{99}Tcm-pertechnetate and the pictures made with a Pho Gamma gamma camera.

In 18 of the 31 patients (58 per cent) the pertechnetate accumulation increased immediately after radiotherapy in the tumour area, in 7 (23 per cent) the uptake was unchanged, and in 6 (19 per cent) it diminished after treatment (*see* Table 5.1). It is remarkable that in 8 of the 18 patients examined at 3 mth the pertechnetate accumulation was unchanged, in one patient the uptake had increased, and in 9 patients decreased as compared with the previous scintigraphy. At this time, all of the 18 patients examined had some uptake of the isotope and none of the patients had symptoms suggesting recurrence of the growth.

At 6 months after therapy 11 out of 14 patients still revealed an uptake in the tumour area, in only 1 case had the uptake disappeared. One patient demonstrated symptoms of recurrent cerebral tumour, the other patients being well.

At 12 months 2 patients out of the 13 examined showed no uptake in the area, 4 of the group developed a recurrent tumour. The mean diameter of the uptake before and immediately after irradiation was measured. The

Table 5.1. Results of $^{99}Tc^m$-Pertechnetate Scintigraphy after Irradiation. Changes in the Accumulation Areas Compared with the Previous Scintigraphy. Of the 6 Cases Marked with an Asterisk, 5 had Recurrences.

After irradiation	*Increased*	*Unchanged*	*Diminished*	*Disappeared*
Immediately	18	7	6	0
(31 patients)	25/31 = 81%		= 19%	
3 mth	1	8	9	0
(18 patients)				
6 mth	2*	7	2	1
(14 patients)				
12 mth	4*	6	1	2
(13 patients)				

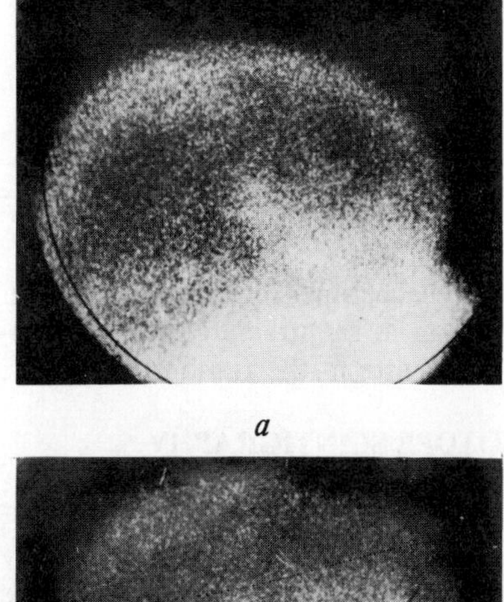

a

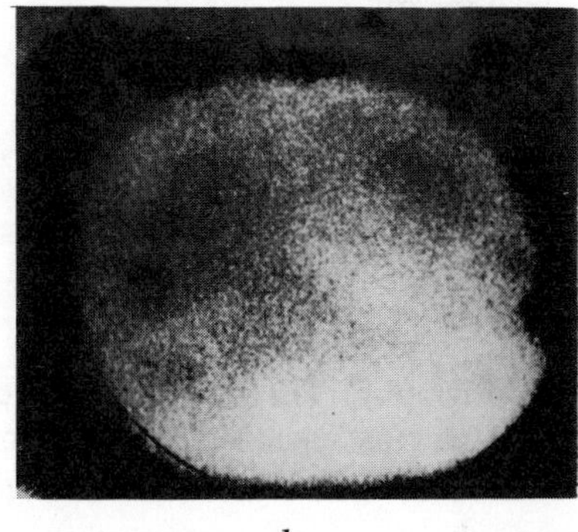

b

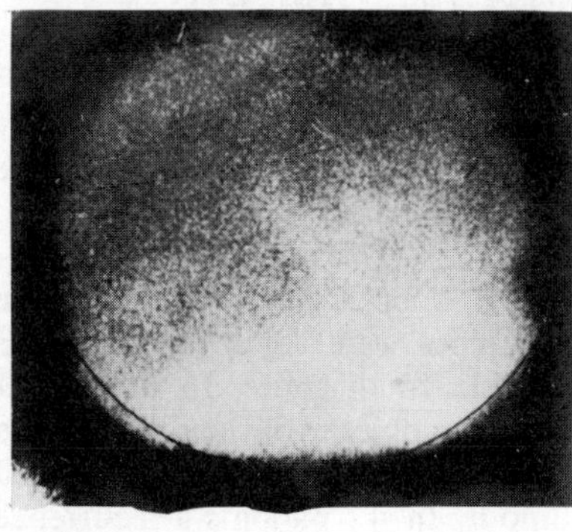

c

Fig. 5.1. a, Patient with a partially operated glioblastoma multiforme before the start of radiation treatment. *b,* At the end of radiotherapy with a dose of 5500 rad an enlarged and intensified accumulation of the isotope in the tumour area is seen. *c,* The uptake has diminished 6 mth after treatment, the patient being quite well.

diameter before irradiation was 5·5 ± 1·5 cm and after therapy 5·9 ± 1·6 cm. An illustrative case is presented in *Fig. 5.1.*

In a recent study [13] examination with $^{99}Tc^m$-citrate after radiotherapy demonstrated an accumulation persisting for at least three months in more than half of the patients.

In an investigation of a tumour-specific radiopharmaceutical, ^{75}Se-sodium selenite, the findings were adverse (Table 5.2). In 16 of the 25 patients scanned before and immediately after irradiation the uptake disappeared, and in 3 patients was diminished; in 6 patients the accumulation of ^{75}Se-selenite was unchanged. Three months after treatment only 1 patient out of 14 had an uptake, and after 6 months not a single patient. Twelve months after therapy one case with recurrence revealed positive

Table 5.2. Results of ^{75}Se-Sodium Selenite Scintigraphy after Irradiation. The Accumulation Areas are Compared with Previous Scintigraphy. One Case, Marked with an Asterisk, had a Recurrence.

After irradiation	*Increased*	*Unchanged*	*Diminished*	*Disappeared*
Immediately	0	6	3	16
(25 patients)		= 24%	19/25 = 76%	
3 mth	0	1	0	13
(14 patients)				
6 mth	0	0	0	7
(7 patients)				
12 mth	1*	0	0	3
(4 patients)				

scintigraphy. The decrease of the selenite accumulation may depend on the fact that irradiation causes an alteration in the irradiated tumour proteins thus affecting the binding of ^{75}Se-selenite in the tumour area [16].

ACCURACY OF RADIOISOTOPE SCINTIGRAPHY IN DIAGNOSIS OF RECURRENCES

Although an accumulation persists in the operation or radiotherapy area of brain tumour patients, the diagnosis of a recurrence is possible only by repeated examination. During follow-up, an increasing accumulation in the cerebral scintigraphy seems to be evidence of a recurrent tumour, as shown in *Fig. 5.2.*

In the material of Kuba et al. [9] 98 brain tumour patients were followed up after operation. All scintigraphies were abnormal 6 months after the operation. The authors were able to diagnose 36 of the 37 recurrences by comparing the follow-up scintigraphies with the preoperative scan. The false positive rate was 32 per cent. Grosch et al. (1975) studied 102 patients operated on for brain tumour. In 42 patients a recurrence developed and 38 (86 per cent) of these were positive. Thirty-one (80 per cent) were correctly diagnosed by angiography. Recurrence after operation was also studied by Schwarz et al. [25]. Of the 45 patients with recurrent tumours 89 per cent were correctly diagnosed by scintigraphy and 95 per cent by angiography.

In all the studies reported repeated examinations were performed and the importance of the comparison of follow-up scintigraphies with pre-operative or pre-irradiation scans was emphasized. Because of a persisting accumulation of isotope resulting from the treatment the number of false positive findings may be high.

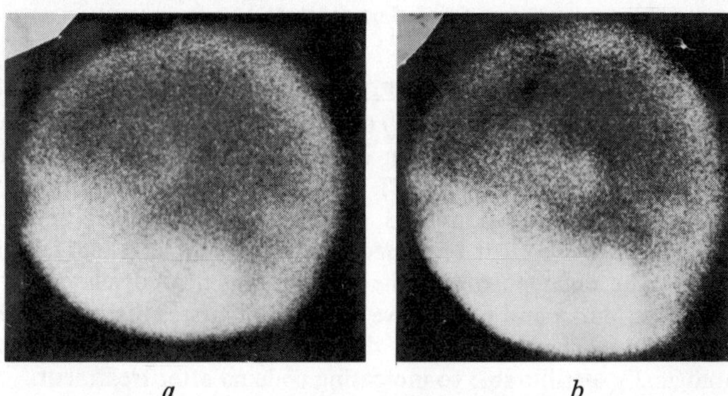

Fig. 5.2. a, Astrocytoma malignum treated with irradiation to a dose of 5230 rad. The gamma picture is taken 1 mth after treatment. *b,* The scintigraphy 10 mth later reveals an enhanced accumulation of the isotope at the site of the tumour. The patient had symptoms of recurrent brain tumour and died 2 wk later.

TRANSIENT ENCEPHALOPATHY AFTER RADIOTHERAPY

Boldrey and Sheline [1] described a deterioration in the clinical status of the patient irradiated for a brain tumour. Three to six weeks after the end of treatment the patient often presents the same cerebral symptoms as originally complained of before treatment. Even palsies and diminished vision may occur. This condition is temporary and most often disappears after some weeks. The enlargement or intensification of the pertechnetate accumulation in the treated area coincides with this delayed radiation reaction, also observed by Wilson et al. [28]. In fact, an incorrect diagnosis of a recurrent brain tumour is often made. This phenomenon is probably due to radiation-induced oedema in the tumour area. No similar oedema has been reported where normal brain tissue is incidentally irradiated in the treatment of a tumour lying outside the brain.

In the irradiation of a mouse cerebral lymphoma Potchen et al. [21] demonstrated an increase of 200 per cent in the capillary permeability of the tumour tissue, the increase in the muscle tissue being only 80 per cent. According to Boldrey and Sheline [1], if a craniotomy is performed at this time abundant oedema of the brain tissues is found.

The regression of a brain tumour after irradiation may take several months as Marks and Gado [14] have pointed out. It would be of interest to find a radiopharmaceutical which would be reliable in the evaluation of an irradiated brain tumour. ^{75}Se-selenite is not recommended for routine use because of the high dose given to the liver and kidney [10]. In addition, the picture quality with ^{75}Se is poor because of the low pulse statistics (about 25 000 counts/picture). The cyclotron-produced ^{73}Se-selenite is under investigation at present [6] but its possible value in diagnosing tumour recurrences remains to be demonstrated.

COMPUTERIZED TOMOGRAPHY

The computerized tomography (CT) of brain tumours has evoked considerable interest. According to Hyman et al. [8] the tumour may appear to enlarge after radiotherapy in the CT picture. In Hyman's report out of 25 irradiated patients the lesion in 3 (8 per cent) was larger than before treatment, in 39 per cent it remained unchanged and in 53 per cent it was diminished. The enlargement of the tumour was not correlated with the clinical status. Marks and Gado have shown similar results in the CT scan after irradiation. They point out that the increase in the lesion size is morphologically attributable to increasing oedema after treatment.

Pendergrass et al. [20] compared computed tomography and radioisotope scintigraphy in brain studies of 538 patients. Their series included 97 patients with neoplasms, 23 of these being recurrent tumours; positive CT scan was obtained in all 23 cases. Only 11 positive findings were found in brain scintigraphy. The results of this study appear to have been based on single studies without follow-up investigations. In the report by Christie et al. [2] of 657 patients with intracranial disease six recurrent brain tumours were detected; all these patients were correctly diagnosed both by computed tomography and by scintigraphy.

Computed tomography seems to be a fairly reliable method in the diagnosis of recurrent brain tumours, affording more detailed information than does radioisotope scintigraphy. However, CT scanners are not available in all centres and in addition the studies are rather expensive for regular follow-up.

SUMMARY AND CONCLUSIONS

Reliable diagnostic tests for recurrent brain tumours are difficult to present. Angiography in the follow-up of brain tumours may be exacting for both the patient and hospital staff. As the delayed reaction to radiation coincides with an enlarged area of uptake of ^{99}Tc^{m}-pertechnetate and with an enhanced density of the tumour area in the CT scan, the diagnosis of a recurrence is based chiefly upon the clinical neurological status of the patient during the first six months after surgical and/or radiation treatment. If a tumour specific radiopharmaceutical could be found in the future, the differential diagnosis of the accumulation in the tumour area would be easier.

At present, as the ^{99}Tc^{m} accumulation persists during the follow-up, it is pertinent to perform the examinations with isotopes or CT scan both before and at the end of the treatment in order to make comparisons with the subsequent examinations.

REFERENCES

1. Boldrey E. and Sheline G. (1966) Delayed transitory clinical manifestations after radiation treatment of intracranial tumours. *Acta Radiol.* **5**, 5–10.
2. Christie J. H., Mori H., Go R. T. et al. (1976) Computed tomography and radionuclide studies in the diagnosis of intracranial disease. *Am. J. Roentgenol. Ther. Nucl. Med.* **127**, 171–174.
3. Deeley T. J. (1974) The treatment of recurrent tumours. In: Deeley T. J. (ed.), *Modern Radiotherapy and Oncology. Central Nervous System Tumours.* London, Butterworths, pp. 264–269.
4. Flipse R. C., Vuksanovic M. and Fonts E. A. (1968) Sequential brain scanning in radiation therapy of malignant tumors of the brain. *Am. J. Roentgenol. Ther. Nucl. Med.* **102**, 93–96.
5. Grosch G., Borchard U., Deckart H. et al. (1975) Hirnszintigraphische Dispensaire in der Früherfassung vor Rezidivtumoren. *Radiobiol. Radiother.* **16**, 795–802.
6. Guillaume M. (1978) Personal communication.
7. Harper P. V., Lathrop K. A., McCardle R. J. et al. (1964) The Use of Technetium-99m as a Clinical Scanning Agent for Thyroid, Liver and Brain. In *Medical Radioiosotope Scanning Vol. 2.* Vienna, IAEA, pp. 33–45.
8. Hyman R. A., Loring M. F., Liebeskind A. L. et al. (1978) Computed tomographic evaluation of therapeutically induced changes in primary and secondary brain tumors. *Neuroradiology* **14**, 213–218.
9. Kuba J., Koutný V. and Klaus E. (1972) Hirnszintigramm in der Diagnostik von Rezidiven intrakranieller Raumforderungen. *Fortschr. Geb. Röntgenstr. Nuklearmed.* **117**, 179–186.
10. Kuikka J. and Nordman E. (1978) Measurement of ^{75}Se-sodium selenite in the human body. *Int. J. Nucl. Med. Biol.* **5**, 30–34.
11. Léveillé J., Pison C., Karakand Y. et al. (1977) Technetium-99m glucoheptonate in brain-tumor detection: an important advance in radiotracer techniques. *J. Nucl. Med.* **18**, 957–961.
12. Mallard J. R. (1971) In: Belcher E. H. and Vetter H. (eds.), *Radioisotopes in Medical Diagnosis.* London, Butterworths, p. 681.
13. Mäntylä M., Rekonen A. and Nordman E. (19) Value of ^{99}Tc^{m}-citrate in diagnosis of brain tumours. Personal communication.
14. Marks J. E. and Gado M. (1977) Serial computed tomography of primary brain tumors following surgery, irradiation and chemotherapy. *Radiology* **125**, 119–125.
15. Nordman E. and Holsti L. (1973) Roentgen and telecobalt therapy of tumors of the brain. *Radiol. Clin. Biol.* **42**, 199–211.
16. Nordman E., Jászági-Nagy E. and Rekonen A. (1976) Changes in tumour cell selenite (^{75}Se) affinity due to irradiation. *Ann. Clin. Res.* **8**, 43–47.
17. Nordman E. and Rekonen A. (1975) Interpretation of ^{99m}Tc-pertechnetate scintigraphy after irradiation of brain tumours. *Int. J. Nucl. Med. Biol.* **2**, 25–29.
18. Oldendorf W. H. and Iisaka Y. (1969) Interference of scalp and skull with external measurements of brain isotope content: Part 2. Absorption by skull of gamma radiation originating in brain. *J. Nucl. Med.* **10**, 184–187.
19. Otto H.-J., Koch R. D., Abraham U. et al. (1974) Ergebnisse nuklear-medizinischer und elektroencephalographischer Verlaufuntersuchungen nach Hirntumoroperationen. *Radiol. Diagn. (Berl.)* **1**, 47–66.
20. Pendergrass H. P., McKusick K. A., New P. J. F. et al. (1975) Relative efficacy of radionuclide imaging and computed tomography of the brain. *Radiology* **116**, 363–366.

21. Potchen E. J., Kinzie J., Curtis C. et al. (1972) Effect of irradiation on tumor microvascular permeability to macromolecules. *Cancer* **30**, 636–642.
22. Ramsay R. and Quinn J. L. III (1972) Comparison of the accuracy of initial and delayed ^{99m}Tc pertechnetate brain scan. *J. Nucl. Med.* **13**, 131–134.
23. Ryeson T. W., Spies S. M., Singh N. B. et al (1978) A quantitative clinical comparison of three ^{99m}Technetium labelled brain imaging radiopharmaceuticals. *Radiology* **127**, 429–432.
24. Schneider C., Prevot H. and Tzonos T. (1968) Szintigraphie mit ^{203}Hg und ^{99m}Tc in der Diagnostik von Hirntumoren. *Dtsch. Med. Wochenschr.* **93**, 285–290.
25. Schwarz G., Schreyer H. and Argyropoulos G. (1976) Radiology for detecting brain tumor recurrences. *Acta Radiol.* [*Diagn.*] (*Stockh.*) **17**, 193–199.
26. Voutilainen A. (1974) Scanning after irradiation. In: Deeley T. J. (ed.), *Modern Radiotherapy and Oncology. Central Nervous System Tumours.* London, Butterworths, pp. 292–310.
27. Wende S. (1966) Verlaufsuntersuchungen bei Hirntumoren mit radioaktiven Isotopen. *Acta Radiol.* [*Diagn.*] (*Stockh.*) **5**, 928–935.
28. Wilson C. B., Grafts D. and Levin V. (1977) Brain Tumors: Criteria of Response and Definition of Recurrency. In: *Modern Concepts in Brain Tumour Therapy.* National Cancer Institute Monograph No. 46; December 1977, 197–203.
29. Winkelmann H. and Deckart H. (1973) Die Bedeutung der Hirnszintigraphie bei Rezidivtumoren. *Radiol. Diagn.* (*Berl.*) **1**, 95–99.
30. Witcofski R. L., Maynard C. D. and Roper T. J. (1967) A comparative analysis of the accuracy of the Technetium-99m pertechnetate brain scan: follow-up of 1000 patients. *J. Nucl. Med.* **8**, 187–196.

Stanley Dische

6 Hypoxic Cell Sensitizers in Clinical Radiotherapy

INTRODUCTION

In the treatment of malignant disease by radiotherapy there is a variable pattern of success and failure. Failure when it occurs may be due to re-growth of tumour in the primary site and or in the lymphatic drainage included in the original field of treatment, or it may occur at a distant site. In the latter situation we must look to methods for the successful eradication of distant metastases in an early stage by regimens of cytotoxic chemotherapy.

When failure occurs within the volume irradiated we must try to determine the reason. In some cases tumour is obviously recurring at the margin of the area irradiated and the volume chosen for treatment was inadequate. In an occasional case it is possible to find that recurrence has occurred in a low dose region present because the original plan was inadequate, or due to difficulties in its daily reproduction through the course of therapy. In a number of cases the original plan of treatment as regards total dose, fractionation and overall time was not achieved, most commonly due to troublesome local tissue reactions which caused interruption in the course of treatment. In some instances failure is related to a low planned dose which had been decided because of the close proximity of a highly radiosensitive structure such as the spinal cord or kidney while in other cases the large volume to be irradiated also necessitated a reduction in dose in order to prevent an undue level of morbidity.

In most cases of local failure, however, it is not possible to implicate any of these reasons, and one has to conclude that despite the achievement of the original plan of therapy viable tumour cells remained. We can add that local tumour failure is more commonly seen with larger than with smaller tumours, in well-differentiated as opposed to poorly-differentiated tumours and with sarcomas and with adenocarcinomas compared with squamous carcinomas.

The history of radiotherapy includes many attempts to increase the rate of local cure. Simple elevation of dose may give us an improved cure rate but only at the expense of an increasingly high morbidity and mortality due to radiotherapy. The protracted fractionation of radiotherapy has been found to improve the therapeutic ratio, i.e. the chance of local cure compared with the chance of normal tissue damage. The benefit to be obtained by extending fractionation beyond 10 or 15 remains controversial. There is now some evidence that with a fewer number of fractions there may be some increase in the incidence of late damage compared with tumour control and early morbidity [30, 87]. The addition of cytotoxic agents and hyperthermia are among the methods more recently introduced [17]. Unfortunately an increase in normal tissue reactions is associated with the use of these techniques and a true improvement in the therapeutic ratio has yet to be proved in randomized controlled clinical trials. It is generally true that most of the methods introduced into radiotherapy in order to increase local cure have led to some increase in morbidity.

The importance of the curve relating oxygen tension and radiosensitivity to clinical radiotherapy was first established by L. H. Gray [46]. Under conditions of hypoxia it may be necessary to multiply the dose required for a biological effect under fully oxic conditions by a factor of three in order to achieve it. Thomlinson and Gray [75] suggested that most malignant tumours seen in clinical practice contain hypoxic cells which might therefore be protected from radiation injury. As most normal tissues contain few, if any, hypoxic cells a method for enhancing the radiosensitivity of resistant hypoxic cells does give the possibility of an enhancing effect upon tumour without significant enhancement in normal tissues. This chapter is concerned with the methods which have been proposed to improve the results of radiotherapy by restoring the radiosensitivity of hypoxic skin.

METHODS TO OVERCOME THE RADIORESISTANCE OF HYPOXIC CELLS

The Fractionation of Radiotherapy

By careful clinical observation the early workers in radiotherapy found that the therapeutic ratio could be improved by extending the number of occasions on which radiotherapy was given. Thomlinson [73] was the first to show in the laboratory that a benefit of fractionation was the reoxygenation of hypoxic cells in tumours during the course of radiotherapy. As tumour cells die after doses of radiation given earlier in the course the demand for oxygen is reduced and as the tumours begin to shrink the flow and distribution of blood is improved. A proportion of the cells which were hypoxic become oxygenated and thus more sensitive to the radiation given in the next treatment. The use of the best fractionation regimen can, in animals, lead to significant improvement in local control. However, the problems involved in optimizing fractionation to facilitate re-oxygenation in clinical radiotherapy are enormous because of the widely varying characteristics of human tumours. There is, at this time, no means of deciding the optimum fractionation for any individual case.

The Use of Densely Ionizing Radiation

When cells are irradiated with densely ionizing radiation such as neutrons and π-mesons the magnitude of the oxygen effect decreases. In effect a greater dose can be expected to be delivered to hypoxic tumour cells without a proportional increase of damage to normal tissue. Clinical trials of fast neutron therapy are underway and trials with negative π-mesons have now commenced. Particularly difficult problems must be overcome in order to make effective use of densely ionizing radiation. The machinery remains expensive and it is still difficult to deliver effective and homogenous dosage to a planned tumour volume. Although the effect upon hypoxic cells is improved the resistance is not entirely eliminated. Because of the differences in relative biological efficiency in different tissues it is difficult to compare the normal tissue effects with those achieved with photons and, therefore, to precisely determine any alteration in the therapeutic ratio. Because of these problems it is unlikely that densely ionizing radiation will be widely available, at least not for a number of years to come [64].

Hyperbaric Oxygen and Chemical Sensitizing Agents

These two methods will be considered in detail below.

HYPERBARIC OXYGEN

Development and Technique

In the original description by Gray et al. [46] of the importance of hypoxia as a cause of radiation failure, Scott contributed the results of an experiment in a mouse tumour system which clearly showed an improved

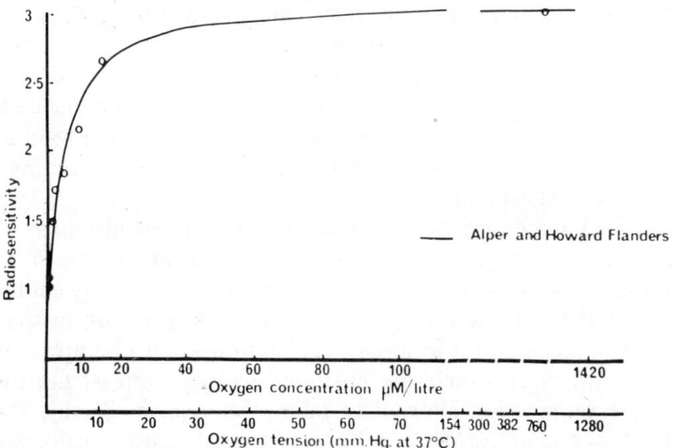

Fig. 6.1. The relationship between oxygen concentration and radiosensitivity. (Prepared by R. H. Thomlinson from T. Alper and P. Howard–Flanders, 1957, *Nature, Lond.* 178, 978.)

tumour control with radiotherapy using hyperbaric oxygen compared with treatment under normal conditions. By raising the oxygen tension throughout all tumour and normal tissues to a high concentration in the upper almost horizontal portion of the curve similar sensitization by oxygen is reached (*Fig. 6.1*).

The hyperbaric oxygen chamber was shortly afterwards introduced into clinical radiotherapy by Churchill-Davidson and his colleagues at St Thomas's Hospital, London. In 1955 in the first publication of clinical work the technique was described and also the result achieved in 8 patients where, using single doses of radiation, half the tumour was treated in the normal fashion and half using hyperbaric oxygen [22]. In 7 of the 8 patients there was histological evidence of increased effect when the tumour was biopsied or removed shortly afterwards. In the remaining case there was so much radiation change that no comparison was possible. Churchill-Davidson went on to explore the use of hyperbaric oxygen in fractionated radiotherapy increasing the number of treatments finally to 6 [21]. Soon other radiotherapy centres were using hyperbaric oxygen to treat patients and there were reports of improved results with tumours at various sites [6, 11, 60, 84].

The original hyperbaric chamber was a modified naval compression chamber and using orthovoltage radiation the whole technique was extremely cumbersome. Improvements in the method followed, the greatest advance being the introduction of the Vickers chamber which incorporated a transparent perspex wall. With this chamber patients could be compressed to 3 atmospheres absolute without use of general anaesthesia [37]. Daily treatment and conventional dose fractionation became possible.

Pressure is gradually raised to 3 atmospheres absolute over a period of 5–10 min. The rise in pressure may cause pain and discomfort in the ears due to inadequate equalization of pressure through the eustachian tubes. Although in some centres this problem is prevented by routine myringotomy with the introduction of polythene grommets under local anaesthesia for treatment, in most it was found using a slow rise in pressure, particularly at the time of the first treatment: problems were minimized and grommets rarely required.

After the chamber pressure reaches 3 atmospheres absolute 15 min is allowed before radiotherapy so that oxygen tension can rise in the deep areas of the tumour. The chamber is wheeled beneath the radiotherapy machine and the patient set up for treatment. Absorption in the wall of the chamber is allowed for in dosage calculation. Radiotherapy commonly takes 5–10 min after which the chamber is moved out of the treatment room and decompression allowed to take place over 5–8 min. The whole procedure takes approximately 40 min. At some centres a doctor and at least two radiographers or technicians are present throughout; in other centres a nurse or radiographer manages the patient in the chamber with the aid of a technician, medical staff remaining on call.

Oxygen toxicity, as manifested by oxygen convulsions will occur in 2–3 per cent of the patients submitted to hyperbaric oxygen treatment. Although some patients are aware that a convulsion has taken place most have little or no recollection and a full recovery is invariable. Some patients will continue their treatment in hyperbaric oxygen although there remains an increased chance of a further convulsion taking place, while others decline further treatment in the chamber. Some patients, particularly those with a history of claustrophobia, refuse to enter the chamber either from the very beginning or after the first treatment. Even when much encouragement is given the patients, 10 per cent of those selected for this treatment may refuse or default.

Stringent precautions against the risk of fire in the chamber and careful maintenance of machinery is essential to prevent risk of explosive decompression. This latter accident is recorded with one American designed chamber when the patient was unharmed but the radiotherapist sustained minor injuries. To date there is no record of these two events occurring with use of the standard Vickers hyperbaric oxygen chamber.

Because each treatment using the hyperbaric oxygen chamber is a considerable procedure there is a natural desire to keep the number of treatments to a small number. Churchill-Davidson in establishing the technique started with 1 and finally settled on 6 treatments as constituting a course and Van den Brenk followed a similar progression to 6, to what he also felt was an optimum number [10, 21]. With use of the Vickers chamber and the giving of treatment without anaesthesia it was possible to treat patients as many as 40 times in a course of radiotherapy so simulating their standard treatment in air [14]. Other centres, however, using the Vickers chamber felt that even without anaesthesia treatment in hyperbaric oxygen presented a considerable stress upon the patient and upon the radiotherapy centre and the number of treatments in hyperbaric oxygen should be reduced below those normally employed.

Although a number of centres established facilities for use of hyperbaric oxygen in the early years only a limited number of prospective controlled trials were established. There was the comparative study performed by Churchill-Davidson and his colleagues at the beginning of their work and report on the short term responses in carcinoma of bladder and head and neck tumours by Van den Brenk [21], but the favourable view was based upon consecutively treated cases compared with those managed before the introduction of hyperbaric oxygen. The benefit of hyperbaric oxygen was considered unproven by most radiotherapists who felt that, although the initial results were promising, the complex, expensive and potentially hazardous technique should not be established widely until there was conclusive evidence as to its value. Some who had taken up the method with enthusiasm and reported their initial experience favourably later recorded their disillusionment [82, 85].

It also became evident that there were increased effects in normal tissue especially the larynx but also the spinal cord and the gastrointestinal tract [12, 13, 21, 24, 27]. This increment in normal tissue effect had to be balanced against the improvement in tumour control. This was obviously a situation where only randomized controlled long term clinical trials could lead to a definitive answer as to the value of hyperbaric oxygen.

The Medical Research Council's Steering Committee on the Evaluation of Different Methods of Cancer Therapy established a working party concerned with hyperbaric oxygen and radiotherapy in 1962, under the chairmanship of Sir Hedley Atkins and later Sir Brian Windeyer. The majority of the randomized controlled clinical trials which have now been recorded were performed under the aegis of this body. Until 1971 the working party acted mainly to co-ordinate the studies in different centres and only a limited standardization of protocol was agreed between the centres. The most stringent criteria agreed was that similar treatment should be given to patients randomized to oxygen as those to air. The head and neck, the bronchus, the uterine cervix and the bladder were all regarded as sites of carcinoma suitable for clinical trials.

In 1971 when the first set of trials were reaching initial evaluation it was agreed that the use of similar treatments for oxygen and air cases was not necessarily the best way to test the efficacy of hyperbaric oxygen. A further series of trials was established when the dose and fractionation regimen considered best in air was to be assessed against that thought to be best in hyperbaric oxygen. At this time it became possible for centres to agree upon a much stricter standardization of treatment by radiotherapy and in the handling of data. Centres contributing at that time to the Medical Research Council trial in the UK were Cardiff, Portsmouth, Glasgow, Mount Vernon and Oxford; they were joined by the Groote Schuur Hospital, Cape Town. In the late 1960s in the USA studies were initiated in carcinoma of the cervix; a multi-centre randomized controlled trial was established by the Radiation Therapy Oncologic Group and Fletcher and his colleagues set out to perform a trial at the MD Anderson Hospital, Houston, Texas.

Results of Randomized Controlled Trials

The results of the randomized controlled trials have now been reported either in final or interim form. These are considered first according to the tumour site studied and then generally.

Head and Neck Cancer

The first Cardiff trial, in head and neck cancer, was carried out in association with the MRC working party [50]. In this trial a dose between 3500 and 4600 rad was given, depending on the field size, in 10 fractions over 22 days in hyperbaric oxygen or in air. A total of 295 patients were admitted and a significantly higher local tumour control rate was obtained with hyperbaric oxygen, 53 per cent compared with 30 per cent in air ($P<0{\cdot}001$) (Table 6.1). This resulted in a reduced necessity for salvage surgery but not in a significant improvement in survival. There was significantly higher morbidity when the larynx was included in the treatment volume.

In the second trial, begun in 1971, the identical dose and fractionation

Table 6.1. Medical Research Council Hyperbaric Oxygen Trials:
Head and Neck (1)

		Fractions	*Number of cases*	*% Survival* 2 yr	4 yr	*P*
Cardiff I	Oxygen	10	125	50	37	
	Air	10	151	50	37	
Cardiff II }	Oxygen	10	60	74	62	0.001
Leeds }	Air	conventional	67	50	24	

Head and neck (2)

		Fractions	*Number of cases*	*% Local recurrence-free* 2 yr	4 yr	*P*
Cardiff I	Oxygen	10	125	57	55	0.0005
	Air	10	151	34	31	
Cardiff II }	Oxygen	10	60	72	69	0.01
Leeds }	Air	conventional	67	44	41	

was retained for hyperbaric oxygen except where the larynx was in the field of treatment when the dose was reduced by 10 per cent [51]. The control group received a conventional daily fractionation scheme in air. By June 1976, 104 patients had been entered at Cardiff where the control group was treated in air using 30 fractions over a period of 6 weeks with tumour doses up to 6400 rad. At Leeds 23 patients were included in the trial, the air cases being treated with the daily fractionation regimen normally used by the referring consultant (Berry, 1978). Preliminary results assessed from 1 to 4 years after treatment indicate not only a significant improvement in local control ($P<0{\cdot}001$) but also in survival ($P<0{\cdot}01$); figures for local control with hyperbaric oxygen show an improvement in local control compared with treatment in air by 21–28 per cent [56]. Despite the reduction in dose for the larynx cases, treatment in hyperbaric oxygen remained superior for these cases. No excess morbidity has been seen in this second trial.

The trials indicate that hyperbaric oxygen can improve the results of the radiotherapy of head and neck cancer. There has, however, been much criticism of these results by those who feel that the air control patients at Cardiff fared rather poorly compared with those managed with other regimen of conventional radiotherapy. Even if it is conceded that only an improvement in result of a less adequate scheme of radiotherapy has been demonstrated, it is still a highly significant biological result and there is the probability that even with the best of conventional radiotherapy a further margin of improvement will be obtained using hyperbaric oxygen combined with it. When a conventional technique has been taken to the limits of its possibilities it is no doubt more difficult to show further improvement and an even larger number of cases would be required in any clinical trial.

Although there have been many contributions on this subject, only 3 prospective randomized controlled trials in head and neck cancer have been reported apart from the MRC studies. Van den Brenk [10] showed a significant increase in local clearance of tumour after radiotherapy with hyperbaric oxygen as compared with air in a series of 29 cases. Follow-up of these cases has not been reported. Chang et al. [19] included 51 patients in a trial of hyperbaric oxygen in oropharyngeal cancer. Six fractions were employed in oxygen, 7 or 30 in air. The margin of benefit lay with hyperbaric oxygen both for local control and survival, but these did not achieve statistically significant levels. Shigematsu et al. [71] obtained a similar result when they randomized 42 cases of antral carcinoma to either 4000–5000 rad in 8–10 fractions in hyperbaric oxygen or to 6000–7000 rad in 12–14 fractions in air; in both groups they used twice weekly treatments and 500 rad for individual treatments. The margin of benefit both for local control and survival was in favour of hyperbaric oxygen, but did not achieve statistical significance. It must be pointed out that the limited number of cases included in both trials would have prevented even the substantial margin shown at Cardiff from reaching significance.

We can conclude that all the evidence available is in keeping with the view that hyperbaric oxygen is of benefit in the radiotherapy of head and neck cancer.

Carcinoma of the Bladder

In the first MRC trial in carcinoma of bladder no benefit was shown with hyperbaric oxygen [16]. An examination of the results in the 236 cases which were assessed showed no margin favouring oxygen. Morbidity was not recorded centrally in this early trial. Van den Brenk [10] randomized 16 patients to treatment, either in oxygen using 6 fractions and a total dose of 3000 rad or air using 6 fractions and 3300 rad. There was a considerable margin of benefit in terms of local clearance but this was not of statistical significance and long term follow-up was not reported. Plenk [63] randomized 40 patients to either 4800 rad in 12 fractions in hyperbaric oxygen or to 6000 rad in 24–30 fractions in air. Survival at 2 years was 37 per cent for oxygen and 19 per cent for air. The difference in the survival curves was significant at the $P = 0{\cdot}05$ level. There is no report of the morbidity although this is important, particularly in a trial where different dose and fractionation regimen were employed in oxygen compared with air.

The first MRC trials were performed mainly, although not entirely, using a large number of small fractions, rather more than in the work of Van Den Brenk and of Plenk. In the second trial 6 fractions are being employed in hyperbaric oxygen and this is being compared with 14 in air.

Entry to the trial has been concluded, follow up is continuing and an assessment will soon be made.

We may conclude that, so far, the bulk of evidence suggests that hyperbaric oxygen does not improve the result of radiotherapy in cancer of the bladder.

Carcinoma of the Bronchus

In a series of trials in carcinoma of bronchus performed at Portsmouth in collaboration with the MRC's working party in hyperbaric oxygen a total of 280 patients were randomized between January 1964 and October 1976 [15]. Using conventional small daily fractions, 40 fractions over 8 weeks to a dose of 6000 rad and 30 fractions over 6 weeks to 4500 rad, the trial did not show any improvement in survival using hyperbaric oxygen. When 6 fractions each of 600 rad maximum tissue dose in 18 days were employed, however, hyperbaric oxygen led to improved survival. This improvement was most clearly shown in the 123 patients with squamous cell carcinoma. Survival at 2 years after treatment in hyperbaric oxygen was 24·6 per cent compared with 12·4 per cent in air and at 4 yr 15·9 per cent compared with 2·5 per cent in air. This trend does not reach statistical significance.The trial is to be continued but with an intensified investigation prior to treatment, employing stricter criteria for entry to exclude patients with occult metastasis. Cade and McEwen suggest that a group of patients may emerge where the results of radiotherapy when combined with hyperbaric oxygen may equal that of surgery. The controlled trials at Portsmouth using hyperbaric oxygen in carcinoma of the bronchus are alone in the field.

Carcinoma of the Cervix

Here there is a complex situation. Benefit has been shown in the MRC study which included 4 centres in the UK [83] (Table 6.2). Including all 320 cases randomized, there was an increase in local tumour control by 20–24 per cent at 2–5 years after treatment and this was highly significant ($P<0{\cdot}001$). The greatest benefit was seen in stage III where there was also a significant improvement in survival. This benefit in tumour control was achieved with some increase in morbidity. A remarkable finding in the UK trials was that the main benefit seems to be achieved in patients below the age of 55 (Table 6.3). As yet no significant improvement has been shown at Cape Town and results in subgroups given different regimens of fractionation show a rather different pattern from that which has emerged in the UK trials.

At Leeds an analysis of 75 cases in a trial in stage IIb and III disease has shown no benefit to oxygen and no increase in morbidity [81]. The external beam therapy was given in 10 fractions in both oxygen and air. The technique included a large contribution from 3 intracavitary applications of radiocobalt using the cathetron and this may have weighed the

Table 6.2. Medical Research Council Hyperbaric Oxygen Trials: Cervix
Actuarial local recurrence-free rates according to stage (all patients)

Stage	Treatment series	Total patients	% surviving by years since entry to trial 1	2	3	4	5	Probability of difference between curves due to chance
IIb	Oxygen	12	91	81	61	61	61	0.83
	Air	11	73	73	64	64	64	
III	Oxygen	119	82	77	76	76	71	<0.001
	Air	124	67	50	47	47	44	
IV	Oxygen	30	71	71	71	71	48	0.81
	Air	24	77	53	53	53	53	
All Patients	Oxygen	161	80	76	73	73	67	<0.001
	Air	159	68	52	49	49	47	
Actuarial survival rates according to stage								
IIb	Oxygen	12	92	67	58	42	42	0.34
	Air	11	91	73	73	73	73	
III	Oxygen	119	77	57	49	45	37	0.012
	Air	124	70	49	34	30	25	
IV	Oxygen	30	47	30	20	16	16	0.76
	Air	24	38	17	17	17	17	
All Patients	Oxygen	161	73	53	44	40	33	0.08
	Air	159	67	46	34	31	27	

Table 6.3. Medical Research Council Hyperbaric Oxygen Trials: Cervix
Actuarial local recurrence-free rates according to age (stage III patients only)

Age yr	Treatment series	Total patients	% local recurrence-free by years since entry to trial 1	2	3	4	5	Probability of difference between curves due to chance
Under 35	Oxygen	3						
	Air	2						
35–44	Oxygen	17	88	81	81	81	73	0.12
	Air	10	50	50	50	50	38	
45–54	Oxygen	42	90	90	90	90	85	0.001
	Air	52	70	54	51	51	51	
55–64	Oxygen	38	69	65	65	65	57	0.50
	Air	38	71	50	47	47	42	
65 +	Oxygen	19	76	59	49	49	49	0.53
	Air	22	63	40	40	40	40	
All patients	Oxygen	119	82	77	76	76	71	<0.001
	Air	124	67	50	47	47	44	

trial against showing benefit from a modification in the external beam therapy.

An extensive trial of hyperbaric oxygen in carcinoma of the cervix has been performed at Houston [38]. A total of 223 patients in stages IIb, III and IVa was randomized from September 1968 to March 1974. A complex protocol was employed featuring in some cases exploratory laparotomy and lymphadenectomy and in others extension of radiotherapy to the para-aortic nodes. No significant benefit and also no significant increase in morbidity was reported; however, the margin of local control in the pelvis was in favour of hyperbaric oxygen – 20 of 109 (18 per cent) failing in oxygen compared with 29 of 124 (23·5 per cent) in air: further, the margin of morbidity lay with hyperbaric oxygen: 26 cases compared with 15.

Smaller series have been reported by Glassburn et al. [45] and Glassburn et al. [44] containing 40 and 33 cases, where there has been no benefit in terms of survival but increased morbidity was noted with hyperbaric oxygen. With such small numbers no firm conclusions can be drawn. A multi-centre study in stages IIb and III carried out by the Radiation Therapy Oncologic Group (RTOG) has shown a margin of benefit in favour of oxygen.

When considering the overall results when the hyperbaric oxygen chamber is used in radiotherapy of carcinoma of the cervix we cannot draw any simple conclusions.

General Interpretations

When we look at the results of the trials we need to find some explanation for the differences encountered. Why should hyperbaric oxygen contribute in head and neck tumours but not in bladder tumours? We know that hypoxia is a problem in nearly all the solid tumours which have been studied in animals, although the percentage of hypoxic cells and the biological characteristics of these tumours vary from one to another. In man we have little data to guide us, but it seems unlikely that human tumours are greatly different. Hypoxia is likely to be a problem in all human cancer, including bladder cancer; perhaps it is such a severe problem in the bladder that hyperbaric oxygen is not able to influence it sufficiently to improve the results. We must, of course, recognize that causes other than hypoxia exist for radiation failure, and if other factors dominate then this might account for the findings in carcinoma of bladder.

A possible explanation for the inconsistencies in the results of different trials of hyperbaric oxygen in carcinoma of the cervix may lie in the existence of differing types of tumour at this one site. It is conceivable that biological differences may exist between such tumour types so that hyperbaric oxygen may be beneficial in some patients but not in others.

Aitken-Swan and Baird [3] suggested that there are two types of carcinoma of cervix, one which appears after an *in situ* phase and usually in middle-life and one which appears *de novo* often in older patients. When we compare the UK series with those in Cape Town and Houston we find that the pattern of development of metastasis is rather different. The actuarial metastasis-free rate at 4 years at Glasgow and Mount Vernon is identical at 52 per cent whereas at Cape Town it is 77 per cent. This much lower metastasis rate at Cape Town is very similar to that reported from Houston [18]. This difference in the incidence of distant metastasis may be associated with other biological differences in the primary tumours. Considerable differences in the distribution of tumours among the anatomical sites are seen when comparing racial groups; however, we assume a biological similarity regardless of racial origin when a tumour originates in a single site such as the cervix. This assumption may not be true. A dissimilarity may be relevant to the hyperbaric oxygen trials because the racial composition of the patients included in Cape Town and Houston was different to that in the UK.

If this explanation for the discrepancies in the results is substantiated it may have considerable significance in oncology. We will need to make careful studies to determine the biological characteristics of tumours under treatment and to try and correlate them with the radiation effects achieved. In this way we may be able to determine the optimum conditions for total dose, fractionation, overall time and means of sensitization or adjuvant therapy in each individual case so as to produce the best result.

Hyperbaric Oxygen and the Therapeutic Ratio

The results of the MRC trials leave no doubt that hyperbaric oxygen applied in the radiotherapy of certain malignancies does increase the response observed in the tumour. We have, however, also seen evidence for an increased effect upon normal tissue. It is right, therefore, to question whether all could have been achieved by a simple elevation of radiation dose.

One approach towards an answer to this question is to determine either the amount by which the dose given under normal conditions in air must be raised so as to give the increment of normal tissue damage found with hyperbaric oxygen, or else the reduction of dose in oxygen so that the morbidity associated with normal treatment in air is produced. In the second Cardiff trial the dose given in hyperbaric oxygen was reduced by 10 per cent when the larynx was included in the field of treatment [51]. This reduction is a large one and we should not be misled into thinking that this is a generally applicable figure. The larynx, as Churchill-Davidson in his pioneer work has shown, is a special site with an unusually high percentage of *normal* cells which are hypoxic [21]. Although morbidity was generally slightly greater in hyperbaric oxygen in the first Cardiff trial, no significant increase in effect upon other normal tissues was detectable and in the second trial no reduction in dose has been made when the larynx was not included in the treatment field.

Different normal tissues have different thresholds of radiation dose before damage becomes apparent, and the steepness in the rise in incidence of morbidity with dose from that point also varies from tissue to tissue. For example, we may attempt to give a second course of treatment where the tumour is in certain sites in the head and neck region, but not when it is intimately related to intestine. The intestine is a sensitive normal structure and certainly when we irradiate the bladder or cervix in the treatment of carcinoma this is the main site of morbidity. There was a high incidence of morbidity in patients with carcinoma of cervix given radiotherapy at Cape Town in 10 fractions over 5 weeks to a dose of 4500 rad given either in oxygen or in air, and it has been shown how much this is reduced by bringing the total dose down to 4000 rad [8].

We at Mount Vernon, in co-operation with Cape Town, also attempted to give the dose of 4500 rad in 10 fractions, but abandoned the attempt because of morbidity. Of the 6 patients in whom we attempted to achieve this dose, 3 suffered severe morbidity and 2 of these patients died as a result of it. The other 3 suffered a moderate level of morbidity. In the next 8 patients where the dose was reduced to 4000 rad, as in South Africa, we had 1 case of severe morbidity, 1 slight and 6 who experienced none whatsoever.

We can see that an increment in dose of about 12 per cent leads, in this sensitive situation, to a very great increase in morbidity. In another experience we were able to observe in the clinic an increase in immediate reactions when patients were inadvertently given only a 3 per cent increase in dose when irradiated for pelvic tumours. The increased bowel morbidity with hyperbaric oxygen reported in the MRC cervix trial was only detected by a long term analysis of late morbidity and this was not apparent in the departments concerned with the patients on a day-to-day basis. It seems likely, therefore, from this evidence that the increment of morbidity in hyperbaric oxygen is, in terms of the increment of dose given under normal conditions in air, not likely to exceed 3 per cent.

We can examine the published data to estimate the benefit in tumour control to be expected from an elevation in dose of 3 per cent [28]. A range of increment in control between 3–14 per cent is obtained according to the author and the level chosen on the published curves. All these values fall considerably short of the benefit seen with hyperbaric oxygen in both head and neck and the cervix trials where local control was improved by figures ranging from 21 to 41 per cent according to site and time interval after treatment.

We may conclude that the evidence suggests that a true improvement in the therapeutic ratio may be achieved with hyperbaric oxygen.

The Future of Hyperbaric Oxygen in Radiotherapy

As a method introduced to improve radiotherapy, hyperbaric oxygen is the only one which has been found to be effective in clinical trials where the conditions of test may be regarded as fully acceptable. During the past decade, while the hyperbaric oxygen trials were being performed, other methods for improving the local results of radiotherapy have been introduced. These include the addition of cytotoxic chemotherapy, modifications in the fractionation as to total number and time relationships, the use of heavy particles such as neutrons and pions, and the use of chemical agents as hypoxic cell sensitizers. The benefits which have been shown in the hyperbaric oxygen trials will now have to be measured against these more recently introduced techniques. In the meantime those centres presently equipped with hyperbaric chambers are likely to continue to use them for those tumours where benefit has been shown. An increase in the number of centres with hyperbaric chambers will only follow if the technique is shown to be superior to the other methods now under trial.

CHEMICAL HYPOXIC CELL SENSITIZERS

Laboratory Development

A further approach to the problem is the use of chemical agents which selectively increase the radiosensitivity of hypoxic cells without affecting the radiation sensitivity of well-oxygenated cells. Oxygen is, of course, the best known and also the most effective radiosensitizer of hypoxic cells, but because it is rapidly metabolized in the cells through which it diffuses it does not reach the cells distant to the capillaries. The rationale for the use of the sensitizing drugs is that despite being less active than oxygen they are, for practical purposes, not metabolized in the cells through which they diffuse and they are, therefore, able to reach the distant hypoxic cells in tumours.

In 1963 Adams and Dewey [1] suggested that on the basis of the few radiosensitizing compounds then available and their effects upon hypoxic bacteria that the electron affinity of these compounds and their ability to sensitize was directly related. Subsequent work with bacterial systems and mammalian cells and experience with a large number of radiosensitizing drugs has fully substantiated this proposition and has aided the search for more active sensitizers.

In the early years of the work despite the discovery of a number of radiosensitizing compounds none presented characteristics which enabled progression to the *in vivo* situation.

In 1972 Chapman et al. [20] reported that drugs of the nitrofurans group were potent sensitizers for mammalian cells. This was an important development because a number of compounds in this group were already in clinical use as antibacterial agents (e.g. furadantin). However, it was not possible to achieve hypoxic cell sensitization *in vivo* with these compounds. The concentration necessary to achieve worthwhile sensitization was too highly toxic to the animals being studied.

The real advance towards the clinic occurred when metronidazole (Flagyl), a drug familiar in medicine as a trichomonacide, was found to be a very active sensitizer [5]. The low toxicity of this compound combined with its relatively long metabolic half-life led to dramatic radiosensitization of animal tumours known to contain hypoxic cells [43]. In 1973 metronidazole was first given to patients in doses likely to reach radiosensitization [26, 80]. In order to give serum concentration comparable with those obtained in mice, where radiosensitization was achieved, doses of the order of 10–12 g were required. This single dose can be compared with 200–400 mg given 3 times a day when the drug is used as a trichomonacide or in the treatment of anaerobic infections.

On theoretical grounds based on electron affinity, it was anticipated that the 2-nitroimidazoles would be more efficient sensitizers than a 5-nitroimidazole such as metronidazole [43]. In further work it was shown that the compound Ro 07-0582 synthesized by Roche Products Ltd., a 2-nitroimidazole, was in fact a more efficient sensitizer of hypoxic cells *in vitro* [43].

This led to its test in many different experimental animal tumours using a variety of end points including tumour re-growth delay, local control and cell survival assays *in vitro* or *in vivo* after *in vivo* irradiation. The degree of sensitization achieved depended upon the dose of drug administered (*Fig. 6.2*) [43]. All tumours containing hypoxic cells were sensitized most

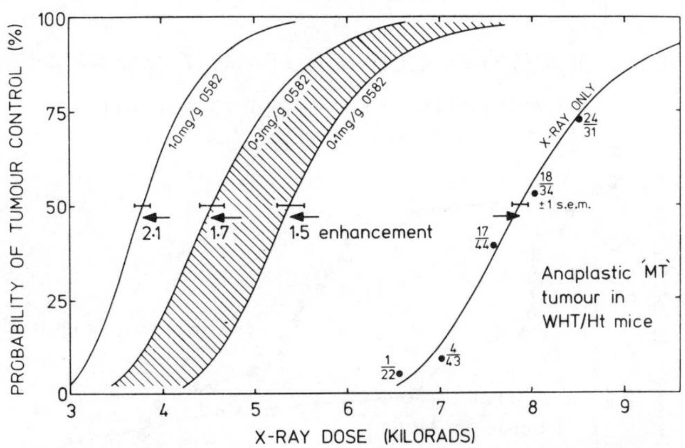

Fig. 6.2. The relationship of dose of misonidazole (Ro 07-0582) and enhancement of tumour control probability. Experiment performed by P. W. Sheldon and S. A. Hill *Br. J. Cancer* **35**, 795–808 (1977).

considerably using single doses of radiation; often an enhancement ratio of 2·0 was obtained. Normal tissues which were well oxygenated were not sensitized in these studies. It was shown in these experiments that the time of administration of the drug relative to irradiation was critical; it must be present at its maximum concentration just at the moment of radiotherapy [43]. The situation is much more critical in the mouse where the biological half-life is 90 min compared with 13 hours in man.

Experiments have also been performed with animal tumours using fractionated doses of drug and radiotherapy and these, including recent studies involving 20 fractions of radiotherapy with misonidazole, have shown considerable improvement in tumour cure probability [43, 70].

Clinical Experience with Metronidazole

In the original administration of metronidazole 12 g, to patients at Mount Vernon and by Urtasun at Edmonton, Alberta, up to 30 tablets of the drug had to be administered either in intact form or crushed into a suspension. Nausea and vomiting was troublesome but no other problem was encountered [26, 80]. Urtasun established a regimen in which radiotherapy was given with metronidazole on 3 occasions in the week for 3 wk. He performed a randomized controlled clinical trial in the management of glioblastoma [77]. Thirty-one patients were randomized into two groups but all received a total tumour dose of 3000 rad in 9 fractions given 3 times a week over an overall time of 18 days, using large parallel opposed fields. Fifteen patients received radiotherapy alone and 16 were given metronidazole, 6 g/m^2 surface area, orally, 4 hours before each treatment by radiotherapy. A statistically significant difference in survival was demonstrated (*Fig. 6.3*). It is reasonable to explain the improved survival

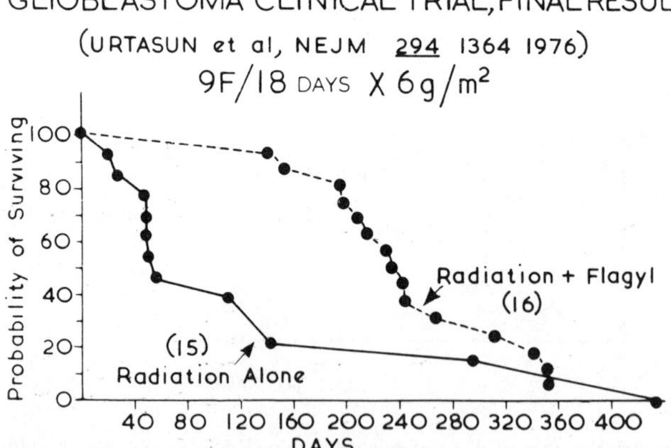

Fig. 6.3. The survival of patients with glioblastoma treated by Urtasun et al. [77] in a randomized controlled trial of metronidazole combined with radiotherapy. A significant prolongation of survival was obtained with use of the sensitizer.

of the patients receiving metronidazole due to increased cell kill because of increased sensitivity of the resistant hypoxic cells. The study can be criticized, however, on the grounds that the control group fared less well than the patients treated by other schemes of radiotherapy. It remains to be seen, therefore, whether metronidazole can improve upon the results of the best of conventional radiotherapy when used either in an unusual fractionation regimen such as the one used by Urtasun in his trial or when added to the conventional regimen. The radiobiological importance of this study for the use of chemical hypoxic cell sensitizers in radiotherapy remains despite this criticism.

There have been other reports of the use of metronidazole with radiotherapy but there is no other record of a randomized controlled clinical trial. A number of groups are presently exploring the use of metronidazole and there has been a suggestion that metronidazole may be a safer drug to employ. The neurotoxicity observed with other nitroimidazoles can be seen with metronidazole, particularly when the drug administration is prolonged and high doses accumulate [23]. Safety probably lies in the dose limitation caused by the nausea and vomiting it provokes [54].

As an hypoxic cell sensitizer in clinical practice misonidazole is likely to be more effective than metronidazole by a factor between two and four. For this reason work with metronidazole is currently being performed in only a few centres.

Clinical Experience with Misonidazole

Early Experience in Administration of Misonidazole to Man

In 1974 the efficacy of misonidazole as an hypoxic cell sensitizer had been demonstrated in many animal tumour models [42]. It was felt that the time had come to see whether it was possible to administer the drug to man so as to achieve radiosensitization of hypoxic cells. Prior clinical experience with this drug was limited to a few pilot studies as a possible trichomonacide in 1967–68 when comparatively low doses were given. It was, effectively, a new drug as opposed to metronidazole which had received extensive use as a trichomonacide though in rather lower dosage to that required for radiosensitization. In 1974 we administered the drug in doses of between 1–4 g to 6 normal volunteers [41]. A linear relationship was shown between drug dose and serum level. No side-effects were encountered. Permission was then granted to give the drug to a limited number of patients suffering from advanced malignant disease. In a series of 8 patients given single doses between 4–10 g satisfactory serum concentrations were achieved similar to those seen in animals where radiosensitization had been clearly demonstrated [47]. There were some gastrointestinal disturbances particularly in the patients given high doses, but otherwise in the single dose study tolerance was good. Promising results were obtained from studies of skin reaction in hypoxic skin and in the response of tumour in patients where multiple nodules were irradiated with or without the sensitizer (*see below*).

Encouraged by the study we moved on to give the drug in multiple doses. It was anticipated that three major problems might be encountered. Firstly there had been some nausea and vomiting in the single dose study, particularly when the larger doses were being given. A reduction in the total amount to be given in a single dose down to a maximum of 120 mg/kg body weight (approximately equal to 5 g/m^2 surface area) seemed advisable. It was not known whether gastrointestinal symptoms would lessen or become more severe with repeated dosage. Secondly, there was a suggestion that in primates repeated administration led to a reduction in peak serum values, possibly through enzyme induction, leading to a more efficient destruction of the drug (Johnson et al., 1976). However, it was suggested by other workers that with the dose and frequency of administration likely to be used in man this would not occur [58]. Finally, there was the evidence in toxicological work in dogs [67] and in primates [57] that misonidazole was neurotoxic, in common with the other nitroimidazoles: convulsions occurred with repeated high dosage. The dosage and frequency of administration planned for patients was set well below those levels giving toxic effects in primates and from these studies a dose giving a good margin of safety was calculated for trial in man.

The result of our further experience with the administration of misonidazole to man has now been extended to over 180 cases [31, 33, 34, 35, 65]. Reports upon the use of misonidazole have now been made [52, 55, 61, 68, 78, 79, 86], recording the international experience of the drug in Austria, Canada, the USA and South Africa as well as further experience in the UK.

The Tolerance of Misonidazole in Man

Gastrointestinal disturbances

The anorexia, nausea and vomiting noted in our first group of patients given large single doses of the drug was certainly dose related and troublesome to those given the highest doses. These patients were all suffering from widespread malignant disease and were receiving considerable radiotherapy in association with the drug. Misonidazole was given to these patients always on an empty stomach. A considerable bulk of material had to be given – up to 20 tablets either in their intact form or crushed and made into a suspension in fruit juice. The drug itself has an unpleasant taste and this has certainly contributed to anorexia and nausea. In subsequent work the patients have on the whole been fitter, the dose given has been smaller and capsules are now used. Further, patients have been allowed a light breakfast and the drug usually given at about 10 a.m. or later. No gastrointestinal disturbance of any significance has since been observed by us. Nausea and vomiting has been reported by other workers [55, 61, 68, 79] and also constipation [68].

Neurotoxic Effects

CONVULSIONS. Convulsions have occurred in 2 of our patients, the one given the largest dose and also in another patient given 2 large doses totalling 16 g where the doses were separated by a period of 3 days. In the latter patient there was an unusually high serum concentration for the dose administered and a prolonged half-life. In both cases convulsions commenced at 20 hours after administration of the last dose, followed by considerable impairment of brain function which showed only a partial improvement before each of the patients died. Both were suffering from advanced malignant disease and death was primarily due to this though the neurological damage contributed [35, 65]. Man seemed particularly sensitive to the neurotoxic effects of misonidazole and a halving of the original plan of dosage was necessary.

PERIPHERAL NEUROPATHY. In a series of 14 patients given misonidazole in 4, 5, 6 or 15–20 doses over a period of between 17–28 days and where the total dose given was approximately 15–16 g/m^2 surface area, 11 suffered peripheral neuropathy. This was of onset between 15–30 days after the beginning of treatment and in some caused the drug to be discontinued during the course of radiotherapy. It took the form of numbness and paraesthesia in the hands and feet with the most troublesome symptoms persistent in the feet. Some patients went on to suffer cramp-like pains in the feet extending up into the calves. Objectively sensory impairment to light touch and pinprick was observed in the toes in most of the patients and this extended up into the lower leg in some cases. Usually the symptoms gradually subsided after a period of several weeks, but in some they persisted until death and one patient remained troubled at 2 years. We have not been able to demonstrate clinically any motor loss in our patients, but this has been reported by other workers (Phillips et al., 1979). Electromyography has shown in our patients a sensory peripheral neuropathy with a mild motor component.

In our subsequent work a reduction of dose of 12 g/m^2 surface area given over a period of at least 17 days resulted in a reduction of peripheral neuropathy to 30 per cent. With monitoring of the serum concentration and appropriate reduction of dose in some cases this has now been reduced to 12 per cent and in nearly all the cases it is of such mild severity as to be of no great clinical importance.

It might be that a larger total dose can be given either when the period of treatment exceeds 4 weeks or when the drug is given in a single weekly dose. Further work is required to show whether this is so. A collaborative effort involving 5 centres where work with misonidazole is proceeding may, by pooling of data, lead to an early answer to this question [32].

TRANSIENT NEUROLOGICAL DISTURBANCES. We have observed in 5 patients following one up to 3 administrations of misonidazole in large doses the appearance of a transient peripheral neuropathy which appears about 12 hours after administration of the drug and which disappears after about 24 hours. The symptoms do not occur with other identical doses given to the same patients. The appearance of this transient disturbance does not seem to be related to later occurrence of established peripheral neuropathy and seems of no clinical importance. We have observed in one patient aged 66, a mild confusional state associated with transient changes in the plantar response and deep reflexes of the legs. The episode was associated with a fall in the Hb concentration to 9 g. Recovery was complete.

Urtasun [76] reported that a man aged 85 who received 8 doses of 2 g ($1{\cdot}5/m^2$ surface area) over a period of 19 days convulsed on day 21 and died on day 44. Post mortem showed evidence for a drug-induced toxic effect. Professor Sealy has reported a transient episode of ataxia in one of his patients and vertical nystagmus in another, but alcohol in excess may have been responsible in both cases. Jentzsch et al. [52] have reported the appearance of a drug related organic psychosyndrome, but in both cases where this was observed all manifestations disappeared within one week of cessation of administration of the drug.

Confusional disturbances are not uncommon in elderly patients with advanced neoplasms and if such patients are given misonidazole it may be difficult to determine if the drug is contributing. It is possible that elderly patients who are suffering some degree of cerebral anoxaemia due to impairment of vascular supply and anaemia may suffer a neurotoxic effect given doses well within the range considered safe and when the plasma concentrations of drug reach normal levels. It is probably wise not to administer the drug to any patient showing evidence for cerebrovascular insufficiency, paticularly when there is anaemia, and to discontinue a course if confusion develops. If the drug is discontinued at the stage of confusion full recovery appears to occur.

Skin Rashes

Hypersensitivity skin rashes considered due to misonidazole have been recorded in 3 of our patients. A maculopapular rash appeared between 8 and 17 days after beginning radiotherapy with misonidazole after a dose of between 6·5–7 g of drug had been given. The maculopapular rash appeared on the arms, hands, feet and legs and also on the trunk in 2 cases. In one, misonidazole was re-administered and provoked recrudescence of the rash. In our 3 cases the rashes were not especially troublesome but did lead to the premature cessation of misonidazole administration. In 4 other cases rashes appeared, not dissimilar in type, during courses of radiotherapy with misonidazole but in all 4 the cautious re-administration of misonidazole did not provoke recrudescence of the rash and it was possible that the misonidazole may not have been responsible. A similar rash also appeared in one of the control cases in a clinical trial who was not given misonidazole.

Similar cases have been observed by Sealy in Cape Town and Kogelnik in Vienna. All these cases have now been recorded [66]. Two further cases have been reported by Partington et al. [59].

Auditory Symptoms

Auditory disturbances have been reported [55, 61]. These workers tend to use large doses on a weekly basis and this may account for the appearance of such symptoms in their patients, but not those treated at other centres. The symptoms are apparently transient and no permanent damage results.

Normal Values in Man

Repeated administration of the drug gives similar curves of plasma concentration on each occasion and no evidence for increased destruction of the drug in man.

Misonidazole is readily absorbed from the stomach and a peak level in the plasma is achieved normally between 1–2 hours after oral administration. After the peak there is a period of slowfall which extends to about 5 hr and this has been called the plateau period (*Fig. 6.4*).

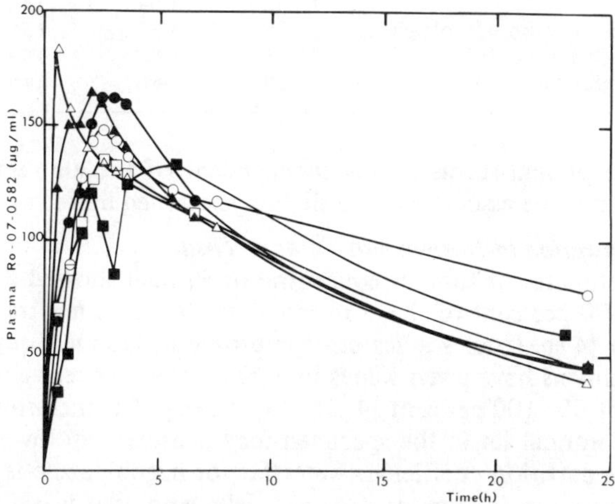

Fig. 6.4. The plasma concentrations of misonidazole (Ro 07-0582) determined in the first patient given 6 doses of misonidazole [35].

The subsequent nitroimidazole clearance is logarithmic, with a mean half-life of 12·8 hours (SD 3·0 hours). The mean plateau concentration achieved per gram of misonidazole given is 23·4 μg/ml. The variance is reduced by correcting for body weight and still further by correcting for surface area. This confirms the general use of surface area when calculating the dose for any one patient (Table 6.4). We have found that the plateau concentration achieved per gram of misonidazole given is lower in men than in women but on the other hand the half-life of the drug in women is shorter than in men. These differences remain after correction for body size. There is a linear relationship between dose given and plasma concentration at the plateau period in both men and women. The half-life of

Table 6.4. Half-life and plateau concentration of misonidazole in 159 patients. The values have been corrected for patient's size in each case by multiplying the patient's weight over the mean weight and by the patient's surface area over the mean surface area.

Measurement	*Mean*	*SD*	*Cases*	*OBS*
Males				
Half-life	13·39	2·86	81	156
Plasma conc/g misonidazole given	21·24	4·53	90	448
(Conc/g) (WT/mean WT)	21·31	4·29	90	448
(Conc/g) (SA/mean SA)	21·34	4·01	84	433
Females				
Half-life	11·94	3·10	61	103
Plasma conc/g misonidazole given	26·22	5·69	69	328
(Conc/g) (WT/mean WT)	25·94	6·07	69	328
(Conc/g) (SA/mean SA)	26·07	5·40	61	315
All Cases				
Half-life	12·82	3·04	142	259
Plasma conc/g misonidazole given	23·35	5·62	159	776
(Conc/g) (WT/mean WT)	23·11	5·02	159	776
(Conc/g) (SA/mean SA)	23·18	4·66	145	748

the drug in plasma seems largely independent of the amount given but small doses may be associated with slightly shortened half-lives.

The Concentration in Normal and Tumour Tissue

The first estimates of tumour concentration in man showed a wide range from 13–100 per cent of the corresponding plasma concentration at time of estimate [47]. Later studies using improved techniques for preparation of the specimens have given values in excess of 40 per cent and usually in the range of 60–100 per cent [4, 25, 35, 79, 86]. The inclusion of a small amount of normal fat in the specimen may considerably lower the result because the partition coefficient water/fat for misonidazole is about 2:1. The concentration in tumour rises and falls with that in plasma with in some cases only a slight delay. An exception may be in brain where concentrations may not rise to plasma levels until 4 or 5 hours after administration. In general radiotherapy should begin 4 hours (± ½ hour) after administration of misonidazole. Estimates of the concentration of misonidazole in normal tissues have been performed [4, 78] showing similar findings to those in tumour tissue.

Misonidazole levels rise rapidly after oral administration in the cerebrospinal fluid [78, 86], with a peak concentration occurring soon after that in the plasma. Usually levels are nearly at the height of those in the plasma but some lower values have been recorded [4, 55].

Metabolism of Misonidazole

Studies have been performed in mice, rats, baboons and in man [39]. There are large differences between man and the animals studied as regards the half-life of the drug in plasma: in the mouse this is between 1 and 1·5 hours, in the rat 1·7 hours, and the baboon 4·5–5·5 hours compared with 12·8 hours in man.

In all species examined small amounts of the breakdown product desmethylmisonidazole may be detected after 4 hours in the plasma but this rarely exceeds 20 per cent of the misonidazole level. This compound is also active as a radiosensitizer. Approximately 10 per cent of the drug is excreted in the urine within the first 24 hr as unchanged misonidazole and 8 per cent as desmethylmisonidazole, but there is a wide variation. Further studies including the use of C^{14} labelled misonidazole in man performed at Mount Vernon Hospital, in collaboration with Roche Products Ltd. have shown a continued excretion of drug unchanged and desmethylmisonidazole for at least 10 days after administration and up to 50 or 60 per cent may be accounted for by urinary excretion.

Extensive faecal excretion does not occur with this nitroimidazole in man in contrast to other species such as the mouse and with other nitroimidazoles given to man such as metronidazole. No loss in respired air has been found in either mice or man.

The remainder of the drug currently unaccounted for is, we believe, broken down by hepatic enzymes and the products excreted only slowly [40]. There is no evidence for significant loss in other tissues.

Direct Diffusion into Tumours

The ability of misonidazole to diffuse deeply into tissues has led to attempts at direct diffusion of the drug into tumours. Awwad et al. [7] reported their findings following the introduction of misonidazole into the bladder 2 hours before cystectomy for carcinoma secondary to schistosomiasis. In 5 of 7 cases concentrations of the order of 400 μg/g were detected in tumour, but not in normal bladder tissues. We have repeated this work in 5 patients with carcinoma of bladder; 2 underwent cystectomy and 3 endoscopic biopsy. Although very high concentrations were achieved in one case, lower levels were reached in others and the normal tissue concentrations approached these concentrations in some. Further work concerned with direct diffusion is proceeding.

Plasma Concentration Measurements and Misonidazole Toxicity

It was shown in the first series of cases given multiple doses of misonidazole that the incidence of peripheral neuropathy was related to the tissue exposure as estimated from the curve of plasma concentration given after each dose of the drug [29]. Further work has confirmed this observation. In a series of 45 patients planned for identical misonidazole therapy, 6 doses over 17–18 days to a total of 12 g/m^2, those who suffered peripheral neuropathy showed significantly higher plateau values and tissue exposure as indicated by the product of the plasma concentration at the plateau period multiplied by half-life. We believe, therefore, that it is important to monitor the plasma concentration not only to pick up those few patients who show unusually high values and who must, therefore be specially at risk for development of misonidazole toxicity, but also to pick up those who show values in the upper part of the normal range when a small reduction of misonidazole dose may appreciably reduce the risk of peripheral neuropathy. Because in any one patient fairly consistent readings are obtained through a course of treatment only a limited number of examinations is necessary.

The high plateau concentration seen in women is partly compensated for as regards tissue exposure by a shorter half-life. However, the mean of the exposure indices for women is 10 per cent greater than for men. We have not seen an overall increase in neurotoxicity in women compared with men but this may be related to differences in the numbers of men and women in the different dose groups. Among the 45 patients given 6 doses of misonidazole and referred to above there were only 8 women, but 4 developed peripheral neuropathy compared with 11 of the 37 men.

The Ability of Misonidazole to Sensitize Hypoxic Cells in Man

In our original study of the administration of the drug to man we attempted to determine whether the drug could sensitize hypoxic cells in man using a technique whereby normal and artificially hypoxic skin was irradiated [29, 36]. With a radio strontium plaque doses ranging from 800–1100 rad were given to areas of skin 15 mm^2 with the limb surrounded by a bag of oxygen. Although the erythema that followed was poorly related to dose the subsequent pigmentation usually at 6–8 weeks was, in most cases, closely related. For irradiation under hypoxia an Esmarch's bandage, a sphygmomanometer cuff at 200 mmHg and the replacement of the oxygen in the bag by nitrogen were employed. Under these hypoxic conditions approximately 2000 rad was required to produce the pigmentation which follows a 1000 rad dose given under oxic conditions. The drug greatly increased the radiation response of skin made temporarily hypoxic but did not significantly alter the response in oxic skin. The relative sensitizing efficiency is a measure expressing as a percentage the restoration of the sensitivity of the hypoxic cells to that of those under oxic conditions. In 6 patients given misonidazole in a range of doses the efficiencies extended from 27–71 per cent. These values can be compared with 11–14 per cent in the 3 patients given metronidazole [36].

A further study was made to determine whether any difference could be detected in the response of tumours in patients with multiple, observable or measurable metastases [74]. Seven patients, all of whom gave their informed consent, took part in the study. The main method employed was the measurement of subcutaneous nodules treated under different conditions. Observations were made in the period of regression after treatment and if the patient survived long enough when re-growth occurred. The most satisfactory situation for study occurred in a young woman with multiple subcutaneous metastases from carcinoma of cervix. Measurement of two groups each of 7 nodules with a mean diameter of 12·6 mm showed a significant difference ($P = 0{\cdot}05$) of the time of re-growth after single doses of 960 and 1120 rad, thus giving a measure of the ability of the system to discriminate. Re-growth seen in the third group of 7 nodules treated with a lower radiation dose of 800 rad, combined with a dose of misonidazole, was similar to that seen after 960 rad alone, indicating a dose enhancement factor of 1·2 (*Fig. 6.5*).

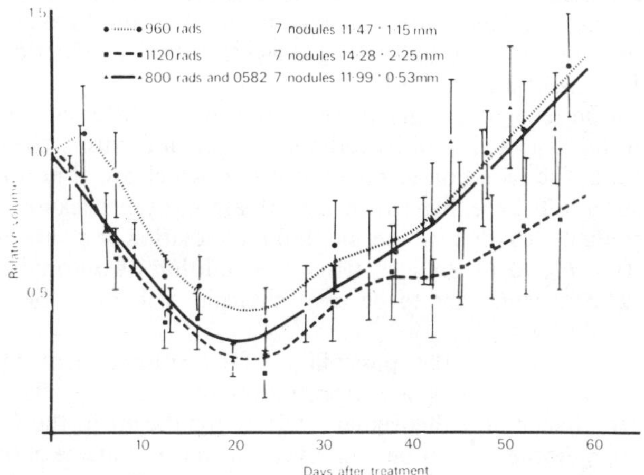

Fig. 6.5. Regression and re-growth seen in a patient with multiple subcutaneous nodules due to carcinoma of cervix [74]. A significant difference exists between the curves for 960 and 1120 rad. Using misonidazole with 800 rad the response is at least as good as 960 rad without sensitizer suggesting an overall enhancement of response of 1·2.

In a second patient with metastases in lung from a primary carcinoma of breast no enhancement was detected. In a third case there was a fairly clear evidence of enhancement though this did not reach significance in the period of survival of the patient while in the fourth with diffuse infiltration of tumour in wide areas of skin there was delay of re-growth when misonidazole was added to the standard dose. In the other cases it was not possible to make any estimate of effect.

Further studies in patients with multiple deposits of tumour have been reported by Dawes et al. [25] and Ash et al. [4]. In both series a majority of cases studied gave evidence for increased response when misonidazole was given with radiotherapy. In one of the cases reported by Ash radiotherapy was given in 10 fractions using less than 200 rad dose increments and in this study increased delay in tumour re-growth was demonstrated.

These studies demonstrate that misonidazole can lead to increased kill of hypoxic cells in man as in animals. They give great encouragement towards the use of the drug in man, but only randomized controlled clinical trials can show whether a significant improvement in cure can result from their use.

Effect upon Normal Tissues

In animal study some enhancement of normal tissue effects has been observed but only when high doses of radiation and misonidazole have been combined, and tissue known to contain a small concentration of hypoxic cells irradiated. With reference to this data and to experience with hyperbaric oxygen there has been a suggestion that a reduction of dose is required for clinical trials [49].

It must be recognized that there is an essential difference between the effects to be expected with hyperbaric oxygen and with a chemical sensitizing agent. The radiation response of tissues which are at normal levels of oxygenation will be enhanced in hyperbaric oxygen because of the continued gradual elevation of the line linking radiation response and oxygen tension (*see Fig. 6.1*). In such tissue the addition of misonidazole in the concentrations which are to be used clinically will result in virtually no increment of effect [2].

There is, however, the possibility of an enhancement of effect in normal tissues containing a concentration of hypoxic cells. It remains to be seen if such an enhancement will be significant in the fractionated courses of radiotherapy to be employed. So far we have seen in all tissues immediate radiation reactions which have been similar to those which we would normally expect with the dose and fractionation regimen employed. It is too early to make any observations as to long term effects.

A problem of interpretation of results with regard to normal tissue effects may present in clinical trials using misonidazole combined with an unusual fractionation regimen and it is essential that such trials incorporate two control groups – the unusual regimen without sensitizer as well as a conventional scheme of radiotherapy.

The larynx presents a special problem because it contains a considerable concentration of hypoxic cells but using misonidazole in the planned dosage in fractionated radiotherapy it is unlikely that increased normal tissue effects will be observed.

We must pursue all clinical trials with extreme care and caution but apart from the larynx there is no evidence to justify reduction of dose and even there we would recommend a cautious use of unaltered dose but initially inclusion only of the patients with more advanced disease.

The Optimum Regimen for the Administration of Misonidazole

The neurotoxicity of misonidazole in man limits the dose which can be given. We must, therefore, consider carefully how best to use this drug in clinical radiotherapy. Among the possibilities are that it may be given:

1. With every treatment in a multi-fraction course given over a number of weeks.
2. With each of a reduced number of fractions so that a higher radiation dose is combined with a high dose of sensitizer.
3. With some of the treatments in a multi-fraction course of radiotherapy, the remaining treatments being given without administration of the drug.
4. Combined with multiple radiation treatments in one day taking advantage of the relatively long half-life of the drug in man.

If using the last three schemes we give 6 doses then we can hope to achieve 50–60 μg/g in the tumour at the time of radiotherapy (*Fig. 6.6*) when an enhancement ratio of 1·6 or greater can be achieved, an enhancement similar to that achieved with neutrons.

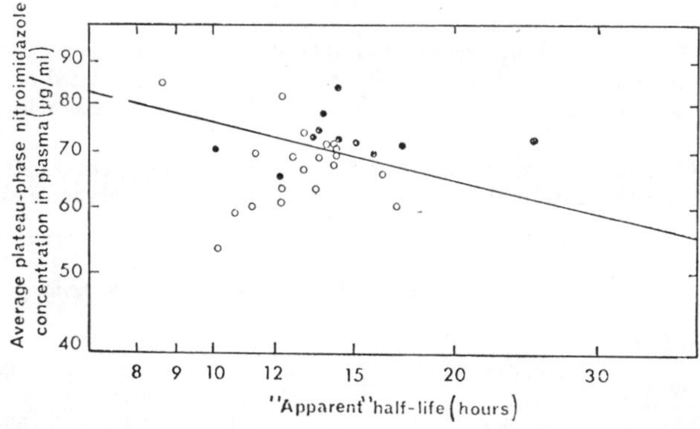

Fig. 6.6. Chart employed for adjustment of dose when patient given 6 doses based on a total of 12 g/m² surface area. The • indicates a patient who developed neuropathy and ○ a patient who did not, using the same regime.

If we give misonidazole daily in a mult-fraction course given over 4–6 weeks we may be dividing our dose into 20 or 30 fractions. Tumour concentrations of around 24 and 20 μg/g may be achieved, giving us enhancement ratios of about 1·25 and 1·3. Because of the shape of the curve linking enhancement ratio with dose and the steep rise in enhancement at low doses we have only just over half the degree of radiosensitization by dividing the dose for daily fractionation (*Fig. 6.7*). On the other hand biological evidence suggests that the reverse is true with radiation dose because of the shape of the survival curves for oxic and hypoxic cells. Particularly when doses start falling below 400 rad the amount of sensitization of hypoxic cells may also fall steeply. Below 200 rad the curves are often drawn so close together that there may not be a theoretical advantage in altering cells from the hypoxic to the oxic state. The con-

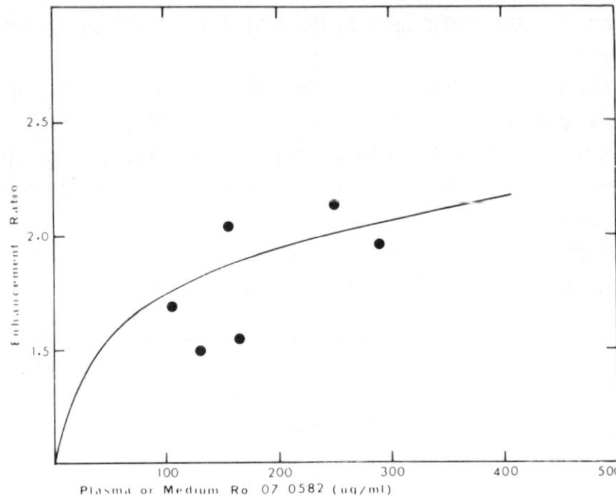

Fig. 6.7. The sensitizing efficiency of Ro 07-0582. Continuous line: Date for sensitization of hypoxic Chinese hamster V79 cells cultured and irradiated *in vitro* [2]. ●: Data for sensitization of hypoxic human skin. (Adapted from Dische et al. [29].)

Table 6.5. Medical Research Council Trials in Hyperbaric Oxygen: Cervix Stage III Results at centres using multiple fractions in both hyperbaric oxygen and in air.

		Fractions	*Total*	*% Local recurrence-free* 2 *yr*	5 *yr*	*P*
Glasgow	Oxygen	20	58	87	80	0·01
	Air		69	64	57	
Mount Vernon	Oxygen	27	31	81	69	0·04
	Air		25	46	40	
	Taken together $P<0{\cdot}001$					

ditions applying at this dose level are difficult to exactly simulate in the laboratory.

We have now the results of the hyperbaric oxygen trials giving evidence to suggest that an oxygen effect does, in fact, occur at around the 200 rad dose level (Table 6.5). This does encourage us to believe that an hypoxic cell sensitizer might give benefit when added to a conventional course of radiotherapy where daily fractionation is employed and treatment times of 4, 5, 6 or more weeks are employed.

Finally there is the independent cytotoxic effect of the nitroimidazoles [48]. It remains to be seen whether, at the level of dose possible in man, this effect is going to be an important one with misonidazole and if it is then, because of the importance of duration of exposure, continuous daily administration of misonidazole may lead to the greatest cell kill of hypoxic cells when compared with more intermittent dosage schemes. We need careful biological study in man to increase our knowledge.

When misonidazole is given with only some of the treatments in a course of radiotherapy it is usually combined with a greater radiation dose than that used in fractions given without it. As a result a number of 'unorthodox' regimens of radiotherapy are being employed. The regimen itself without sensitizer needs to be tested as well as conventional therapy. This leads to three limbed trials and ethical problems with use of the unorthodox regimen without sensitizer.

It is important that we explore all the possibilities of combination of the hypoxic cell sensitizers with radiotherapy. We must, of course, be careful not to have too many trials and too many different regimens. Collaboration between radiotherapy centres at national and international level is essential if we are to learn the value of the drug at an early time.

Dose Regimens

Misonidazole is presently supplied by the Roche Company in capsules containing 500 mg and 100 mg. A scheme for administration of misonidazole has been devised based on the total allowed dose of 12 g/m^2 surface area and the strength of these preparations.

We often employ a 6-dose regimen given twice weekly for 3 weeks. We divide the permitted dose (12 g/m^2 surface area) by 6 and if the dose falls between half gram levels give the lower dose using 500 mg capsules. If the plasma concentration permits we can later elevate the dose to the higher dose level. The plateau and 24-hour concentrations are determined after the first dose and the half-life calculated. If initial readings are above the line in *Fig. 6.6* we make appropriate reductions in dose [65]. Subsequently we take plateau levels only at the second, fourth and sixth doses to monitor the course.

Because of the relatively long half-life of the drug some 10–30 per cent of the plateau concentration remains at 24 hours. This means that in daily administration the dose on the second day will result in a higher level. When the drug is continued on every day the concentration on the second and subsequent days tends to remain constant. In an effort to obtain uniform concentration at every treatment the dose on the first day can be increased.

Although the adjustment of dose does give a more even concentration at time of treatment the variations are relatively small and sometimes may not be easily discernible among the variations which must be expected from day to day. We have concluded that the complications which may result from varying the dose due to confusion on the part of the patient do not make this variable dosage worthwhile and recommend a uniform dose throughout treatment. The following scheme based upon the 12 g/m^2 surface area is now being employed.

Misonidazole in Radiotherapy using Daily Treatment
Calculate patient's surface area. Read daily dose from chart according to number of doses planned for patient

	Number of doses			*Daily dose mg*
	20	*24*	*30*	
	2·0			1200
Surface	1·8			1100
area	1·7	2·0		1000
in	1·5	1·8		900
square	1·3	1·6	2·0	800
metres	1·2	1·4	1·8	700
	—	1·2	1·5	600
			1·3	500

Monitor the plasma concentration on first 3 days during plateau period (3½–4½ hours after administration when radiotherapy is given)
Plasma level should not exceed

Number of doses		
20	24	30
Plasma concentration μg/ml		
30	28	25

Proportional reductions should be made in daily dose if necessary when it would also be necessary to make further daily checks. Subsequently the plateau plasma concentration should be monitored once a week, preferably on a Thursday or Friday, in order to make certain that there is no accumulation of drug concentration. In our experience, however, such accumulations are very uncommon.

The Place of Misonidazole in Clinical Radiotherapy
We have had favourable impressions based on our clinical experience with the drug. At Mount Vernon in carcinoma of cervix we showed that the regression observed at the end of a course of radiotherapy directly correlated with the long term local control. We were able to predict the benefit which was later to be seen in follow-up because we noted a greater number of good regressions in the patients treated in hyperbaric oxygen [27]. Apparent complete regression has been noted in all 8 cases which

have now been given misonidazole with radiotherapy for carcinoma of the cervix and so here also we have promise of benefit.

When a new method is introduced into cancer treatment initial experience is often fallacious and judgement is always influenced by the enthusiasm which accompanies a new exploration. Only randomized controlled clinical trials can give the answer. Many such clinical trials are now underway in all parts of the world. In the UK the Medical Research Council has set up a Steering Committee to co-ordinate work with the chemical sensitizing agents under the overall control of the Cancer Therapy Committee. Three randomized controlled clinical trials in glioblastoma, grades III and IV, in carcinoma of cervix, stage III and in advanced head and neck tumours have now been established on a multi-centre basis. These employ between 10–24 fractions of misonidazole combined with radiotherapy. Other trials are proceeding in Europe, Canada, the USA, South Africa and Australasia. We must patiently wait the results of these studies before deciding the place of misonidazole in clinical radiotherapy.

CONCLUSIONS

There has been some success in the treatment of certain tumours using hyperbaric oxygen and also using neutrons. An increase in effect upon tumour has been shown with chemical sensitizers in patients with multiple nodules of tumour. These observations all confirm that radioresistant hypoxic cells exist in human tumours as they do in animals.

The multiple fractionation used in clinical radiotherapy is obviously successful in overcoming this radioresistance in a considerable number of cases. It seems, however, that at least in some tumour sites hypoxia remains as a common cause of radiation failure. The extent of the problem can only be guessed at and only a controlled trial of a totally effective sensitizer of all hypoxic cells is likely to give this information.

The recently reported trials using hyperbaric oxygen have aroused a new interest in this method which has now been in clinical use for over 27 years. An extension of the use of hyperbaric oxygen will depend on the comparison with other methods now introduced to improve radiotherapy, especially the chemical sensitizing agents which might be expected to be effective in the same type of case. Recent animal studies suggest that in a fractionated course of treatment hyperbaric oxygen may be more effective than misonidazole but only when anaesthesia is used [72]. Sealy has explored the use of a combination of hyperbaric oxygen and misonidazole in groups of patients with advanced oral cancer and has achieved some remarkable responses [69]. There are, therefore, further ways in which hyperbaric oxygen may be used with radiotherapy.

With the chemical sensitizers a considerable effort is now being made, especially in the USA, but also in the UK, to develop new agents which might be better tolerated than misonidazole and which will give a greater degree of sensitization. The ability of misonidazole and other sensitizers to act as cytotoxic agents for hypoxic cells without radiation has widened the possibilities of their use in oncology to their administration in combination with cytotoxic drugs. Many hundreds of compounds are in various stages of study. Their ability to radiosensitize and to act as cytotoxic agents is more easily tested than their toxicological properties. The process of development is a long and expensive one. Even if the experience gained with misonidazole is fully utilized the development of a new drug to the stage of a randomized trial will take 3 years or more. It is important to explore the potential of misonidazole and by collaborative effort see whether we can benefit those patients now coming for treatment. If misonidazole does prove to be effective then we can expect it to be used with the normal control patients in the study of the next drug introduced as a radiosensitizer.

SUMMARY

Among methods to improve the results of radiotherapy are those to sensitize radioresistant hypoxic tumour cells. These give a real possibility of an enhanced effect upon tumour with little or no effect upon normal tissues. Hyperbaric oxygen has been tested with randomized controlled trials and found to give benefit in certain situations. The benefit has to be measured against the effort by patient and department and compared with that obtained using other methods.

Chemical sensitizing agents are simple to employ and there is good evidence both in the laboratory and in man for an effect upon hypoxic cells. Unfortunately, misonidazole, the first agent with real promise to reach the clinic, has proved neurotoxic and the total dose must be limited. Randomized controlled clinical trials are now underway and a great effort is being made to find new agents which may be less toxic and be more effective.

Acknowledgements

I wish to thank Dr M. I. Saunders and past and present research staff for all their work and support. My colleagues in Radiobiology have given me much advice and encouragement, in particular Professor G. E. Adams, Professor J. F. Fowler and Dr O. C. A. Scott. Mrs Eileen Davies has kindly prepared the manuscript.

The support of the Medical Research Council is gratefully acknowledged.

REFERENCES

1. Adams G. E. and Dewey D. L. (1963) Hydrated electrons and radiobiological sensitization. *Biochem. Biophys. Res. Commun.* **12,** 473–477.
2. Adams G. E. and Dische S. (1979) Care with radiosensitizers. *Br. J. Radiol.* **52,** 920–921.
3. Aitken-Swan J. and Baird D. (1966) Cancer of the uterine cervix in Aberdeenshire: aetiological aspects. *Br. J. Cancer* **20,** 642–659.
4. Ash D., Smith M. R. and Bugden R. D. (1979) The distribution of misonidazole in human tumours and normal tissues. *Br. J. Cancer* **39,** 503–509.

5. Asquith J. C., Foster J. L., Willson R. L. et al. (1974) Metronidazole ('flagyl'). A radiosensitizer of hypoxic cells. *Br. J. Radiol.* **47,** 474–481.
6. Atkins H. L., Seaman W. B., Jacox H. W. et al. (1965) Experience with hyperbaric oxygenation in clinical radiotherapy. *Am. J. Roentgenol. Radium Ther. Nucl. Med.* **93,** 651–663.
7. Awwad H. K., El-Merzabani M. M. and Burgers M. V. (1978) Penetration of misonidazole after intravesical administration in cases of carcinoma of the Bilharzial bladder. *Br. J. Cancer* **37,** Suppl. III, 297–298.
8. Bennett M. B., Sealy R. and Hockly J. (1977) *The Treatment of stage III squamous carcinoma of the cervix in air and hyperbaric oxygen. A preliminary report.* British Institute of Radiology, MRC Oxygen Working Party, London, on 14 April 1977. *Br. J. Radiol.* **51,** 68.
9. Berry G. H. (1978) A clinical appraisal of hyperbaric oxygen in head and neck cancer. *Br. J. Radiol.* **51,** 150.
10. Brenk Van den H. A. S. (1968) Hyperbaric oxygen in radiation therapy. An investigation of dose-effect relationships in tumour response and tissue damage. *Am. J. Roentgenol. Radium Ther. Nucl. Med.* **102,** 8–26.
11. Brenk Van den H. A. S., Kerr R. C., Madigan J. P. et al. (1966) Results from tourniquet anoxia and hyperbaric oxygen techniques combined with megavoltage treatment of sarcomas of bone and soft tissue. *Am. J. Roentgenol. Radium Ther. Nucl. Med.* **96,** 760–776.
12. Brenk Van den H. A. S., Kerr R. C., Richter W. et al. (1965) Enhancement of radiosensitivity of skin of patient by high pressure oxygen. *Br. J. Radiol.* **38,** 857–864.
13. Brenk Van den H. A. S., Richter W. and Hurley R. H. (1968) Radiosensitivity of the human oxygenated cervical spinal cord based on analysis of 357 cases receiving Mev X-rays in hyperbaric oxygen. *Br. J. Radiol.* **41,** 205–214.
14. Cade I. S. and McEwen J. B. (1967) Megavoltage radiotherapy in hyperbaric oxygen. A controlled trial. *Cancer* **20,** 817–821.
15. Cade I. S. and McEwen J. B. (1978) Clinical trials of radiotherapy in hyperbaric oxygen at Portsmouth (1964–1976). *Clin. Radiol.* **29,** 333–338.
16. Cade I. S., McEwen J. B., Dische S. et al. (1978) Hyperbaric oxygen and radiotherapy: a Medical Research Council trial in carcinoma of the bladder. *Br. J. Radiol.* **51,** 876–878.
17. Cade Memorial Symposium (1978) Interaction of radiation and antitumor drugs. *Int. J. Radiat. Biol.* **4,** 1–179.
18. Carlson V., Delclos L. and Fletcher G. H. (1967) Distant metastases in squamous-cell carcinoma of the uterine cervix. *Radiology* **88,** 961–966.
19. Chang C. H., Conley J. J. and Herbert C. (1973) Radiotherapy of advanced carcinoma of the oropharyngeal region under hyperbaric oxygenation. *Am. J. Roentgenol. Radium Ther. Nucl. Med.* **117,** 509–516.
20. Chapman J. D., Reuvers A. D., Borsa J. et al. (1972) Nitrofurans as radiosensitizers of hypoxic mammalian cells. *Cancer Res.* **32,** 2616–2624.
21. Churchill-Davidson I., Foster C. A., Wiernik G. (1966) The place of oxygen in radiotherapy. *Br. J. Radiol.* **39,** 321–331.
22. Churchill-Davidson I., Sanger C. and Thomlinson R. H. (1955) High-pressure oxygen and radiotherapy. *Lancet* **1,** 1091–1095.
23. Coxon A. and Pallis A. (1976) Metronidazole neuropathy. *J. Neurol. Neurosurg. Psychiatry* **39,** 403–407.
24. Coy P. and Dolman C. L. (1971) Radiation myelopathy in relation to oxygen level. *Br. J. Radiol.* **44,** 705–707.
25. Dawes P. J. D. K., Peckham M. J. and Steel G. G. (1978) The response of human tumour metastases to radiation and misonidazole. *Br. J. Cancer* **37,** Suppl. III, 290–296.

26. Deutsch G., Foster J. L., McFadzean J. et al. (1975) Human studies with 'high dose' metronidazole: a non-toxic radiosensitizer of hypoxic cells. *Br. J. Cancer* **31**, 75–80.
27. Dische S. (1974) The hyperbaric oxygen chamber in the radiotherapy of carcinoma of the uterine cervix. *Br. J. Radiol.* **47**, 99–107.
28. Dische S. (1978) Hyperbaric oxygen. The Medical Research Council trials and their clinical significance. *Br. J. Radiol.* **51**, 888–894.
29. Dische S., Gray A. J. and Zanelli G. D. (1976) Clinical testing of the radiosensitizer Ro 07-0582. II. Radiosensitization of normal and hypoxic skin. *Clin. Radiol.* **27**, 159–166.
30. Dische S., Martin C. M., Saunders M. I. et al. (1979a) Spinal cord damage and fractionation in the treatment of carcinoma of the bronchus. In preparation.
31. Dische S. and Saunders M. I. (1978) Clinical experience with misonidazole. *Br. J. Cancer* **37**, Suppl. III, 311–313.
32. Dische S., Saunders M. I., Anderson P. et al. (1978b) The neurotoxicity of misonidazole. The pooling of data from five centres. *Br. J. Radiol.* **51**, 1023–1024.
33. Dische S., Saunders M. I. and Flockhart I. R. (1978a) The optimum regime for the administration of misonidazole and the establishment of multi-centre clinical trials. *Br. J. Cancer* **37**, Suppl. III, 318–321.
34. Dische S., Saunders M. I., Flockhart I. R. et al. (1979b) Misonidazole. A drug for trial in radiotherapy and oncology. *Int. J. Radiat. Biol.* **5**, 851–860.
35. Dische S., Saunders M. I., Lee M. E. et al. (1977) Clinical testing of the radiosensitizer Ro 07-0582: Experience with multiple doses. *Br. J. Cancer* **35**, 567–579.
36. Dische S. and Zanelli G. D. (1976) Skin reaction – a quantitative system for measurement of radiosensitization in man. *Clin. Radiol.* **27**, 145–149.
37. Emery E. W. and Lucas B. G. (1964) The irradiation of conscious patients under high pressure oxygen. *Br. J. Radiol.* **37**, 475–477.
38. Fletcher G. L., Lindberg R. D., Caderao J. B. et al. (1977) Hyperbaric oxygen as a radiotherapeutic adjuvant in advanced carcinoma of the uterine cervix. Preliminary results of a randomized trial. *Cancer* **39**, 617–623.
39. Flockhart I. A., Large P., Troup D. et al. (1978a) Pharmokinetics and metabolic studies of the hypoxic cell radiosensitizer misonidazole. *Xenobiotica* **8**, 97–105.
40. Flockhart I. A., Troup D. and Marten T. R. (1978b). Unpublished observation.
41. Foster J. L., Flockhart I. R., Dische S. et al. (1975) Serum concentration measurements in man of the radiosensitizer Ro 07-0582 – some preliminary results. *Br. J. Cancer* **31**, 679–683.
42. Fowler J. F. (1975) Cancer Research Campaign Gray Laboratory, Mount Vernon Hospital, Northwood, Middx. Annual Report.
43. Fowler J. F., Adams G. E. and Denekamp J. (1976) Radiosensitizers of hypoxic cells in solid tumours. *Cancer Treat. Rev.* **3**, 227–256.
44. Glassburn J. R., Brady A. W. and Plenk H. P. (1977) Hyperbaric oxygen in radiotherapy. *Cancer* **39**, 751–765.
45. Glassburn J. R., Damsker J. I., Brady L. W. et al. (1974) Hyperbaric oxygen and radiation in the treatment of advanced cervical carcinoma. In: *Fifth International Hyperbaric Congress Proceedings, II,* 813–819 (Simon Fraser University).
46. Gray L. H., Conger A. O., Ebert M. (1953) The concentration of oxygen dissolved in tissues at the time of irradiation as a factor in radiotherapy. *Br. J. Radiol.* **26**, 638–648.
47. Gray A. J., Dische S., Adams G. E. (1976) Clinical testing of the radiosensitizer Ro 07-0582. I. Dose tolerance, serum and tumour concentration. *Clin. Radiol.* **27**, 151–157.

48. Hall E. J. and Biaglow J. (1977) Ro 07-0582 as a radiosensitizer and cytotoxic agent. *Int. J. Radiat. Biol.* **2,** 521–530.
49. Hendry J. H. and Sutton M. L. (1978) Care with radiosensitizers *Br. J. Radiol.* **51,** 927–928.
50. Henk J. M., Kunkler P. B. and Smith C. W. (1977) Radiotherapy and hyperbaric oxygen in head and neck cancer. *Lancet* **2,** 101–103.
51. Henk J. M. and Smith C. W. (1977) Radiotherapy and hyperbaric oxygen in head and neck cancer. Interim report of 2nd clinical trial. *Lancet* **2,** 104–105.
52. Jentzsch K., Karcher K. H., Kogelnik H. D. et al. (1977) Initial clinical experience with the radiosensitizing nitroimidazole Ro 07-0582. *Strahlentherapie,* **153,** 825.
53. Johnson R., Gomer C. and Pearce J. (1976) An investigation of the radiosensitizing effects of Ro 07-0582 on hypoxic skin in primates. *Int. J. Radiat. Biol.* **1,** 593–599.
54. Karim A. B. M. F. (1978) Prolonged metronidazole administration with protracted radiotherapy. *Br. J. Cancer* **37,** Suppl. III, 299–301.
55. Kogelnik H. D., Meyer H. J., Jentzsch K. et al. (1978) Further clinical experience of a phase I study with the hypoxic cell radiosensitizer misonidazole. *Br. J. Cancer* **37,** Suppl. III 281–285.
56. Medical Research Council (1978) A report of the Medical Research Council's Working Party on Radiotherapy and Hyperbaric Oxygen. *Lancet* **2,** 881–884.
57. Parkes M. W. (1974) Personal communication.
58. Parkes M. W. (1975) Personal communication.
59. Partington J., Koziol D., Chapman D. et al. (1979) A new side effect of the hypoxic cell sensitizer misonidazole. *Cancer Treat. Rep.* **63,** 123–125.
60. Phillips D. L., Morris S. and Orr J. S. (1966) Report on the first year's use of hyperbaric oxygen in supervoltage radiotherapy at the Western Infirmary, Glasgow. *Clin. Radiol.* **17,** 173–176.
61. Phillips T. L., Wasserman T. H., Johnson R. J. et al. (1978) The hypoxic cell sensitizer programme in the United States. *Br. J. Cancer* **37,** Suppl. III, 276–280.
62. Phillips T. L., Wasserman T. H., Johnson R. J. (1979) Initial clinical and pharmacologic evaluation of misonidazole (Ro 07-0582), an hypoxic cell sensitizer. *Int. J. Radiat.* **5,** 775–786.
63. Plenk H. P. (1972) Hyperbaric radiation therapy. Preliminary results of a randomized study of cancer of the urinary bladder and review of the 'oxygen experience'. *Am. J. Roentgenol. Radium Ther. Nucl. Med.* **114,** 152–157.
64. Proceedings of Third Meeting of Fundamental and Practical Aspects of Fast Neutrons and other High LET Particles in Clinical Radiotherapy. Held at The Hague, Amsterdam, 13–15 September, 1978.
65. Saunders M. I., Dische S., Anderson P. et al. (1978) The neurotoxicity of misonidazole and its relationship to dose, half-life and concentration in the serum. *Br. J. Cancer* **37,** Suppl. III. 268–270.
66. Saunders M. I., Dische S., Kogelnik H. D. et al. (1980) Skin rashes associated with misonidazole *Cancer Treatment Rep.* Awaiting Publication.
67. Scharer K. (1972) Selective alterations of Purkinje cells in the dog after oral administration of high doses of nitroimidazole derivatives. *Verhandlungen Dtsch. Ges. Pathol.* **56,** 407–410.
68. Sealy R. (1978a) A preliminary clinical study in the use of misonidazole in cancer of the head and neck. *Br. J. Cancer* **37,** Suppl. III 314–317.
69. Sealy R. (1978b) Personal communication.
70. Sheldon P. W. and Fowler J. F. (1978) Radiosensitization by misonidazole (Ro 07-0582) of fractionated X-rays in a murine tumour. *Br. J. Cancer* **37,** Suppl. III, 242–245.

71. Shigematsu Y., Fuchihata E., Makino T. et al. (1973) Radiotherapy with reduced fraction in head and neck cancer, with special reference to hyperbaric oxygen radiotherapy in maxillary sinus carcinoma (A controlled study). In: Sugahara T., Révész I. and Scott O. (eds.), *Fraction Size in Radiobiology and Radiotherapy*. Tokyo, pp. 180–187.
72. Suit H. D., Maimonis P., Rich T. A. et al. (1979) Anesthesia and efficacy of hyperbaric oxygen in radiation therapy. *Br. J. Radiol.* **52,** 244.
73. Thomlinson R. H. (1969) In: Proceedings of Carmel Conference on time and dose relationship in radiation biology as applied to radiotherapy. *Brookhaven Natn. Lab. Report No. 50203,* p. 242.
74. Thomlinson R. H., Dische S., Gray A. J. et al. (1976) Clinical testing of the radiosensitizer Ro 07-0582. III. Regression and re-growth of tumour. *Clin. Radiol.* **27,** 167–174.
75. Thomlinson R. H. and Gray L. H. (1955) The histological structure of some human lung cancers and the possible implications for radiotherapy. *Br. J. Cancer* **9,** 539–549.
76. Urtasun R. C. (1978) Personal communication.
77. Urtasun R. C., Band P., Chapman J. D. et al. (1976) Radiation and high dose metronidazole in supratentorial glioblastomas. *New Engl. J. Med.* **294,** 1364–1367.
78. Urtasun R. C., Band P. R., Chapman J. D. et al. (1977) Clinical phase I study of the hypoxic cell radiosensitizer Ro 07-0582, nitro-imidazole derivative. *Radiology* **122,** 801–804.
79. Urtasun R. C., Chapman J. D., Feldstein M. L. et al. (1978) Peripheral neuropathy related to misonidazole incidence and pathology. *Br. J. Cancer* **37,** Suppl. III, 271–275.
80. Urtasun R. C., Sturmwind J., Rabin H. et al. (1974) 'High-dose' metronidazole: A preliminary pharmacological study prior to its investigational use in clinical radiotherapy trials. *Br. J. Radiol.* **47,** 297–299.
81. Ward A. J., Dixon B. and Stubbs B. (1978) A clinical appraisal of hyperbaric oxygen in cervix cancer (Abstract). *Br. J. Radiol.* **51,** 150–151.
82. Watson T. A. and Banerjee P. (1969) Clinical experience with hyperbaric oxygen in radiotherapy. *J. Can. Ass. Radiol.* **20,** 132–137.
83. Watson E. R., Halnan K. E., Dische S. et al. (1978) Hyperbaric oxygen and radiotherapy: A Medical Research Council trial in carcinoma of the cervix. *Br. J. Radiol.* **51,** 879–887.
84. Wildermuth O. (1965) The case for hyperbaric oxygen radiotherapy. *JAMA* **191,** 986–990.
85. Wildermuth O., Warner G. A. and Marty R. (1969) Clinical hybaroxic radiotherapy after five years. *Radiology* **93,** 1149–1154.
86. Wiltshire C. R., Workman P., Watson J. V. et al. (1978) Clinical studies with misonidazole. *Br. J. Cancer* **37,** Suppl. III, 286–289.
87. Withers H. R., Thames H. D., Flow B. L. et al. (1978) The relationship of acute to late skin injury in 2 and 5 fraction/week gamma ray therapy. *Int. J. Radiat. Biol.* **4,** 595–601.

W. H. Sutherland

7 Accuracy in Radiotherapy: a survey of some effects of human fallibility

INTRODUCTION

In the treatment of cancer by radiation the primary objective is the delivery of the correct amount and distribution of absorbed energy to the target volume of tumour-bearing tissue. Expressed thus, the process seems straightforward, but in practice every treatment is the end product of a long sequence of steps, each involving the manipulation, interpretation and recording of data. When data are handled, whether in the form of tabulated figures, slide rule or keyboard calculations, readings from meters, settings on scales and timers, or entries in treatment records, mistakes are certain to arise from the fallibility of the human operator. In order to achieve the above primary objective every radiotherapy department should actively pursue a secondary objective of avoiding the effects of human fallibility.

The literature of industrial psychology contains many examples of investigations of the mistake rates due to human fallibility in repetitive tasks of all kinds. Minor and Revesman [16] found a mistake rate of 1–2 per cent amongst trained operators entering 10 digit numbers into keyboards under 'good' conditions, while Klemmer and Lockhead [15] found slightly lower rates for experienced card punch operators in the New York Federal Reserve Bank. A study by Hill and Wigmore [11] of mistakes in drug prescribing and administration showed a rate of 15·3 per cent dropping to 4·2 per cent with the introduction of redesigned drug sheets. Blake [1] and Colquhoun [3] both found average mistake rates around 2–5 per cent during extensive research on the effects of environment and time of day on human performance in a variety of tasks requiring attention to mathematical and visual detail.

A mistake rate of 1–2 per cent in the highly quantitative speciality of radiotherapy could lead to an unacceptable number of incorrect treatments per year. Several groups in the USA have published results from retrospective or concurrent mistake surveys. Herring et al. [10] found mistakes in accumulated tumour dose of 5 per cent or more in 48 per cent of all treatments in one centre, and in 7·8 per cent of 308 treatments reviewed retrospectively in a second centre in which special steps had already been taken to guard against numerical mistakes. Kartha et al. [14] analysed 1200 patient records and found tumour dose mistakes of 5 per cent or more in 10 per cent of all treatments given with two cobalt machines up to 1972. In a later study, covering 4688 patients treated during the period 1971–75, Kartha [13] reported a revised mistake rate of 7·2 per cent. No comparable reports have been published yet from centres outside the USA. ICRU Report 24 [12] contains a short review of the frequency of errors and mistakes in radiotherapy.

At this point it is useful to distinguish between the terms 'error' and 'mistake'. An error is the difference between the actual value and the recorded value of any quantity such as the reading of a meter, the setting on a timer or the dose at a point in a patient. All measurements and settings of physical quantities involve errors. These can be subdivided into systematic errors associated with such factors as imperfect calibration, linearity and scaling of meters, time lags in the operation of relays, small irregularities in tabulated data etc. and random errors caused by factors such as parallax on a meter reading, temperature and pressure effects on dosemeter readings, etc. Random and systematic errors combine to produce a certain total uncertainty in the recorded value of any quantity. Sometimes larger uncertainties are present which are difficult to estimate at the present state of our knowledge, such as biological variation in the response of different patients to the same absorbed dose.

Mistakes, on the other hand, are quite unpredictable and are generally caused by inattention, misunderstanding, misjudgement or just plain carelessness. For example, an actual dose of 213·81 rad may be read as 215 by an operator partly because the dosemeter indicates slightly high at that particular part of the scale, and partly because the operator uses the left eye for reading meters and therefore biases all readings upwards by parallax. These are examples of errors, but if the same operator then enters the result into the treatment record as 251 rad he/she has made a plain (but quite common) mistake involving a reversal of the order of two or more adjacent figures in a number.

It is generally very easy to distinguish between errors and mistakes, but there may be some overlap, particularly when the magnitudes are small. For example, if the actual dose of 213·81 rad mentioned above was recorded as 212 it would be impossible to tell whether the operator had made an error in the other direction (e.g. by reading the meter with the right eye) or a plain mistake by writing down 212 instead of 215. Although very little has been written about mistakes, the literature on the effects of errors in radiotherapy would fill many volumes. For a recent comprehensive analysis of errors, see Campion et al. [2]. In this chapter I shall deal only with the effects of mistakes resulting from human fallibility.

METHODS AND RESULTS

Numerical mistakes can be detected and corrected at an early stage in each treatment by means of a twice-weekly check through all treatment prescriptions and records, before they have a significant effect on the tumour dose. Although a relatively simple regular manual check of this kind practically eliminates the effect of numerical mistakes throughout the department, in principle it is better to seek ways to prevent the occurrence of the mistakes at source. Any action of this kind must be based on a detailed knowledge of the nature of the mistakes. The purpose of this report is to present an analysis of the mistakes that have been picked up in one particular centre over a period of 9 years. A full check of the records of all patients on treatment takes about a half-day by one person, and the task is rotated amongst the three or so medical physicists directly concerned with radiotherapy treatments.

Mistakes are entered on a check list (*Fig. 7.1*) and generally fall into one of three main categories:

A. Mistakes in the recording of Given Dose (GD) or Tumour Dose (TD). At the time of discovery of the mistake, the patient was receiving the prescribed dose, but the wrong value was being entered in the treatment record.
B. Mistakes which, if uncorrected, would cause the final Tumour Dose to be wrong by less than ±5 per cent at the completion of the course of treatment.
C. Mistakes which, if uncorrected, would cause the final Tumour Dose to be wrong by ±5 per cent or more at the completion of the course of treatment.

Mistakes of type A are nearly always simple slips by the radiographer in the addition of the daily Given Dose or Tumour Dose to the cumulative total during the filling in of the entries on the lower half of page 2 of the treatment record (*see Fig. 7.3*). Because each course of treatment provides a large number of opportunities for mistakes of type A, they outnumber all others in the final analysis. Even in the absence of a system of regular checking, they are normally self-correcting, since the appropriate column fails to reach the expected total at the end of treatment, and a quick check reveals and corrects the wrong entry without any effect on the actual dose received by the patient. Nevertheless, mistakes of this kind could affect the tumour dose if a course of treatment is interrupted and re-prescribed on the basis of the last entry in the Cumulative Given Dose or Cumulative Tumour Dose column, which may be carrying an undetected numerical mistake at that particular time. No instance has been recorded of this actually occurring.

Mistakes of type A are entered by a tick in line 7 of *Fig. 7.1* accompanied by a tick either in line 8 or line 9 according to the nature of the mistake. The second and fourth examples in *Fig. 7.1* are typical. In most cases the cause of the wrong entry is failure to notice that the Daily Given Dose or Daily Tumour Dose has been changed during the course of the treatment; the original dose from the top of the column is added in as the contribution from a subsequent fraction, instead of the new dose which appears as a correction further down the column. However, sometimes the mistake is only a simple arithmetical slip in the addition, and because this is just as likely to occur in the 'thousands' position it can lead

DATE/PHYSICIST	12/4/77 W.H. Sutherland			
NAME OF PATIENT	DICKENS	JONES	POOLE	NEWBERRY
HOSPITAL No.	77/3057	77/3281	76/4103	77/3165
MACHINE	Co	Co	LA	LA
Mistake made by	MO	R	C	R
Initials	L.S.M	W.G.	A.U.F	V.T.
TD O.K. at end of T		×		×
CUM. GD mistake				×
TD TO DATE mistake		× ×		
TD ± % by end of T	−14%		+5%	
MO – misread % d.d. chart			×	
MO – wrong % d.d. chart				
MO – bad maths	×			
MO – 100% TD/GD i/o % on plan				
MO – TD% for 1 field i/o both				
MO – TD% full sep i/o half-sep				
MO – wrong data on T/plan				
MO – wrong transfer, plan to TS				
MO – KX10 cut-out factors				
MO – STAB cut-out factors				
Cervix wedge chart mistake				
FSD/SSD factor mistake				
STAB/KX10 output chart mistake				
R – wrong wedge used on LA				
R – wrong MD used on LA				
R – Co60 calculator misread				
R – LA correction factor				
R – bad maths				
R – muddle after T/alterations				
R – wrong transfer, p1 to p2 TS				
R – used T/time of 'other' Co60				
R – could not read MO's writing				
R – could not read own writing				
R – unclassified mistake				
	May have been worked for TD 3000 i/o 3500	(a) 3450 i/o 2450 for "TD TO DATE" ON 7th FRACTION AND 4500 i/o 3500 AT END. EXCESS NOT NOTICED. (b) DITTO IN 2nd COLUMN BUT 3625 i/o 2625 AND 4750 i/o 3750	121 % i/o 127 %	466 i/o 456 THO' CORRECT in adjacent column carrying same figures

Fig. 7.1. **All treatment record sheets are checked for potential mistakes twice per week, and details are recorded on this form for later analysis.**

to a mistake that is numerically very large, as in the second example in *Fig. 7.1*. Table 7.1 shows a summary of a representative 'run' of type A mistakes made by one radiographer during a 4-month period.

Mistakes in category B are often the result of incorrect interpolation between columns or rows of tabulated data, failure to allow for the effects

Table 7.1. Summary of Type A Mistakes
Examples of type A mistakes made by one radiographer in adding up the Cumulative GD or TD-to-Date columns of the treatment records during a 4-mth period. In all instances the actual dose to the patient was correct at the time of the check

Added 1000 rad too much		*Added 100 rad too little*	
30/1/73	entered 2855 instead of 1855	17/1/73	entered 2837 instead of 2937
11/4/73*	entered 3450 instead of 2450	23/1/73	entered 818 instead of 918
11/4/73*	entered 3625 instead of 2625	13/2/73**	entered 965 instead of 1065
24/4/73	entered 2143 instead of 1143	18/4/73	entered 1028 instead of 1128
Added 100 rad too much		*Other addition mistakes*	
12/1/73	entered 3700 instead of 3600	12/1/73	entered 2050 instead of 2000
17/1/73	entered 4150 instead of 4050	23/1/73	entered 250 instead of 375
13/2/73**	entered 1731 instead of 1631	13/2/73**	entered 2640 instead of 2650
13/2/73**	entered 424 instead of 324	13/2/73**	entered 1069 instead of 1068
		27/2/73	entered 1705 instead of 1765
		1/5/73	entered 199 instead of 189

of reduced area when calculating a shadow tray treatment, or just deliberate 'rounding off' by the person carrying out the calculation. In many instances it is not possible to determine the exact reason and it is entered in the mistake record simply as 'bad math'.

Mistakes of type C are analysed fully for magnitude, distribution, causation, etc. By reworking the calculation backwards an attempt is made to find the most likely cause of the mistake so that a full record can be made at the time of detection. An appeal to the person who made the mistake rarely produces a satisfactory explanation; since he is unaware of having made a mistake he is also *ipso facto* unaware of the reasons why he did so. Mistakes of type C, particularly those involving large percentages, are referred at the time of correction to the consultant in charge of the patient.

Table 7.2 shows the yearly rates since 1969 of type C mistakes per 100 patients treated, and corresponding totals published by the American groups are included for comparison. The lower rate in Cardiff may be due partly to differences of interpretation. For example, the Cardiff rates in Table 7.2 are confined to type C mistakes as defined above, and do not include those type A mistakes which were greater than ±5 per cent since the latter were unlikely to have any real effect on the actual tumour dose received by the patient. Their inclusion would bring the Cardiff yearly rates into reasonable agreement with the American figures. The progressive decrease in the Cardiff yearly mistake rate is the result of a number of small improvements in data presentation and handling, introduced as a result of accumulating experience in recognizing and eliminating steps and situations which are particularly mistake-prone.

Table 7.2. Yearly Rates of Type C Mistakes
Yearly rates of type C mistakes per 100 patients treated (mistakes of ±5 per cent or more in the final TD if not corrected). Comparable average rates are included from four similar surveys in the USA.

	1969	*1970*	*1971*	*1972*	*1973*	*1974*	*1975*	*1976*	*1977*	*1978*
Cardiff	4·0	4·4	4·0	4·0	3·4	3·4	2·7	2·2	2·7	2·1
Kartha (1976) Chicago					7·2					
Kartha et al. (1972) Chicago					10					
Herring et al. (1970) Centre A					48					
Herring et al. (1970) Centre B					7·8					

Table 7.3 presents a summary of 4122 potential mistakes picked up in the 10 years during which the twice-weekly check has been in operation. The category of staff responsible for the mistakes is coded as follows: R = radiographer; MO = medical staff below the rank of consultant radiotherapist; C = consultant radiotherapist; P = physicist. On average a mistake of some kind was found in the records of 17·9 per cent of all patients treated (neglecting the small effect of the occasional occurrence of multiple mistakes in the records of a single patient). However, more than half of these (2381) were type A mistakes by radiographers which at the time of detection were not affecting the actual tumour dose in any way, and would be extremely unlikely to do so even if they remained hidden right to the end of the course of treatment.

Radiotherapists (C + MO) were responsible for 66·6 per cent of the type B mistakes and for 73·8 per cent of the type C mistakes. The larger numbers of mistakes made by medical staff below consultant rank are in direct proportion to the larger numbers of treatments prescribed, and do not reflect any real difference in mistake rates between consultants and their more junior colleagues. A random sample of treatment records showed a MO : C ratio of 4·3 : 1 in the numbers of treatments prescribed, close to the corresponding 4·0 : 1 ratio in the mistakes of types B and C made by medical officers and consultants respectively in Table 7.3. The small numbers of mistakes attributed to physicists in Table 7.3 indicates only the lack of opportunities for making the kind of mistakes that would show up in this survey, and carries no suggestion that physicists are in any way better at avoiding human fallibility mistakes.

The rest of this chapter will concentrate mainly on the 742 type C mistakes represented by the bottom block of Table 7.3. If these were really caused by human fallibility we should expect to find them randomly

Table 7.3. Summary of Potential Mistakes
Yearly summary of the 4122 mistakes which were detected and corrected before they could affect the final Tumour Dose of 23 089 patients treated during 1969–78

		1969	*1970*	*1971*	*1972*	*1973*	*1974*	*1975*	*1976*	*1977*	*1978*		*Total*	
TYPE A TD not changed	R	198	183	160	196	212	214	260	388	332	238			
	MO	5	1	–	4	1	–	–	–	–	–			
	C	–	2	1	–	–	–	2	–	1	–			
	P	–	–	–	1	–	–	–	–	–	–			
	Total	203	186	161	201	213	214	262	388	333	238		2399 10·4%	
TYPE B TD change <5%	R	36	32	32	21	35	37	53	27	35	8			
	MO	33	45	44	64	74	70	63	36	63	33			
	C	8	16	17	7	12	16	18	17	6	11			4122 17·9%
	P	–	4	–	2	–	1	–	–	4	1			
	Total	77	97	93	94	121	124	134	80	108	53	981 4·2%		
TYPE C TD change ⩾5%	R	26	26	20	23	20	21	15	3	12	15			
	MO	36	47	46	58	54	41	32	34	51	30		1723 7·5%	
	C	17	6	17	12	8	14	12	14	7	11			
	P	–	7	1	–	2	–	–	2	–	2			
	Total	79	86	84	93	84	76	59	53	70	58	742 3·2%		
Patients treated		1954	1933	2124	2309	2500	2243	2209	2456	2555	2806		23 089	

distributed between overdoses and underdoses. Any significant departure from a random distribution should be traceable to an excess of particular mistakes always operating in one direction, and it should then be possible to eliminate these particular mistakes by finding and removing the causes. Table 7.4 shows a subdivision of the type C mistakes into those that would have caused overdoses and those that would have caused underdoses if not

Table 7.4. Summary of Subdivided Type C Mistakes
742 mistakes that would have changed the final TD by ±5 per cent or more if not corrected (type C) (all years, 1969–1978. 23 089 patients)

	Overdose				*Underdose*			
	MO+C	*R*	*P*	*Total*	*MO+C*	*R*	*P*	*Total*
5%–10%	150	37	3	190	175	37	6	218
10%–20%	64	18	1	83	89	37	1	127
20%–30%	25	10	–	35	10	19	–	29
30%–40%	8	1	–	9	6	5	–	11
40%–50%	4	1	–	5	3	5	–	8
50%–60%	2	1	1	4	1	3	1	5
60%–70%	2	2	–	4	–	–	1	1
70%–80%	–	1	–	1	1	–	–	1
80%–90%	–	–	–	–	–	–	–	–
90%–100%	2	3	–	5	3	–	–	3
>100%	2	1	–	3	–	–	–	–
				339				403

corrected. The small excess of underdoses in Table 7.4, particularly those around 10 per cent in the MO + C column, occurred mainly during 1977 and was the result of an increased misuse of linear accelerator instead of cobalt percentage depth dose figures.

Table 7.4 also shows that there is an approximately inverse-exponential relationship between magnitudes and numbers of mistakes. An analysis of the main causes of the mistakes during the 10 year period should provide valuable data for modifying the system in order to reduce the mistake making opportunities. It could be argued that such an analysis provides the *only* valid basis for modifying the system, and that any attempt to design an automated system to prevent mistakes without the back-up of a prior survey of the kind described here is likely to be ineffective. In particular, a good system must set out to reduce the type C mistakes.

In this centre it is the responsibility of the consultant or his registrar to enter all relevant prescription details on page 1 of the treatment record, *Fig. 7.2.* This includes any data look-up and calculations that are required in working out the prescription. Most of the type B and type C mistakes made by the radiotherapists could be avoided by rearranging the system to eliminate numerical manipulation by the radiotherapist during prescribing. To some extent this would just transfer the mistake-making opportunities

TELE-COBALT

SOUTH WALES RADIOTHERAPY & ONCOLOGY SERVICE	SURNAME MR./MRS./MISS	Unit No.
DIAGNOSIS	FIRST NAMES	Date of Birth
	ADDRESS	Tel. No.
		Occupation

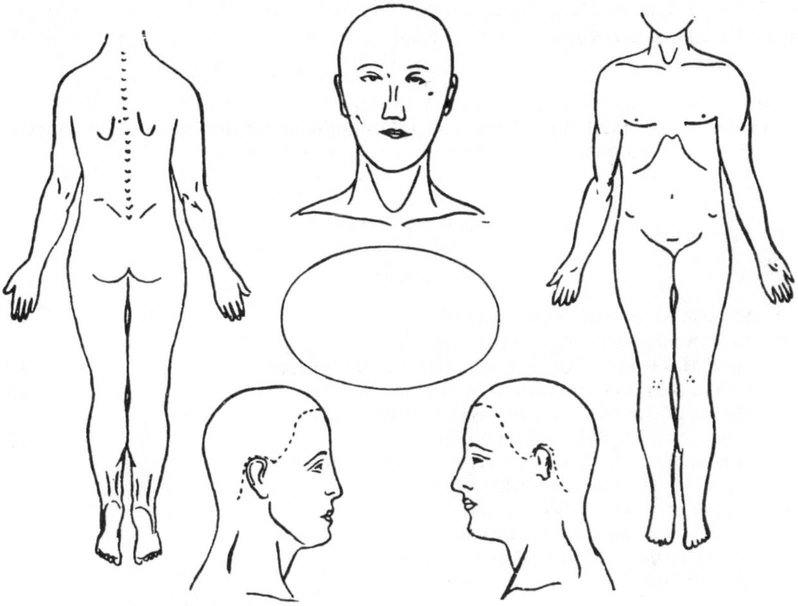

METHODS OF: BEAM DIRECTION / COMPENSATION

MEASUREMENTS:

PROPOSED:— NUMBER OF FRACTIONS / FRACTIONS/WEEK / DURATION

INTENTION RADICAL / PALLIATIVE

PRESCRIBED BY— / DATE

FIELD	FIELD SIZE	WDG	SSD / RADIUS	TUMOUR DOSE	% T.D.	% G.D.	GIVEN DOSE	SKIN/Sub. Dermal MAX DOSE	REMARKS

SUMMARY DURATION TOTAL TUMOUR DOSE MAX. SKIN/SUBDERMAL DOSE

NUMBER OF FRACTIONS FROM TO

Fig. 7.2. Page 1 of the standard treatment record sheet used in Velindre Hospital for patients receiving telecobalt therapy.

to a different category of staff. More important, it would remove a vital training element from the work of a teaching centre, where the junior radiotherapist must be trained to take full responsibility for his own prescription, which includes responsibility for selection and manipulation of the appropriate data. It should also include responsibility for his own mistakes!

Table 7.5 presents a breakdown of type C mistakes by radiotherapists into 12 main categories, with a final 'unclassified' section for the small

Table 7.5. Summary of Causes of Type C Mistakes
Summary of causes of type C mistakes by radiotherapists that would have changed the final TD by ±5 per cent or more if not corrected (all years, 1969–78)

1.	Bad maths	(a)	unclassified	159	254
		(b)	'half sep.' errors	56	
		(c)	3500/4000 error	25	
		(d)	multiply/divide	14	
2.	Misread percentage depth dose chart				141
3.	Read wrong percentage depth dose chart				49
4.	Used 100% instead of %TD or %GD marked on plan				17
5.	Wrong data transfer: plan to treatment sheet				15
6.	Misuse of Cut Out/Air Gap factors (superficial)				12
7.	Misuse of FSD/SSD correction factors				11
8.	Misuse of Cut Out/Air Gap factors (orthovoltage)				10
9.	%TD for full instead of half separation				9
10.	Misuse of cervix wedge correction factors				6
11.	Wrong data marked on planning request				5
12.	%TD for one field instead of two fields				5
13.	Unclassified				13
	Total				547

number of miscellaneous mistakes that defy classification. The numbers in group 1(a) are probably too high since this category tends to be a 'rubbish bin' for dumping all those unexplained mistakes that have no apparent cause. Group 1(b) reveals a rather unexpected weakness in dividing the patient thickness by 2, preparatory to looking up the central percentage depth dose value for a parallel-opposed pair of beams. Many variations turn up, but the tendency is to produce an answer that is 1 cm too small when the thickness is an odd number (e.g. 17/2 = 7·5). This bias is another contributing factor to the small excess of potential underdoses around 10 per cent in Table 7.4.

Group 1(c) represents the situation where the radiotherapist fills in the intended Tumour Dose or Given Dose (e.g. 3500 rad) and then apparently calculates for a quite different value (e.g. 4000 rad). The two numbers often differ by multiples of 500 rad which can be in either direction. For example, this mistake occurred 7 times during 1977 with the following pairs of numbers: 4320/4000, 3000/5000, 3975/4500 and 3500/4000 repeated four times. The checking physicist never sees the real cause of this mistake, which might be interruptions by phone or otherwise between the entry of the intended dose and the completion of the calculation, or a distracting conversation nearby which 'imprints' the wrong number. Group 1(d) involves multiplying instead of dividing, or dividing instead of multiplying by a factor, usually when calculating percentage tumour doses or percentage given doses. The frequency of this mistake has increased since the introduction of electronic calculators because the operations make use of adjacent keys.

Table 7.6. Summary of Type C and Type A Mistakes in One Session
A short run of 4 type C and 2 type A mistakes picked up during one checking session. The figures indicate the percentage effect on the final Tumour Dose if the mistakes were not corrected

Pt. No.	*Made by*	*Unit*	*Effect on TD*	*Cause*
1.	MO	^{60}Co	+100%	Used %TD for one field instead of both fields of parallel/opposed pair.
2.	MO	^{60}Co	+100%	Used %TD for one field instead of both fields of parallel/opposed pair.
3.	MO	^{60}Co	+36%	Used percentage depth dose for full separation instead of half separation of parallel/opposed pair.
4.	MO	^{60}Co	+28%	Given Dose read from wrong column of cervix wedge table.
5.	R	^{60}Co	–	Cumulative Given Dose entered as 2393 instead of 1393.
6.	R	^{60}Co	–	Cumulative Given Dose entered as 2140 instead of 2240.

Group 2 mistakes often arise from interpolation between the adjacent pairs of numbers rather than the correct pair of numbers in a percentage depth dose table, and are usually difficult to distinguish from mistakes in group 1(b). Group 3 is similar to group 2 but is a special case where the percentage depth dose table is read correctly, but for the wrong treatment machine. Group 4 mistakes are usually caused by failure to make use of the percentage Given Doses or percentage Tumour Dose entered on the treatment plan, the prescription being calculated as if all percentages are 100 per cent.

Mistakes in groups 9 and 12 are relatively rare, but constitute a special problem because they contribute to the potential overdoses of large magnitude in Table 7.4. As an example containing both of these categories, Table 7.6 lists a short run of mistakes picked up during a single afternoon checking session. The same person was responsible for the first three entries.

Table 7.7 contains an analysis of the 181 type C mistakes made by radiographers during the years 1969–78. These occur mainly when the entries on the top of page 2 of the treatment record (*Fig. 7.3*) are filled in by the radiographer. The calculation of the given dose per fraction and the treatment time or accelerator monitor dose for each field is carried out by the radiographer in charge of the particular treatment machine. The calculation includes various machine-associated correction factors for items such as field size, shadow tray or table attenuation, non-standard FSD, etc.

Table 7.7. Summary of Causes of Type C Mistakes
Summary of causes of type C mistakes by radiographers that would have changed the final TD by ± 5 per cent or more if not corrected (all years, 1969–78)

1.	Bad maths	53
2.	Misread cobalt treatment time calculator	19
3.	Misread output chart for superficial or orthovoltage machine	18
4.	Used output for area of applicator instead of area of cut-out (superficial machine)	16
5.	Mistakes resulting directly or indirectly from prescription changes during the course of treatment	14
6.	Misuse of accelerator correction factors	8
7.	Wrong data transfer from page 1 to page 2 of the treatment record	8
8.	Interchange of the figures 2 and 3 (*see text*)	6
9.	Used treatment time of 'wrong' cobalt machine	6
10.	Misuse of cervix wedge factors	5
11.	Misread bad writing or figures of MO	5
12.	Misuse of FSD/SSD correction factors	5
13.	Unclassified	18
	Total	181

Again 'bad maths' contributed the greatest number of mistakes, but a smaller percentage of the total than in Table 7.5. (29 per cent and 46 per cent respectively). Arithmetical slips by the radiographers are more varied in character and show no evidence for any recurring patterns that would justify further subdivision within group 1.

Group 2 in Table 7.7 provides one example of a general principle that became evident in the early stages of the work reported here: as soon as a mistake-prone situation has been identified, the introduction of new corrective procedures or new devices will usually reduce the total number of mistakes, but will at the same time give rise to new unexpected mistakes associated with the new procedures. In order to eliminate mistakes caused by misreading of cobalt-60 output charts and the subsequent slide rule or manual calculation of the treatment time to set on the machine timer, a special circular calculator was introduced (*Fig. 7.4*). This stores all the output data for one cobalt machine and provides the radiographer with a direct read-out of the treatment time for any given dose and any field size.

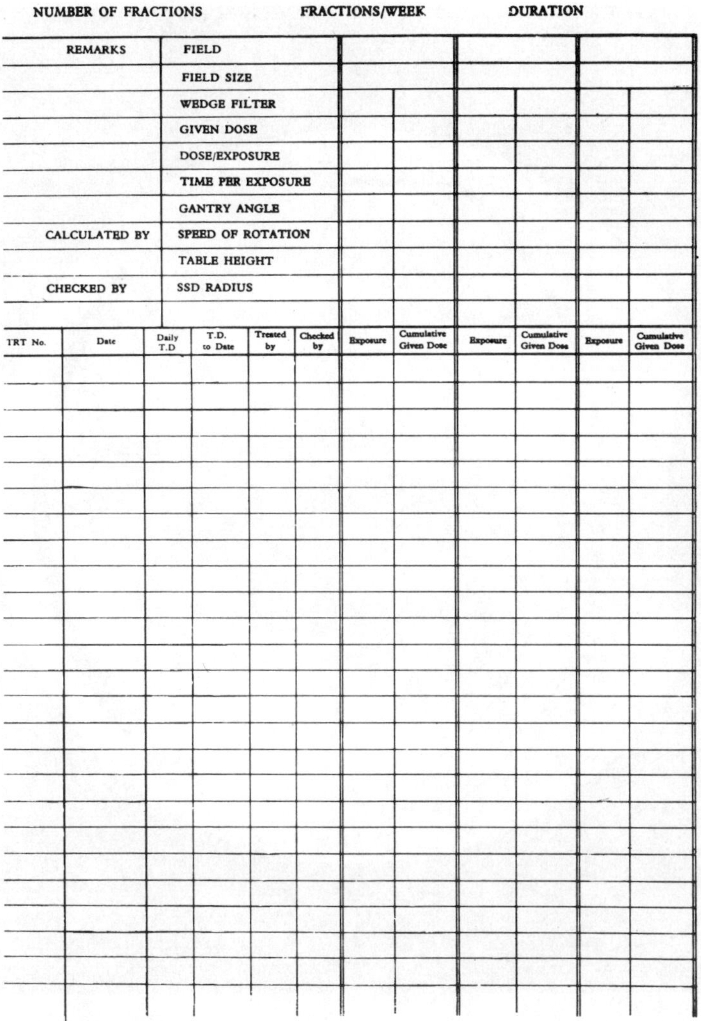

NUMBER OF FRACTIONS FRACTIONS/WEEK DURATION

REMARKS	FIELD						
	FIELD SIZE						
	WEDGE FILTER						
	GIVEN DOSE						
	DOSE/EXPOSURE						
	TIME PER EXPOSURE						
	GANTRY ANGLE						
CALCULATED BY	SPEED OF ROTATION						
	TABLE HEIGHT						
CHECKED BY	SSD RADIUS						

TRT No.	Date	Daily T.D	T.D. to Date	Treated by	Checked by	Exposure	Cumulative Given Dose	Exposure	Cumulative Given Dose	Exposure	Cumulative Given Dose

Fig. 7.3. Page 2 of the standard treatment record sheet used in Velindre Hospital for patients receiving telecobalt therapy.

A simple adjustment each month takes care of the effect of decay throughout the lifetime of a particular source. A full description of the device has appeared [17] and only brief details are included here to illustrate the present point.

These calculators save much time and effort for the radiographers and without doubt have prevented a large number of mistakes, but in turn they

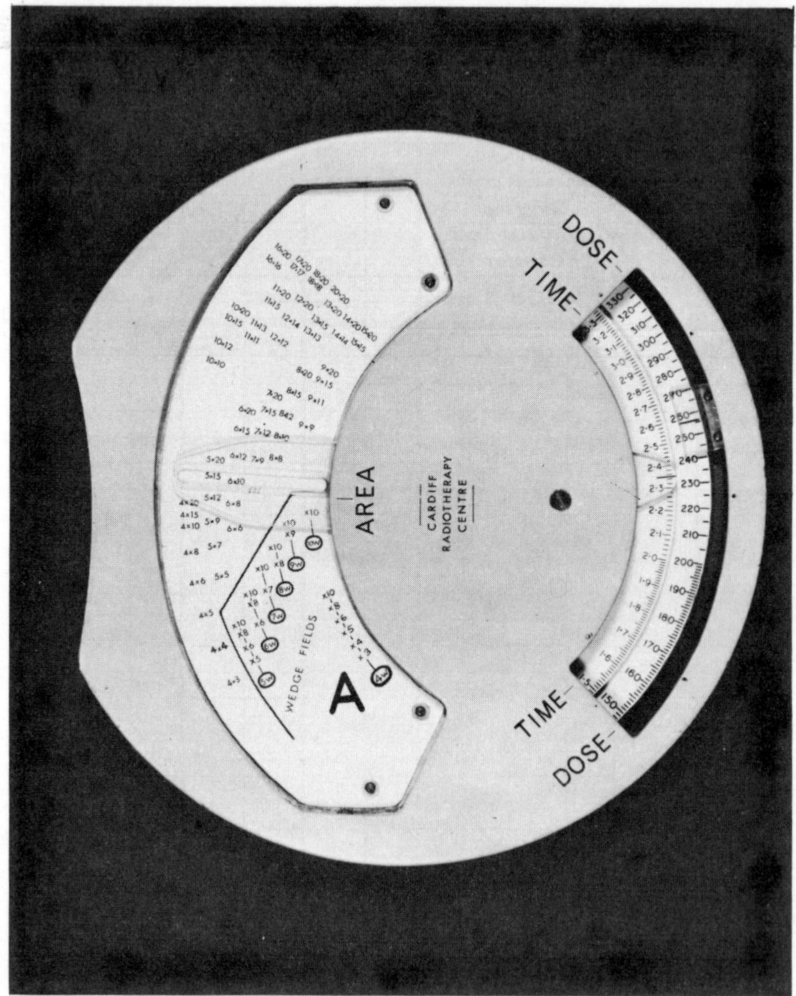

Fig. 7.4. A treatment time calculator, designed to avoid mistakes in treatment parameters in telecobalt therapy. (Reproduced by courtesy of 'British Journal of Radiology'.)

have contributed the second largest category (group 2) of type C mistakes in Table 7.7. These arose from misreading the TIME scale and a selection – by no means complete – of actual examples is shown in *Fig. 7.5.* The figures in brackets show the effect that the mistake would have had on the tumour dose if not corrected before the completion of the course of treatment. The misreading is sometimes associated with the

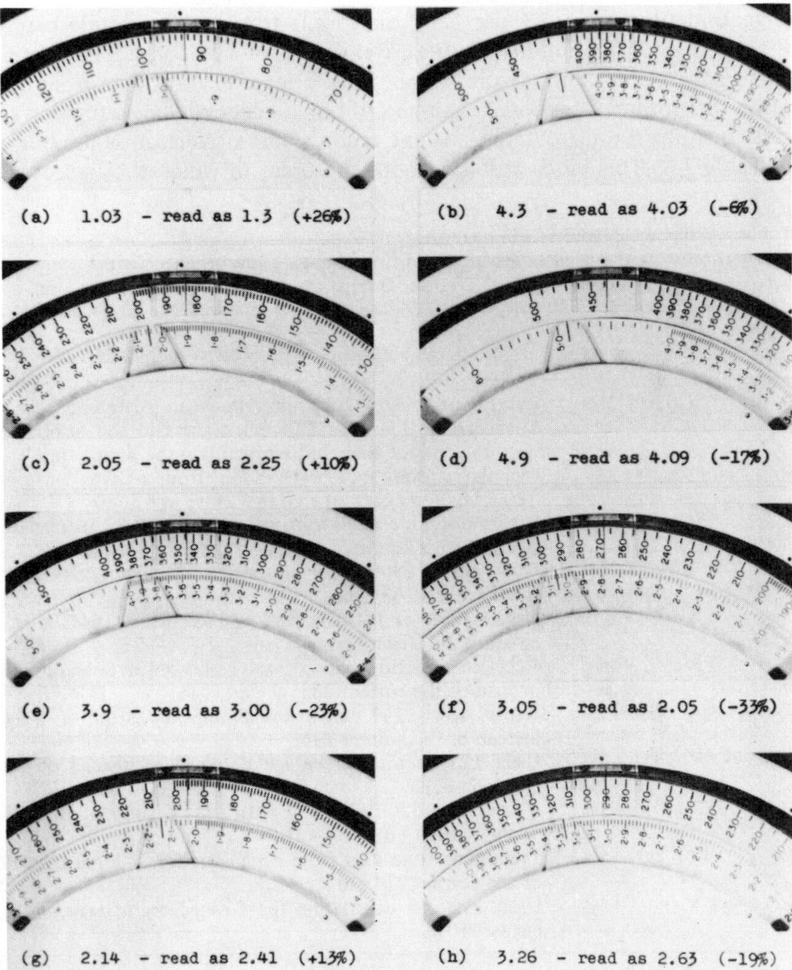

Fig. 7.5. Examples of some mistakes caused by misreading the scales of the treatment time calculator shown in *Fig. 7.4.* The figure in brackets shows the effect on final Tumour Dose if not corrected.

changes that occur in the pattern of subdivision at several places in all logarithmically based scales, for example, *Fig. 7.5(b)* and *Fig. 7.5(c)*. Directly opposite forms of misreading are illustrated in *Fig. 7.5(a)* and *Fig. 7.5(b)*. *Fig. 7.5(c)* represents a slight variation on *Fig. 7.5(a)*. *Fig. 7.5(d)* is a particularly bad version of *Fig. 7.5(b)* not related to any feature of the scale. *Fig. 7.5(e)* arose because the cursor line momentarily covered the bar of the figure 9 and made it look like 0, showing how a relatively large underdose of –23 per cent can result from a very simple cause. Finally, *Fig. 7.5(g)* and *Fig. 7.5(h)* are examples of a common tendency to change the order of the figures when transferring numerical data from one place to another. Occasional examples of this tendency by all categories of staff turn up throughout the mistake records and a selection is presented in Table 7.8. This raises a doubt about the order in which the figures are

Table 7.8. Type C Mistakes when transferring Data
A selection type C mistakes arising from interchanging the order of figures, showing the percentage effect on the final Tumour Dose if the mistakes were not corrected

Made by	*Unit*	*Effect on TD*	*Cause*
R	^{60}Co	–28%	Treatment time of 2·34 min entered in treatment record, but correct time was 3·24 min. (girl said she 'probably used the correct time, but wrote down the wrong time')
R	^{60}Co	+23%	Calculated the 'Dose per fraction' from a Given Dose of 3800 when the prescribed Given Dose was 3080
R	^{60}Co	–20%	Treatment time read from calculator as 2·62 instead of the correct 3·26 min
MO	^{60}Co	–17%	Wrote down 1360 as the prescribed Given Dose instead of the intended 1630 rad
C	LA	+17%	Used a %TD of 140% instead of the correct 104% in calculating the Given Dose
R	LA	+16%	Accelerator strip chart recorder showed a dose of 328 instead of the correct 283
R	LA	+7%	Wrote down 143 when calculating the Monitor Dose instead of the correct 134
MO	^{60}Co	–8%	Used 121 as the percentage depth dose instead of the correct 112%
MO	KX10	+7%	Wrote down 6200 when calculating the Given Dose instead of the correct 6020
R	^{60}Co	+5%	Treatment time read from calculator for 241 rad instead of the correct 214 rad
MO	LA	+5%	Used 110% in calculating the Given Dose instead of the correct 101%

actually entered into digital timers or accelerator dosemeters, and points the need for a recording system as suggested in the Recommendations of the Radiotherapy Apparatus Safety Measures Panel (DHSS, [4]) on all major treatment machines to guard against the drastic effect of an occasional interchange in the order of the figures when setting up a patient treatment.

Some of the calculator mistakes featured in *Fig. 7.5* could probably be avoided by redesigning the scale, but this would undoubtedly introduce a fresh variety of misreading, and in any case would represent a diminishing return from a considerable effort. For example, only two of these mistakes were found in 1977 and none in 1978. The treatment time calculators will drop out of use with the commissioning of a minicomputer system under construction at the time of writing to monitor all treatments on two cobalt machines, with later extension to two linear accelerators. This system will cover most of the known mistake-making situations that have come to light during this work, from the radiotherapist's prescription calculation right through to the confirmation and recording of the machine parameters and the cumulative dose. Advance descriptions are available [6, 7, 8].

Group 8 in Table 7.7 represents a run of very unusual mistakes of a similar type made by the same radiographer. Because of their special interest they are presented in detail in Table 7.9. In each case the figure 2 was substituted for the figure 3, resulting in considerable potential under-dosage. Because the checking routine is rotated amongst several physicists the special nature of the sequence was not noticed until nearly a month had elapsed, covering the first five entries in Table 7.9. When questioned

Table 7.9. Unusual 'Run' of Type C Mistakes
An unusual run of type C mistakes made by the same radiographer and involving the figures 2 and 3. The effect on the final Tumour Dose if the mistakes were not corrected is shown

Date	*Effect on TD*	*Cause*		
5/1/71	–19%	Correct treatment time per fraction	=	3·25 min
		Time entered in treatment record	=	2·25 min
14/1/71	–29%	Correct dose per fraction	=	344 rad
		Treatment time calculated for		244 rad
14/1/71	–31%	Correct dose per fraction	=	325 rad
		Treatment time calculated for		225 rad
26/1/71	–32%	Correct dose per fraction	=	313 rad
		Treatment time calculated for		213 rad
28/1/71	–28%	Correct treatment time per fraction	=	3·24 min
		Time entered in treatment record	=	2·34 min
		(girl said she 'probably used 3·24 min')		
5/8/71	–28%	Correct treatment time per fraction	=	3·52 min
		Time entered in treatment record	=	2·52 min
17/9/71	–29%	Correct dose per fraction	=	350 rad
		Treatment time calculated for		250 rad

immediately after the fifth mistake, the girl claimed that she had probably set the correct time of 3·24 min on the cobalt timer, although she had interchanged the order of the figures when entering the details in the treatment record. She could not remember back as far as the first mistake in Table 7.9. The second, third and fourth entries represent actual mistakes in the calculation of the dose per exposure, which would have affected the final tumour dose if not picked up and corrected in the routine twice-weekly check. Only the figures 2 and 3 were involved, and there was no evidence in the records for an increased incidence of mistakes of other kinds from the same girl during this period. It was soon found that the girl had been

Table 7.10. Summary of Total Mistakes (116) attributed to Physicists from 1969 to 1978

		1969	*1970*	*1971*	*1972*	*1973*	*1974*	*1975*	*1976*	*1977*	*1978*	*Total*
CAUSED	A (TD O.K.)	–	–	–	1	–	–	–	–	–	–	1
by	B (TD<5%)	–	4	–	2	–	1	–	–	4	1	12
physicist	C (TD≥5%)	–	7	1	–	2	–	–	2	–	2	14
												27
MISSED	A (TD O.K.)	1	3	–	3	1	3	2	5	9	6	33
by physicist	B (TD<5%)	1	1	1	–	–	2	3	4	3	1	16
during check	C (TD≥5%)	2	2	2	1	–	2	1	–	1	1	12
												61
Introduced	A (TD O.K.)	–	–	–	1	–	–	–	–	2	–	3
by physicist	B (TD<5%)	1	–	3	1	3	4	3	2	1	–	18
during check	C (TD≥5%)	1	–	1	1	1	–	1	1	–	1	7
												28

working without her glasses ('. . . but I am much prettier without them') and when these were restored to their correct place the mistake sequence came to an end. However, when another two examples turned up 7 months later (last two entries in Table 7.9) no time was lost in verifying that the glasses were again missing. In the last example the girl could not remember which time she had actually set on the cobalt timer. A satisfactory compromise was finally reached in the form of contact lenses!

Mistakes made by physicists (excluding those associated with the routine checks) are listed in the upper block of Table 7.10. In accordance with previous practice in this report, those involving ±5 per cent or more in the final Tumour Dose are analysed further in Table 7.11. As expected,

Table 7.11. Analysis of Physicists Mistakes
Type C mistakes made by physicists that would have changed the final TD by ±5 per cent or more if not corrected, and not associated with the routine check

Misuse of factors in treatment planning	4
Wrong data used in treatment planning	3
Wrong information written on treatment plan	3
Treatment time mistake with radioactive sources	2
Misuse of TLD factors in Cathetron dosimetry	2
Total	14

Table 7.12. Type C Mistakes introduced by the Physicists as a Direct Result of Routine Search for Mistakes

Used data for wrong applicator or wrong FSD	2
Did not use correct data from treatment sheet	2
Misuse of factors caused by wrong entry on treatment sheet	2
Mistake caused by misinterpreting the bad writing of the MO	1
Total	7

most of them occur during some aspect of treatment planning, since this task provides the greatest opportunity for numerical mistakes by physicists.

Because physicists are just as fallible as other categories of staff, it is inevitable that some new mistakes are generated as a direct result of the routine checks. When a mistake that has already been made by somebody else is missed during a check, the omission is recorded as a mistake by the checking physicist, even when it is picked up and corrected by another physicist in the next check. These 'misses' are summarized in the middle block of Table 7.10. New mistakes introduced by physicists during the checking procedure are shown in the lower block, and analysed in Table 7.12.

Mistakes in the middle and lower blocks of Table 7.10 are in a rather special category, since they would not have arisen if the checking physicists had not been engaged in searching for mistakes made by other staff. Therefore, they were not included in Tables 7.2, 7.3 and 7.4, since it would be wrong to allow the fallibility mistake rates that form the subject of this report to be modified by the procedure used for monitoring them. The mistakes attributed to physicists in the earlier tables included only those in the upper block of Table 7.10, which resulted from activities unconnected with the routine checks.

DISCUSSION

It is important to emphasize that the large number of potential mistakes gathered together and presented in this report never became actual mistakes – they were all picked up in the routine checks and corrected during the courses of treatment, otherwise they would not appear in this analysis. They were spread over 10 yr and 23 089 patients, and the majority (82 per cent) were either unimportant (type A) or small in magnitude (type B). Radiotherapy is the most quantitative of the various medical specialities and involves so much data-handling that some mistakes are inevitable. However, judged against the mistake rates of 1–2 per cent common in other comparable fields of activity, the results presented here (a mean rate of 0·5 per cent for all staff per unit of data handled) are encouraging and show that a radiotherapy treatment (in UK at least) is actually a relatively 'mistake-free' procedure even without a check system. With the twice-weekly check in operation, the effect of numerical mistakes is reduced practically to zero.

Nevertheless, there is no cause for complacency, and every effort should be made in radiotherapy departments to eliminate the effects of human fallibility. To do this by full automation of the treatment sequence, thereby effectively eliminating the human operator, represents an over-reaction and would certainly not be acceptable in UK radiotherapy practice. Instead we should reduce the need for data-handling by human operators; with modern technology data-handling is more appropriately assigned to a minicomputer. Where data must be handled by the human, well researched check procedures should be installed to monitor the process. It should be remembered that when the checking system described here was instituted in 1968 the technology for automated 'select and confirm' was not yet available.

The manual checking system has served two related but distinct purposes: it was immediately effective and has remained effective in eliminating most of the results of human fallibility under the conditions applying in this centre, and it has provided a solid basis for the design of an automated system of treatment calculation and verification. The automated systems presently available or under development (including the one mentioned) and [6, 7, 8] will be just as expensive to operate as the manual system, since they will certainly absorb at least as many man-hours in the form of supervision and maintenance.

Manual checking has a number of weaknesses: it is not fully comprehensive, in that at least two important sections of the treatment chain are not included. These are the pre-treatment activities centred around tumour localization, involving diagnostic radiology, mould room, tomography, etc. and also at the other end of the chain, verification of the actual machine parameters during treatment. However, in favour of manual checking is the fact that automated systems will also usually neglect at least the former of these activities, and are unlikely ever to include the low energy machines, orthovoltage and superficial, together with treatments using radioactive sources. The manual system takes in *all* treatment machines and techniques *without any additional expense or complications,* which is an important consideration in view of the mistake-prone nature of the low energy machines with their high outputs, multiple energies, assorted applicators and distances, lead cut-outs, etc.

It is difficult to evaluate the effectiveness of the manual checks, since we do not know how many of the 4122 potential mistakes in Table 7.3 would have been picked up and corrected during normal departmental procedures in the absence of the twice-weekly routine search. However, at the time of detection most of the 742 type C mistakes had already caused wrong doses to be given for one or more fractions, and were therefore more likely to remain hidden throughout the full courses of treatment.

CONCLUSIONS

It is difficult to find firm evidence in the literature of radiotherapy for a minimum value of mistake in tumour dose that would be likely to affect the outcome of a course of treatment. The precision of dose required in radiation therapy has been studied extensively by Herring and Compton [9] in connection with the Prototype Accelerator Project of the Committee on Radiation Therapy Studies of Stanford University School of Medicine. Their findings are summarized in a short extract from Appendix B of Enviro-Med Report 216 [10] :

> The clinical data show that an increase of less than 10% above the tolerance dose produces a readily observable increase in the frequency of necrosis. Moreover, the probability of achieving local control of a potentially curable tumor will be significantly lessened if the radiation dose to the tumor is reduced below the normal tissue tolerance. For example, a reduction of 10% in the radiation dose below the aforementioned levels has been shown to decrease the probability of local control of stage T2 and T3 supraglottic squamous cell carcinoma by a factor as great as seven. The dosimetry system and the radiation functions of a therapy system must perform at a level such that the total uncertainty in the tumor dose and in the critical structures receiving doses close to their tolerance levels is less than ±5%.

The opinions of a number of workers are summarized in ICRU Report 24 [12] leading to a similar general conclusion that the eradication of certain types of tumours requires an accuracy of ±5 per cent in the delivery of the absorbed dose to the target volume. Many radiotherapists would disagree with these opinions. The random and systematic uncertainties which are inherent in the treatment process certainly approach this figure in many situations, and so there is little room left in a well-organized radiotherapy department for fallibility mistakes of the type reported in this survey.

Unfortunately, experience shows that when data are handled by human operators mistakes will continue to arise. Until a comprehensive system of automated treatment calculation and verification is available, designed to eliminate as much as possible of the data handling [6, 7, 8] the best defence at present is a regular and thorough check of treatment records. This view is shared by a number of other workers, as shown by the following quotations:

> Significant errors can occur in the treatment of patients due to the inherent fallibility of the human –
>
> – a review process, in which the patient's record is searched periodically for errors can yield the information such that the effects of errors can, for practical purposes, be eliminated.
>
> Herring et al. [10].

> The occurrence of arithmetic errors in the charts of individual patients was common: a regular, perhaps weekly, review of patient charts to reveal errors is worth the investment of effort.
>
> The most frequent random errors were arithmetic mistakes in patient charts, indicating that charts should be checked weekly.
>
> Golden et al. [5].

> We believe that systematic checking of treatment cards, set-up details and other relevant parameters by a trained clinical physicist or dosimetrist is essential to improve the dosage accuracy and is worth attempting in all radiation centers.
>
> Kartha et al. [14].

REFERENCES

1. Blake M. J. F. (1967) Time of day effects on performance in a range of tasks. *Psychol. Sci.* 9, 349–350.
2. Campion P. J., Burns J. E. and Williams A. (1973) *A Code of Practice for the Detailed Statement of Accuracy.* London, HMSO.
3. Colquhoun W. P. (1972) *Aspects of Human Efficiency: Diurnal Rhythms and Loss of Sleep.* London, English Universities Press.
4. DHSS (1975) Recommendations of the Radiotherapy Apparatus Safety Measures Panel. Scientific and Technical Services, London, DHSS.
5. Golden R., Cundiff J. H., Grant W. H. et al. (1972) A review of the activities of the AAPM Radiological Physics Center in inter-institutional trials involving radiation therapy. *Cancer* 29, 1468–72.
6. Harper M. W. and Smith C. W. (1977) A microcomputer system for treatment calculation and set-up. In: Rosenow U. (ed.), *Proceedings of the Sixth International Conference on the Use of Computers in Radiation Therapy.* Göttingen, Strahlenabteilung, Universitats-Frauenklinik D–3400.
7. Harper M. W., Warren B. C., Caple M. et al. (1976) *Treatment Calculation, Verification and Recording using a Microcomputer.* Annual Report of the South Wales Cancer Research Council.
8. Harper M. W., Warren B. C., Caple M. et al. (1977) *Treatment Calculation, Monitoring, Verification and Recording.* Annual Report of the South Wales Cancer Research Council.

9. Herring D. F. and Compton D. M. J. (1971) The Degree of Precision required in the Radiation Dose delivered in Cancer Radiotherapy. In: Proceedings of the Third International Conference on the Use of Computers in Radiation Therapy. *Br. J. Radiol.* Special Report Series No. 5, pp. 51–58.
10. Herring D. F., Dobson J., Hasterlik R. J. et al. (1970) *A Study of the Automation of Radiation Treatment Machines.* Enviro-Med Report 216, under contract PR 1195 for Stanford University School of Medicine Committee on Radiation Therapy Studies. California Enviro-Med Inc.
11. Hill P. A. and Wigmore H. M. (1967) Measurement and control of drug administration incidents. *Lancet* **1**, 671–674.
12. ICRU Report 24 (1976) *Determination of Absorbed Dose in a Patient irradiated by Beams of X or Gamma Rays in Radiotherapy Procedures.* Washington, ICRU Publications.
13. Kartha P. K. I. (1976) Personal communication.
14. Kartha P. K. I., Chung-Bin A. and Hendrickson F. R. (1972) Dosage accuracy in clinical Radiation Therapy: Part 1 – Clinical Dosimetric Aspects. Paper presented at 1972 AAPM meeting.
15. Klemmer E. T. and Lockhead G. R. (1962) Productivity and errors in two keying tasks: a field study. *J. Appl. Psychol.* **46**, 401.
16. Minor F. J. and Revesman S. L. (1962) Evaluation of input devices for a data setting task. *J. Appl. Psychol.* **46**, 332.
17. Sutherland W. H. (1971) A new treatment time calculator designed to avoid errors in ^{60}Co therapy. *Br. J. Radiol.* **44**, 221–223.

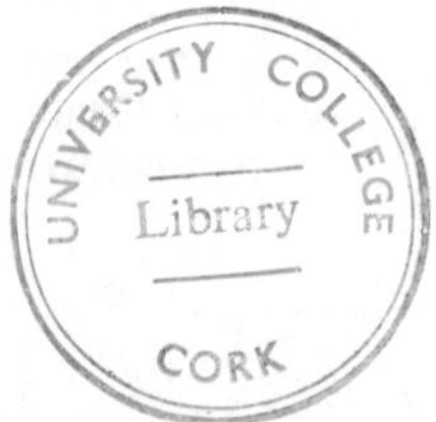

Stephen K. Carter

8 Cancer Chemotherapy–Current Status

Chemotherapy now has several roles to play in the cancer treatment spectrum. Recognizing the diversity of the many different diseases called cancer, this variety of roles is not surprising. Chemotherapy can be either curative in its therapeutic intent or palliative. Within a given kind of cancer, drug treatment may have both roles to play at different times in the course of the disease. This would be reflective of the stage of the cancer at presentation or whether the drug treatment was the initial therapy or a therapy upon relapse after prior drugs. In its curative mode, chemotherapy may involve the use of a single drug, or drugs in multiple combinations. In addition, chemotherapy in combination with surgery and/or radiation is another curative thrust and one which is currently in great primacy in therapeutic research. Chemotherapy as part of a combined modality approach has received a great deal of publicity and needs to be more fully understood as to its potentials, successes, failures and problems.

RATIONALE FOR DRUGS

The rationale for the use of drugs in the treatment of cancer is to achieve the selective killing of tumour cells. Underlying this rationale are the principles of the 'cell kill hypothesis' as elucidated by Skipper et al. [63]. The principles are as follows:

1. The survival of an animal (with L1210 leukaemia) is inversely related to either the number of leukaemic cells inoculated or the number remaining after treatment.
2. A single leukaemic cell is capable of multiplying and eventually killing the host.
3. For most drugs, a clear relationship exists between the dose of drug and its ability to eradicate tumour cells.
4. A given dose of a drug kills a constant fraction of cells, not a constant number, regardless of the cell numbers present at the time of therapy.

This fourth principle means that cell destruction by drugs follows first-order kinetics. For example, treatment reducing a population from 1 000 000 to 10 cells should reduce a population of 100 000 to 1 cell. The clinical implication of first-order cell destruction is that to eradicate a tumour population effectively, it is necessary either to increase the dose of drug or drugs to the maximum limits tolerated by the host or to start treatment when the number of cells is small enough to allow the destruction of tumour at doses of drug that are reasonably tolerated. The implication is not, as often has been stated, that eradication of the last neoplastic cell is not possible with chemotherapy.

The logical conclusion derived from the above hypothesis is that the maximum opportunity for achieving cure exists during the early disease stage. It is more difficult to eradicate disseminated disease than localized cancer, and much easier to control small tumours than larger ones. Therefore, early detection may offer one of the best hopes for cancer control.

Conceptually, tumour cells can be divided into three groups. One group is composed of actively replicating cells; a second involving cells temporarily non-dividing but potentially capable of replication; a third containing cells which no longer have the capacity to multiply and whose ultimate destiny is death and loss from the neoplastic mass.

THE GOMPERTZIAN FUNCTION

The experimental model view of the growth curve of a cancer is that it follows a Gompertzian function. This means that growth at every instant is exponential but with a growth constant which is simultaneously exponentially slowing. Therefore, as a tumour mass increases in size, its mass doubling time becomes progressively longer. This Gompertzian behaviour is attributed to the interplay of three factors. The first is an increase in the average generation time of the actively multiplying cells. The second is a progressively increasing cell loss from the tumour because of cell death and/or cell shedding. The third is an increased proportion of cells going into G_0 or the so-called 'non-replicating compartment'. It must be accepted that the Gompertzian aspect of tumour growth is recognizable only when a tumour is measured in its clinically palpable range. It is assumed that in the clinically indetectable period the growth is exponential. While this may be true in rodent models there are no data that prove that this obtains in the human situation.

If the Gompertzian model were clinically relevant it would have significant clinical implications and this theory has guided a good deal of clinical chemotherapy research over the last decade. As a mass responds to treatment, i.e. gets smaller, it would be assumed that the doubling time would increase as a consequence of a greater number of cells moving into cycle. This larger percentage of metabolically active cells would therefore increase the sensitivity of the neoplastic population to cell cycle specific agents. This has led to the sequential use of cell cycle non-specific agents, e.g. cyclophosphamide, to bring down the mass, to be followed by cell cycle specific agents such as Ara-C or methotrexate. While these sequential combinations have been theoretically attractive, none have proved to be clearly superior, in clinical trials, to other approaches.

Another implication of the Gompertzian growth concept is that metastasis would be expected to be more sensitive to chemotherapy in general, and to cell cycle specific agents in particular, than the primary tumour from which they arise. The smaller the size of the metastatic focus the greater the differential sensitivity will be. Therefore, the insensitivity of a primary tumour to a given drug regimen might not necessarily predict the response of its metastasis to the same regimen. This theoretical construct has made adjuvant chemotherapy highly attractive. It has been assumed that regimens that could shrink clinically evident metastatic growth would be that much more effective against minimal residual disease left after surgical removal of the primary tumour. There is evidence in stage III breast cancer, from Bonadonna's work [22], that chemotherapy can shrink the primary tumour to a higher degree than it can metastatic masses and yet the same kind of chemotherapy is not effective against microscopic residual disease in post-menopausal women. Rosen et al. [59], at the memorial Sloan-Kettering Cancer Center, have shown that chemotherapy can shrink a primary osteogenic sarcoma in nearly every case tried and yet in the adjuvant situation many relapses are still observed. It has been shown in head and neck cancer [13] that preoperative drug treatment can shrink the primary, but data on adjuvant treatment after surgery are still not available. There is therefore some evidence from clinical experience to indicate that either the classic Gompertzian construct is not clinically relevant or that other factors, besides kinetics, are causing chemotherapy to be less effective in the adjuvant situation than would be expected.

A *sine qua non* of the cell kill hypothesis and the Gompertzian growth concept is an inverse relationship between sensitivity to chemotherapy and the tumour burden. This is based not only on a purely kinetic construct but on the basis of biochemical resistance as well. This means that the larger the total malignant mass the higher will be the proportion of the permanently drug resistant variants to any given compound or regimen. This has been estimated to be one in 10^6–10^7 cells by Hutchinson and Schmid [37]. Hutchinson has further shown that it takes only 5–6 doses of cyclophosphamide to induce significant resistance in L1210 and Skipper has data to support as few as 2–3 doses of methylCCNU doing the same in rodent solid tumours.

A third factor besides kinetics and resistance that can explain clinical results differing from experimental models is pharmacology. The higher the cell number, the greater the chances will exist for the existence of sites, either within the tumour, or in selected organs, where tumour cells will be protected from efficient exposure to cytotoxic drugs.

One assumption built into clinical studies is that the period of tumour recurrence is directly related to the number of viable cells which have escaped surgery of the primary. It assumes these cells are acting consistently with the early part of Gompertzian growth curve. In experimental tumours it is possible to obtain estimates of the metastatic tumour exterior present at diagnosis. From data of this kind, Skipper (1975) has attempted to do such an analysis for human breast carcinoma and osteogenic sarcoma. The basis of the analysis is the clinically observed recurrence rates after surgery plus available data indicating that the median doubling time of some metastatic lesions in breast cancer is 30–40 days. The analysis assumes that the limit to clinical detection of a recurrence is 10^9 cells, which corresponds to a spherical mass of 10 mm in diameter. It also assumes exponential growth until this size is reached, which is probably the most unproven assumption in the analysis. His analysis indicates that in women with four or more positive nodes about 85 per cent could be expected to have 10^8 residual cells or less but only about half could be expected to have 10^5 residual cells or less. In node negative women, on the other hand, 86–90 per cent could be expected to have 10^4 residual cells or less. This calculation is very dependent on the assumed doubling time of cells. In osteogenic sarcoma when the estimate is 10–20 days the estimated residual tumour cell burden after amputation would be 10^5 or less in 69 per cent if the doubling time is 10 days. If it is 20 days however, the estimate falls to 38 per cent.

In experimental systems a steep dose-response relationship has been observed for most anticancer drugs. In these systems the maximum dose of drug compatible with host survival appears to be optimal in terms of achieving maximum reduction of the tumour cell population. For many agents twice the dose which kills 10 per cent of the animals (LD_{10}) is lethal to 90 per cent (LD_{90}).

DOSE TECHNIQUES

Skipper and his colleagues have reported that for almost all antitumour agents high-dose intermittent drug treatment was substantially more effective than low-dose, equitoxic daily treatment. As a result of studies such as these in the USA most cytotoxic drug treatment uses high-dose intermittent scheduling. It is worth noting that the superiority of this high-dose intermittent treatment is not clearly established by review of existing clinical data.

Controlled comparisons of chronic daily dosing of a drug vs. high-dose intermittent schedule of the same drug in the same tumour are hard to find. Some drugs do not appear to show a classic dose-response effect. For example, low doses of bleomycin in lymphomas appears equal to high doses in terms of response rate [3, 29]. The same is true for L-asparaginase in childhood leukaemia [57]. The Eastern Cooperative Oncology Group showed that 2·0 mg/kg/dx5 of DTIC was equivalent to 4·5 mg/kg/dx5 in a melanoma trial that has generally been ignored [52]. Young et al. [71] compared the value of intermittent low-dose oral melphalan with very large parental doses of cyclophosphamide in patients with advanced ovarian cancer. The response rates were equivalent but the toxicity of the cyclophosphamide was greater. Creech et al. [18] reported that low doses of cyclophosphamide, methotrexate and 5-fluorouracil (CMF) for breast cancer was equally effective, and less toxic when compared with the usual high-dose approach.

Retrospective analysis of the single agent shows that daily oral cyclophosphamide is comparable with intermittent schedules in breast cancer [10]. The same is true for low-dose daily methotrexate in head and neck cancer [13]. The ovarian cancer literature shows comparable response rates with daily chlorambucil to the intermittent use of other alkylating agents. Trying to draw too many conclusions from these data is hazardous since the data are heterogeneous as to patient selection, response criteria and data reporting.

Durodola [24] reviewed the Burkitt's tumour experience in Ibadan using cyclophosphamide. Various doses were used differing by a factor of over 20-fold, and the drug was administered as an intravenous infusion, a single intravenous injection or multiple intravenous injections. Complete remissions were observed on every dose schedule and no significant difference between any schedule as regards complete remission induction were noted. Long term survivors were independent of cyclophosphamide dosage or the dose schedule even in stage III patients.

Recently Norton and Simon [53] at the National Cancer Institute have suggested a hypothesis which runs counter to some of our older assumptions. This hypothesis assumes that human tumours grow in a Gompertzian fashion; that is, there is an initial exponential growth phase followed by a slowing in the rate of growth. In Gompertzian growth, tumour volume increases until it reaches a plateau. The growth rate of tumour at any instant is assumed to be a complex function which incorporates the net effect of cell birth and cell loss. The growth rate is expressed as the increase in tumour volume per unit of time. The instantaneous growth rate decreases as the volume of tumour increases. In the mathematical model they draw, cell production is slowest at either the beginning or the end of the Gompertz curve, even though the fraction of cells proliferating at any instant will be large at the beginning of the curve. They postulate that the maximum growth rate (and therefore the maximum sensitivity to drugs) will occur when the tumour mass is approximately 37 per cent of its eventual maximum size. Therefore, the most aggressive drug treatment would be indicated when the tumour cell burden is very low. As Devita [23] has pointed out, Norton and Simon's model predicts that a therapeutic regimen which causes regression of an advanced tumour will only be as effective when the foci of tumour are microscopic if doses are not reduced. In fact, the highest doses of drug may be required to eradicate the residual cells in microscopic foci. The very highest doses might be needed toward the end of a regimen. The concept is equivalent to a chemotherapeutic 'booster'. Contrary to the model of Norton and Simon, in most studies of adjuvant therapy, the doses of drugs in therapeutic regimens which are effective in advanced disease have been decreased for patients with less advanced disease in order to make the concept of therapy more palliative to both patient and primary physician.

Since the kinetics of microscopic residual tumour cells in man cannot be measured and the concentration versus time of exposure of these cells to drugs cannot be quantified, the choice and dose schedule of drugs used in adjuvant treatment must be empirical. The choice of drugs, until recently, has been based on the activity the drugs have had against advanced disease. What is currently unknown is whether the level of activity of drugs for advanced disease is correlated with positive effect when the drugs are used as adjuvant therapy [14].

CHILDHOOD TUMOURS

Cancers in children have been in the forefront of many innovative treatments, including the approach that used combinations of different types of therapy. Since chemotherapy has been particularly effective against a wide variety of aggressive neoplasms in children, these diseases have proved to be an appropriate model for the study of adjuvant chemotherapy.

Wilms' tumour is one of the earliest examples of chemotherapy being effective as an adjuvant to surgery and radiation. Surgery alone gives a 2-year relapse free survival rate of 30 per cent [19] which in this tumour is considered to be equivalent to cure. The addition of postoperative radiation increased the 2-year relapse free survival rate to 47 per cent [19]. In 1959, when Klapproth [42] analysed the world literature, the 2-year survival rate was only 21 per cent with surgery, and 25 per cent with surgery plus radiation. When actinomycin D was administered intermittently every three months following surgery plus radiation, Farber [26] was the first to show a 2-year disease free survival of 89 per cent. Vincristine has also been shown to be effective in Wilms' tumour [65] and now both drugs have been used in combination. The Wilms' Tumor Study Group [21] has recently reported a 2-year relapse free survival of 81 per cent with actinomycin D + vincristine as adjuvant therapy as compared with 57 per cent with actinomycin D alone and 55 per cent with vincristine alone. The Medical Research Council in the UK has reported a 2-year disease free survival of 87 per cent with vincristine alone and 62 per cent with actinomycin D alone in stages I–II–III. The current protocols of the Wilms' Tumor Study Group and other investigators is an attempt to improve these results by adding the highly active agent adriamycin to the adjuvant regimens.

Ewing's sarcoma had a dismal prognosis before the utilization of chemotherapy in the adjuvant setting. When clinically localized, disease was treated only with surgery and/or radiation, the 5-year survival was 4–19 per cent [20, 25]. Metastatic recurrence in lungs and bone occurred frequently and 75–85 per cent of patients were dead within 2 years. Pinkel [54] was the first to report on the success of a combination of radiotherapy and chemotherapy. In the last decade cyclophosphamide, vincristine, actinomycin D, and, most recently, adriamycin have been used singly or usually in combination in a variety of adjuvant studies. Surgery is no longer employed [6] and radiotherapy is the major modality used for local control, with new approaches being evaluated [64]. At the National Cancer Institute, Pomeroy and Johnson [56] have studied radiation combined with alternating high-dose pulses of adriamycin, cyclophosphamide, and vincristine. In 43 patients presenting with localized disease they have reported 64 per cent alive after 2 years and 52 per cent after 5 years. In a study from the Memorial Sloan-Kettering Cancer Center in New York [66] 80 per cent of 20 patients were alive and disease-free at 2 years having been treated under a protocol which combines radiation with all four of the drugs (adriamycin, cyclophosphamide, vincristine, and actinomycin D). In Milan, Fossati-Bellani et al. [28] reported on irradiation of the primary site combined with intermittent cyclical courses of adriamycin, cytoxan and vincristine for a total of 18 months. Fourteen of 19 consecutive patients were in constant remission for from 12–40 months. The 2-year disease free survival is in excess of 50 per cent.

Chemotherapy is not only reducing relapses due to metastatic disease, but is also having a positive effect on the local control achieved with radiation [66]. Newer approaches to Ewing's sarcoma include irradiation of both lungs.

Embryonal rhabdomyosarcoma is the most common soft tissue sarcoma which afflicts the paediatric population. The embryonal type is only one of four known histologic types [36, 38]. The tumour can be found in sites as diverse as the head and neck area, pelvis, limbs, and retroperitoneum. At the time of initial diagnosis only 20–30 per cent of children are amenable to radical surgery [34], and the cure by this approach appears to range from 10–50 per cent. The Children's Cancer Study Group [40] in the USA reports cures with surgery in only 5 out of 25 children and Lawrence et al. [43] report 8 out of 32 patients cured with surgery when the tumour was in the head and neck area. When radiation is added to surgery [48], a slight increase in long term survival is seen (10 out of 49). Credit for initially trying chemotherapy in the adjuvant setting again goes to Pinkel [55] who first proposed it in 1961. Additional positive results with chemotherapy added to surgery and radiation have been reported by Kilman et al. [41], using actinomycin + vincristine. They reported a 5-year survival of 71 per cent in 31 patients, with an 86 per cent survival in those children whose tumour was 'completely resectable'. The Children's Cancer Study Group [25] compared surgery alone versus surgery plus actinomycin D and vincristine in a controlled study. Forty-five per cent of patients were relapse free when treated with surgery only, as compared with 83 per cent treated with surgery plus drugs. Ghavimi et al. [31], utilizing the same protocol described previously for treatment of patients with Ewing's tumour, reported that all of 20 patients with loco-regional disease are alive from 4 to 42 months.

One of the benefits of the use of drugs for rhabdomyosarcoma is that less mutilating surgery than was practised in the past can now be contemplated [67]. Heyn [34] has reported a 2-year survival rate of 70·8 per cent in patients with microscopic residual disease in whom radical surgery was not technically feasible. Even when residual disease was gross, the 2-year survival rate was still 43·2 per cent. Currently all of the co-operative groups in the USA who treat solid tumours in children have joined in intergroup study of rhabdomyosarcoma. Their protocol is designed to answer the following questions:

1. Is postoperative radiotherapy routinely indicated in surgically resectable tumours?
2. Is actinomycin D + cytoxan + vincristine superior to actinomycin D + vincristine?
3. Is the optimal duration of chemotherapy in the adjuvant situation 1 or 2 years?

CANCER OF THE BREAST

Breast cancer is a disease which is in the forefront of much that is happening with chemotherapy and can be viewed as the solid tumour for which the most data exists in which to evaluate the various roles for drug treatment.

The traditional role of chemotherapy in the treatment of breast cancer, which has been for the palliation of patients with disseminated disease who have failed hormonal manipulation, would not be applicable. Much of the available chemotherapy literature describes results in patients treated only after primary or secondary hormone treatments had failed and thus were far advanced, often with poor performance abilities, heavily pre-treated and with a large tumour burden. Despite this, a wide range of chemotherapeutic agents have been shown to be active [10] and have served as the building blocks for the development of successful combination approaches.

5-Fluorouracil has been the most extensively studied drug and has probably been the most commonly used non-hormonal drug for breast cancer study. Among the alkylating agent group of drugs all of which have similar activity rates, cyclophosphamide is the most commonly used agent and has been the alkylating agent used in almost all combinations. Adriamycin is perhaps the most active of all the single agents as its response rate in previously untreated patients has exceeded 40 per cent in some series. Methotrexate and the vinca alkaloids have been less commonly used as single agents by the practising oncologists but their clear cut activity has led to their inclusion in combination studies.

The common denominator in the development of almost all successful combination chemotherapy regimens, such as those for leukaemia, lymphoma, and testicular tumours, has been the availability of drugs active as single agents, with independent mechanisms of action and without completely overlapping toxicity patterns. This potential has existed for breast cancer for a long time. Greenspan [33] was probably the first investigator to demonstrate that this potential could be successfully exploited. Cooper [16] in his 1969 abstract reported a response rate of 90 per cent with a 5-drug combination (CMFVP) which in a wide range of published subsequent reports by other investigators has been shown to be effective in about half the cases treated. When 11 different studies were reviewed which utilized the CMFVP regimen in some modified form the response rates ranged from 20 to 70 per cent with a cumulative response rate of 47 per cent in 529 cases [7].

Dissection of the CMFVP regimen has involved removing one or two drugs and most of these 3- or 4-drug combinations have had response rates similar to those reported for the 5-drug approach [7]. At the National Cancer Institute Canellos and others developed a 4-drug intermittent modification in which vincristine was dropped. Subsequently the Eastern Cooperative Oncology Group and the National Cancer Institute, in Milan, have reported on a CMF regimen in which the prednisone has been dropped. This regimen also has activity in excess of 50 per cent and is now one of the major commonly used combinations.

Adriamycin has also been incorporated into a number of successful combinations. Salman and Jones have reported on a combination of adriamycin plus cytoxan with a high response rate. Bonadonna has shown adriamycin plus vincristine to be equivalent to CMF in a controlled study. A variety of groups have combined 5-fluorouracil with cytoxan and adriamycin and achieved high response rates.

Adriamycin still appears to be the most active of the single agents for the treatment of advanced breast cancer with a reported cumulative response rate of 43 per cent for previously untreated patients. The rate falls to 26 per cent for previously treated patients [7]. When pretherapeutic variables are looked at for adriamycin the site of the dominant lesion appears to be the most critical. The response rate is 60 per cent for soft tissue, 42 per cent for visceral and only 10 per cent for bone. In comparison cytoxan gives a 24 per cent response rate in bone and 5-fluorouracil a 28 per cent response rate.

The Southwest Oncology Group has been studying three adriamycin-containing combinations. One regimen is the adriamycin plus cytoxan on the schedule originally reported by Salman and Jones. A second is the FAC regimen originally described by M. D. Anderson in which 5-fluorouracil is added to the two drugs. A third regimen includes adriamycin given 60 mg/m^2 every 21 days for three doses and then followed by CMFVP on the continuous schedule. The complete plus partial response rate, at last report, is 42 per cent (56/134) for the two drugs, 45 per cent (69/152) for the three drugs and 44 per cent (61/138) for the six drugs. The length of response is also equivalent for all three regimens, as is survival [69].

Tormey et al. have reported for cancer and leukaemia group B a study in which a continuous 'Cooper' revision with CMFVP was compared to an intermittent administration of the same five drugs and a regimen in which adriamycin was substituted for methotrexate in the intermittent regimen. The results are as follows:

CMFVP (continuous) 43/86 = 50 per cent
CMFVP (intermittent) 55/104 = 53 per cent
CAFVP 72/100 = 72 per cent

The survival in the adriamycin group was also longer.

Valagussa et al. [70] have gone back and analyzed their chemotherapy experience in 204 women with advanced disease, to see how the traditional prognostic variables of disease free interval, menopausal status, and dominant lesion predicted for positive effeet. The regimens used were CMF ± vincristine and adriamycin + vincristine ± prednisone. In the 204 women the overall response was 53·9 per cent with a median overall survival in all treated of 16 months (responders 24 months vs. 10 for non-responders). When free interval was analyzed the response rate was not affected but median survival was decreased in the subset with a 0–2 year disease free period. The response rate was lower for women 0–2 years post-menopausal (43·4 per cent) as compared with pre-menopausal (64·7 per cent) and 2–10 years post-menopausal (64·2 per cent). Despite this the median survival was not different in the three menopausal subgroups. As might be expected visceral dominant lesions had a lower response rate (43·8 per cent) as compared with soft tissue (61·5 per cent) and bone ± soft tissue (60·7 per cent).

The chemotherapy of advanced disease breast cancer appears to have reached a temporary plateau. The promise of 5-drug Cooper regimen and adriamycin have been confirmed but the ability to increase response rates beyond a 50–65 per cent period appears to be stalled. More critically the complete response rate has not risen and the survival figures in most figures tend to be very similar. It is hard to understand why with six active drug classes to manipulate the oncologists treating advanced breast cancer have not been able to improve results in the last five years.

Today, the exciting new development is adjuvant drug treatment after mastectomy. In 1972 the National Cancer Institute launched a large-scale controlled trial of the use of chemotherapy as an adjuvant to surgical operation in women in whom cancer had already spread. This study was carried out by the National Surgical Adjuvant Breast Project (NSABP), headed by Dr Bernard Fisher. Half of the women were given L-phenylalanine mustard (L-PAM) after radical mastectomy and half were given a placebo [27]. Treatment failures occurred in 22 per cent of 108 patients receiving placebo and in 9·3 per cent of 103 women given L-phenylalanine mustard. This difference was only statistically significant for pre-menopausal women and continued follow-up has shown no meaningful difference for post-menopausal women.

In 1973, Bonadonna at the National Cancer Institute of Milan began a study identical to Fisher's except that the chemotherapy was CMF (cytoxan, methotrexate, 5-fluorouracil), which had been found to be superior to

L-PAM in advanced disease [4]. At the time of this first report, only 5·3 per cent of 207 women who received the CMF had recurrence of cancer, as opposed to 24 per cent of 179 women who had surgery only. However, the patients in the study had been followed for an average of only 14 months. In the most recent analysis of this data (three years after mastectomy), the total failure rate was 45·7 per cent in control patients compared with 26·3 per cent in women given CMF [5]. New disease manifestations were higher in the subgroup having four or more nodes (37·9 per cent vs. 19·1 per cent). After 12 months of analysis, however, there was no difference in the recurrence rate for post-menopausal women. At three years, the failure rate in post-menopausal women was 40·1 per cent in controls vs. 36·2 per cent in the CMF group. When the control group is analysed, it is seen that pre-menopausal patients show a higher incidence of early recurrence compared with post-menopausal patients. In the CMF-treated women, the failure rate was comparable in both the pre- and post-menopausal groups.

Most patients receiving the CMF complained of various degrees of nausea and vomiting within a few hours after the drug injection. In more than two-thirds of the patients, the daily administration of cyclophosphamide caused prolonged nausea and loss of appetite. Some patients showed a repeated tendency to discontinue treatment or diminish the dose to decrease the abdominal discomfort.

In the large majority of patients, myelosuppression has been the signal to limit the dose. Severe leukopenia and/or thrombocytopenia were rare and no one required transfusion of white blood cells or platelets. Stomatitis was observed in 19 per cent, but was mild and promptly reversible. Some degree of alopecia occurred in 69 per cent of the women, but only 5 per cent required a wig. Cystitis secondary to cyclophosphamide occurred in 30 per cent but haemorrhage cystitis was documented in only two cases.

Despite the variety of toxic manifestations CMF was in general fairly well tolerated. All patients were treated as outpatients and the large majority continued to work while on therapy.

The updated results of the CMF study leave us in a difficult position. On the one hand, the overall study in terms of relapse rate still favours the CMF over the control in a statistically significant manner. The same is true of Fisher's L-PAM study. On the other hand, when post-menopausal women with positive nodes are looked at separately, there is no evidence to support adjunctive chemotherapy, at least as prescribed to date. If one reads Bonadonna's original paper carefully, it can be seen that he stated that the 'results should be considered with caution, since, at present the effects of this therapy on survival and possible long term side effects remain unknown' [27]. He indicated that, while the results were 'promising', the optimism should be tempered by the consideration that it is too early to tell whether CMF therapy was merely delaying recurrence or actually lengthening survival. Since breast cancer is a chronic disease which may reappear as many as 20 years after initial surgical operation, there is validity to the above statement. Fisher also cautioned about the preliminary nature of his study. Unfortunately, these cautions were not heeded and the studies were highly publicized in a manner which suggested that a therapeutic triumph had occurred.

It is clear that we cannot meaningfully analyze adjuvant studies for at least several years in terms of making therapeutic recommendations to the public. In the CMF update, there is no statistically significant survival gain overall for the treated group and it will be years before the definitive analysis can be undertaken.

What is urgently needed is continued research. There are a number of possibilities: (*a*) longer treatment with CMF beyond 12 months; (*b*) differing drug combinations; (*c*) the addition of hormonal therapy is highly attractive, especially with our new ability to measure oestrogen receptor site presence; (*d*) immunotherapy offers still another potential choice.

OSTEOGENIC SARCOMA

Osteogenic sarcoma is another tumour in which chemotherapy combined with other therapies is considered more useful than any single approach. Studies at the Sidney Farber Cancer Institute with high doses of methotrexate with Citrovorum Factor Rescue [39] and by the Cancer and Leukemia Group B with adriamycin [17] appear to have dramatic impacts on the disease-free survival after 2 years. In patients with advanced disease, both regimens produce responses in 20–30 per cent of those to whom they are given. The interpretation of these studies using adjuvant therapy is clouded by the fact that only historical controls were used. Perhaps the diagnostic criteria for exclusion of metastases was more stringent in recently selected patients as compared with the historical controls. Similar data from the Mayo Clinic [38] indicated that the 2-year disease-free interval in the patients currently selected for adjuvant therapy may be twice that reported in the series of Marcove [49] or in other series [30]. Preliminary reports of adjuvant effects for such therapies as interferon, transfer factor and anticoagulation lead to the suspicion that almost anything can be seen to be positive when compared with the earlier data base. Therefore, we either need a more careful delineation of the critical factors known to affect survival (e.g. the histology and size of the lesion, etc.) in the current patient series as compared with the older historical controls or we need more controlled studies before we can feel confident about the benefits of adjuvant chemotherapy in this disease.

INTERNAL CANCER

For many years, the standard chemotherapy for advanced large bowel cancer has been 5-fluorouracil (5-FU). In a review of over 2000 cases from the literature, this drug has had attributed to it response in 21 per cent of the patients [11]. There have been five controlled clinical trials utilizing 5-FU as adjuvant to 'curative' surgical resection in patients with Dukes C lesion [51]. None have shown any benefit of the drugs in terms of relapses or survival. In view of the comments above about osteogenic sarcoma, it is of interest that a recent report utilizing an 'historical control' was reported as positive [46]. It is clear that a 21 per cent response rate in advanced disease cannot be interpreted to mean that 5-FU has important efficacy as an adjuntive agent. Recently, the combination of methyl CCNU + 5-FU either as a pair or with vincristine added has been shown to be more active than concurrent controls given only 5-FU. In a study from the Mayo Clinic the 3-drug combination gave a 43 per cent response rate [50] as compared with 19 per cent for 5FU, but it is important to note that survival was not improved. In a study from the Southwest Oncology Group, the 2-drug combination produced a 30 per cent response rate compared with a 9 per cent rate for a low-dose weekly regimen using 5-FU. The latter regimen produced minimal toxicity [2]. There are now at least five major trials under way designed to evaluate the efficacy of methyl CCNU + 5-FU adjuvant treatment after curative surgical resection for Dukes B_2 and C lesions [12].

LUNG CANCER

There have been many trials of the alkylating agents, especially cyclophosphamide, in combination with 'curative surgical resection' for the management of primary lung cancer [44]. Cyclophosphamide alone produces a remission in approximately 30 per cent of patients [47]. Much of the cumulative data comes from earlier studies in which the criteria of response were not as stringent as are used today. Interpretation of data on lung cancer is further complicated by the various histological types of tumour, the extent of the disease when discovered, prior therapy and the fact that shrinkage of tumour based on changes of the X-ray can as readily be due to improvement of pneumonitis secondary to atelectasis as to killing of cells. Some recent studies have reported response rates under 20 per cent, some even less than 10 per cent. Given the paucity of objective responses (and minimal, if any, improvement in survival), it is not surprising that results of trials using single alkylating agents have been discouraging. With the exception of treatment for oat cell cancer, no combination of drugs have been proved superior to the use of single agents. Although oat cell lesions do respond, this disease is now considered to be disseminated when it is first diagnosed. Therefore studies of the effects of surgery combined with chemotherapy are difficult to contemplate. Combination of therapeutic approaches with radiation are being studied. In a controlled setting, none have produced a better result when radiation is used.

END-POINTS

The history of cancer chemotherapy has been that early data reporting was initially all that was possible. Any response to drugs was important and tumour shrinkage independent of duration and survival was worth reporting. As greater success was achieved in tumours such as childhood leukaemia and the lymphomas response alone became an inadequate end-point for a study. Complete response became an important bench mark of progress, and duration of response and impact on survival became essential to include in reports of clinical studies in these diseases. This required longer follow-up and more sophisticated data analysis and data reporting techniques. In the literature of today a report of a drug trial in previously untreated IV Hodgkin's disease which gave only the induction rate would be considered far too early for total evaluation. What would be required before a final judgement could be made would be the length of relapse-free survival and overall survival which would include in it the potential for secondary salvage. In terms of the toxicity the data needed for final evaluation would be not only the acute toxicity but the chronic toxicity which would include besides chronic organ damage, the development of second tumours and the cost to the patient in terms of variety of psychological factors which are only now beginning to be fully appreciated.

In clinical trials of adjuvant chemotherapy the need for long term analysis is a *sine qua non*. In these trials the participating chemotherapist, who in many cases is the study chairman, does not have objective regression or response as an early parameter to gauge what is happening. What he is treating are microscopic foci of metastatic disease, which he assumes to be present based on theoretical assumptions, but which he cannot see, measure, or evaluate except indirectly in terms of ultimate relapse and survival. In this situation, the first end-point which can be looked at in adjuvant drug studies is the relapse rate and from this an actuarial projection of a relapse-free survival curve. The first cost–benefit analysis that can be made is between relapse rate and acute toxicity. What is not yet known is what the minimal duration of follow-up should be in adjuvant trial before we can feel some confidence that an actuarial projection of a relapse-free survival, based on relapse rates at early fixed points in time, will be predictive for ultimate effects. Since new trials need to be designed quickly as case accession to studies reaches estimated required numbers, the need and the pressure for an early analysis is severe.

One of the major assumptions built into the concept that relapse rates are a meaningful end-point for adjuvant studies is the assumption that relapse rates will predict for eventual survival. This assumption in the main appears justified but it ignores the question of secondary therapy upon relapse and its impact on survival. The impact of secondary therapy can be great in two situations. The first situation is where secondary therapy has a significant salvage potential and therefore can have an impact on the number of patients who in the final analysis live or die. The second situation is where final survival differences may not be very great and significant survival prolongation or the lack thereof, by palliative chemotherapy at relapse can be an important hidden variable in the analysis. Since adjuvant protocols do not control or specify in any way for the therapy upon relapse this is a factor which has to make us cautious in our interpretations of carly relapse rate data as absolutely predictive for the overall survival.

CARCINOGENIC POTENTIAL

There is a considerable amount of experimental data which reveals the carcinogenic potential of anticancer agents especially the alkylating agents, procarbazine and the nitrosoureas. Immunosuppression caused by anticancer drugs may also be a factor in second tumour development and the lymphomas and squamous cell carcinomas associated with purine antimetabolites such as immuran may well be due to that effect [61].

Rosner [60] has accumulated 82 cases of acute myelogenous leukaemia, 11 of acute lymphoblastic leukaemia, 12 CML and 37 CLL in patients with Hodgkin's disease. Many of the chronic leukaemias and the ALL occurred simultaneously with or antedated the lymphoma. It is hard to know in this series if this incidence is part of the natural history of the disease or is due to therapy since the treatment was not, in this series, given in a systematic way according to current standards.

Arseneau et al. [1] at NCI have reported a 21-fold increase of second tumours in patients with Hodgkin's disease treated with total nodal irradiation and combination chemotherapy. Canellos [8] and Canellos et al. [9], in more recent reports from NCI, have described 8 cases of a second malignant tumour which included 4 cases of acute myelogenous leukaemia in 65 cases of Hodgkin's disease treated with drugs and radiation.

Coleman et al. [15] reporting for Stanford, have described a study of 680 patients with Hodgkin's disease treated from 1968 to 1975. Six cases of leukaemia occurred in patients in clinical remission with the longest being 7·5 years after diagnosis. Two additional cases occurred in patients with active Hodgkin's disease. In 320 cases treated only with radiation no leukaemia cases were observed and the same was true for 30 patients treated with drugs only. The cases occurred in the group receiving combined radiation and drugs. The actuarial probability of developing leukaemia at 5 and 7 years is 1·5 and 2·0 per cent for the whole group and 2·9 and 3·9 per cent for the 330 patients treated with combined radiation and chemotherapy.

Lerner [45] has reported a small series of 13 women with breast cancer who received long term adjuvant chlorambucil therapy. Three cases of acute myelocytic leukaemia were observed.

Reimer et al. [58] have described a survey of 70 institutions in which alkylating agents were used to treat ovarian cancer. The survey was for cases of second tumours developing. A total of 5455 cases were surveyed. It would be expected that 0·62 cases of acute non-lymphocytic leukaemia might occur in a population of that size. In the survey 13 cases were found for a 21-fold increase in relative risk. Twelve of these 13 cases occurred in women who were followed for more than 2 yr. The relative risk for patients given chemotherapy was 36·1 and rose to 171·4 for those surviving for 2 years with the rate being 13·75 per 1000 patients per year.

The fact that we now are concerned about such long term complications is a manifestation of the great success of cancer chemotherapy in prolonging life. In many situations we treat with curative intent and no therapy is without its risk. The risk of second malignancies is now a fact that will have to be included in the final analysis of many studies.

REFERENCES

1. Arseneau J. C., Sponzo R. W., Levin D. L. et al. (1972) Non-lymphomatous malignant tumors complicating Hodgkin's disease: possible association with intensive therapy. *N. Engl. J. Med.* **287**, 1119.
2. Baker L. H. et al. (1976) Phase III comparison of the treatment of advanced gastrointestinal cancer with bolus weekly 5-FU vs. Methyl CCNU plus bolus weekly 5-FU. *Cancer* **38**, 1–7.
3. Blum R. H., Carter S. K. and Agre K. (1973) A clinical review of bleomycin – a new anti-neoplastic agent. *Cancer* **31**, 903–914.
4. Bonadonna G., Brusamolino E., Valagussa P. et al. (1976) Combination chemotherapy as an adjuvant treatment in operable breast cancer. *N. Engl. J. Med.* **294**, 405–410.
5. Bonadonna G., Rossi A., Valagussa P. et al. (19) The CMF Program for operable breast cancer with positive axillary nodes. Updated analysis on the disease-free interval, site relapse and drug tolerance. *Cancer* (In Press).
6. Boyer C. W., Brickner T. J. and Perry R. H. (1976) Ewing's sarcoma – case against surgery. *Cancer* **20**, 1602–1606.
7. Broder L. E. and Tormey D. C. (1974) Combination chemotherapy of carcinoma of the breast. *Cancer Treat. Rev.* **1**, 183–203.
8. Canellos G. P. (1975) Second malignancies complicating Hodgkin's disease in remission. *Lancet* **1**, 1294.
9. Canellos G. P., Devita V. T., Arseneau J. C. et al. (1975) Second malignancies complicating Hodgkin's disease in remission. *Lancet* **1**, 947–949.
10. Carter S. K. (1974) The chemical therapy of breast cancer. *Semin. Oncol.* **1**, 131–144.
11. Carter S. K. (1976a) Large bowel cancer – the current status of treatment. *J. Natl. Cancer Inst.* **56**, 3–10.
12. Carter S. K. (1976b) Current protocol approaches in large bowel cancer. *Semin. Oncol.* **3**, 433–443.
13. Carter S. K. (1977a) The chemotherapy of head and neck cancer. *Semin. Oncol.* **4**, 413–424.
14. Carter S. K. (1977b) Correlation of chemotherapy activity in advanced disease with adjuvant results. In: Salman S. E. and Jones S. E. (eds), *Adjuvant Therapy of Cancer.* Amsterdam, North-Holland.
15. Coleman C. N., Williams C. J., Flint A. et al. (1977) Hematologic neoplasia in patients treated for Hodgkin's disease. *N. Engl. J. Med.* **297**, 1249–1252.
16. Cooper R. G. (1960) Combination chemotherapy in hormone resistant breast cancer (abstract). *Proc. Am. Ass. Cancer Res.* **10**, 15.

17. Cortes E. P. et al. (1974) Amputation and adriamycin in primary osteosarcoma. *N. Engl. J. Med.* **291**, 998–1000.
18. Creech R. H., Catalano R. B., Mastrangelo M. J. et al. (1980) An effective low-dose intermittent cyclophosphamide, methotrexate and 5-fluorouracil treatment for metastatic breast cancer. In the press.
19. Cross R. E. and Neuhauser E. B. D. (1950) Treatment of mixed tumors of the kidney in childhood. *Pediatrics* **6**, 843–552.
20. Dahlin D. C., Coventry M. B. and Scanlon P. W. (1961) Ewing's sarcoma. A critical analysis of 165 cases. *J. Bone Jt. Surg.* **43**, (A): 186–192.
21. D'Angio G. J., Evans A. E., Breslow N. et al. (1976) The treatment of Wilm's tumor. *Cancer* **38**, 633–646.
22. DeLena M., Zucali R., Viganotti G. et al. (1978) Combined chemotherapy–radiotherapy approach in locally advanced (T_{3b}–T_4) breast cancer. *Cancer Chemother.–Pharmacol.* **1**, 55–61.
23. Devita V. T. (1977) Adjuvant therapy – an overview. In: Salman S. E. and Jones S. E. (eds.), *Adjuvant Therapy of Cancer.* Amsterdam, North-Holland.
24. Durodola J. I. (1976) Burkitt's lymphoma in Ibadan: response to various doses of cyclophosphamide and long-term survivors. *Eur. J. Cancer* **12**, 425–432.
25. Falk S. and Alpert M. (1967) Five year survival of patients with Ewing's sarcoma. *Surg. Gynecol. Obstet.* **124**, 319–324.
26. Farber S. (1966) Chemotherapy in the treatment of leukaemia and Wilm's tumor. *JAMA* **198**, 826–836.
27. Fisher B., Carbone P., Economou S. G. et al. (1975) L-Phenylalanine mustard (L-PAM) in the management of primary breast cancer. A report of early findings. *N. Engl. J. Med.* **292**, 117–122.
28. Fossati-Bellani F., Barni S., Gasparini M. et al. (1946) In: Salman S. S. and Jones S. E. (eds.), *Adjuvant Therapy of Cancer.* Amsterdam, North-Holland p. 646.
29. Friedman M. A. (1978) A review of the bleomycin experience in the United States. *Recent Results Cancer Res.* **63**, 152–168.
30. Friedman M. and Carter S. K. (1972) The therapy of osteogenic sarcoma. Current status and thoughts for the future. *J. Surg. Oncol.* **4**, 482–510.
31. Ghavimi F., Exelby P. R., D'Angio G. J. et al. (1975) Multidisciplinary treatment of embyronal rhabdomyosarcoma in children. *Cancer* **35**, 67–86.
32. Goldin A. J. and Carter S. K. (1974) Screening and evaluating of antitumor agents. In: Holland J. and Frei E. III (eds.), *Cancer Medicine.* Philadelphia, Lea and Febiger.
33. Greenspan E. N. (1964) Regression of metastatic hepatomegaly from mammary carcinoma: cytotoxic combination with 5-FU. *NY State J. of Med.* **64**, 2442–2449.
34. Heyn R. M. (1975) The role of chemotherapy in the management of soft tissue sarcomas. *Cancer* **35**, 291–294.
35. Heyn R. and Holland R. (1970) Treatment of rhabdomyosarcoma in children. *Proc. Am. Ass. Cancer Res.* **11**, 36 (abstr.)
36. Horn R. C. and Enterline H. T. (1958) Rhabdomyosarcoma; a clinico-pathological study and classification of 39 cases. *Cancer* **11**, 181–199.
37. Hutchinson D. J. and Schmid F. A. (1973) In: Minich E. (ed.), *Drug Resistance and Selectivity.* New York, Academic Press, pp. 73–126.
38. Ivins J. E. et al. (1976) Transfer factor versus combination chemotherapy. A preliminary report of a randomized post-surgical adjuvant study in osteogenic sarcoma. *Ann. N.Y. Acad. Sci.* **277**, 558–574.
39. Jaffe N. et al. (1976) Adjuvant methotrexate and citrovorum factor treatment of osteogenic sarcoma. *N. Engl. J. Med.* **294**, 994–997.

40. Johnson D. G. (1975) Trends in surgery for childhood rhabdomyosarcoma. *Cancer* **35,** 916–920.
41. Kilman J. W., Clatworth H. W., Newton W. A. et al. (1973) *Ann. Surg.* **178,** 346–351.
42. Klapproth H. J. (1959) Wilm's tumor. A report of 56 cases and analysis of 1,351 cases reported in the world literature from 1940 to 1958. *J. Urol.* **81,** 633–648.
43. Lawrence W. Jr., Jegge G. and Foote F. W. Jr. (1964) Embryonal rhabdomyosarcoma. A clinico-pathological study. *Cancer* **17,** 361–376.
44. Legha S. et al. (1980) Adjuvant chemotherapy of lung cancer. Review and prospects. *Cancer* (In Press).
45. Lerner H. (1977) Second malignancies diagnosed in breast cancer patients while receiving adjuvant chemotherapy at the Pennsylvania hospital. *Proc. Am. Ass. Cancer Res.* **18,** 340.
46. Li M. C. and Ross S. T. (1976) Chemoprophylaxis for patients with colorectal cancer. *JAMA* **235,** 2825–2828.
47. Livingstone R. B. and Carter S. K. (1970) *Single Agents in Cancer Chemotherapy.* New York, Plenum.
48. Mahour G. H., Soule E. H., Mills S. D. et al. (1967) Rhabdomyosarcoma in infants and children. A clinico-pathologic study of 75 cases. *J. Pediat. Surg.* **2,** 402–409.
49. Marcove R. C. et al. (1970) Osteogenic sarcoma under the age of 21. A review of 145 operative cases. *J. Bone Jt. Surg.* **52,** 411–423.
50. Moertel C. G. et al. (1975) Therapy of advanced colorectal cancer with a combination of 5-fluourouracil, methyl CCNU and vincristine. *J. Natl. Cancer Inst.* **54,** 69–71.
51. Moertel C. G. et al. (1976) Fluourouracil as an adjuvant to colorectal surgery. The breakthrough that never was. *JAMA* **236,** 1935–1936.
52. Nathanson L., Wolter J., Horton J. et al. (1971) Characteristics of prognosis and response to imidazole. Carboxamide in melanoma. *Clin. Pharmacol. Ther.* **12,** 955–962.
53. Norton L. and Simon R. (1977) Tumour size, sensitivity to therapy and design of treatment schedules. *Cancer Treat. Rep.* **61,** 1307.
54. Pinkel D. (1962) Cyclophosphamide in children with cancer. *Cancer* **15,** 42–49.
55. Pinkel D. and Pickren J. (1961) Rhabdomyosarcoma in children. *JAMA* **175,** 293–298.
56. Pomeroy T. C. and Johnson R. E. (1975) Combined modality therapy for Ewing's sarcoma. *Cancer* **35,** 36–47.
57. Rausen A. and Glidewell O. (1970) L-Asparaginase in advanced childhood leukemia: comparative trial of drug schedules singly and in combination. *Proc. Am. Ass. Cancer Res.* **11,** 66.
58. Reimer R. R., Hoover R., Fraumeni J. F. et al. (1977) Acute leukaemia after alkylating-agent therapy of ovarian cancer. *N. Engl. J. Med.* **297,** 177–181.
59. Rosen G., Murphy M. L., Huvos A. G. (1976) Chemotherapy en block resection and prosthetic bone replacement in the treatment of osteogenic sarcoma. *Cancer* **37,** 1–11.
60. Rosner F. (1976) Acute leukemia as a delayed consequence of cancer chemotherapy. *Cancer* **37,** 1033–1036.
61. Sieber S. M. and Adamson R. H. (1975) Toxicity of antineoplastic agent in man. Chromosomal aberrations, effects, congenital malformations and carcinogenic potential. *Adv. Cancer Res.* **22,** 57–155.
62. Skipper H. (1978) Booklet 7 of 1975 from Southern Research Institute. In: Spreafico F. and Garattini S. (eds.), 'Chemotherapy of Experimental Metastasis'. In: Baldwin R. W. (ed.), *Secondary Spread of Cancer.* London, Academic, pp. 101–129.

63. Skipper H. E., Schabel F. M. and Wilcox W. S. (1964) Experimental evaluation of potential anticancer agents XIII on the criteria and kinetics associated with curability of experimental leukemia. *Cancer Chemother. Rep.* **35**, 1–111.
64. Suit H. D., Martin R. G. and Sutow W. W. (1973) In: Sutow W. et al. (ed.) *Medical Pediatric Oncology*. St. Louis, Mosby, pp. 473–496.
65. Sullivan M. P., Sutow W. W., Cangir A. et al. (1967) Vincristine sulfate in the management of Wilm's tumour. *JAMA* **202**, 381–384.
66. Tefft M., Chabora B. M. and Rosen G. (1977) Radiation in bone sarcomas. *Cancer* **39**, 806–816.
67. Tefft M., Fernandez C. H. and Moon T. E. (1977) Rhabdomyosarcoma response with chemotherapy prior to radiation in patients with gross residual disease. *Cancer* **39**, 665–670.
68. Tormey D., Leone L., Perloff M. et al. (1978) Evaluation of intermittent vs. continuous and of adriamycin vs. methotrexate 5-drug chemotherapy regimens for breast cancer. *PAACR–ASCO* **19**, 320.
69. Tranum B., Hoogstratem B. and Heilbrun L. (1978) Treatment of advanced breast cancer: update, A 3-arm prospective study. *PAACR–ASCO* **19**, 340.
70. Valagussa P., Brambilla C. and Bonadonna G. (1978) Advanced breast cancer: are the traditional stratification parameters still of value when patients are treated with combination chemotherapy. *PAACR–ASCO* **19**, 363.
71. Young R. C., Canellos G. P., Chabner B. A. et al. (1974) Chemotherapy of advanced ovarian cancer: A prospective randomized comparison of phenylalanine mustard and high dose cyclophosphamide. *Gynecol. Oncol.* **2**, 489–497.

Thomas J. Deeley

9 Cancer Information for Workers in Oncology

This chapter will deal with the imparting of knowledge of those people who are actively working in the cancer field. I have purposely selected the word 'information' rather than 'education' because I think this more aptly covers the wide spectrum of people involved who need degrees of knowledge. The Oxford English Dictionary reveals the difference: information implies the imparting of knowledge whereas education suggests a more organized system of instruction. The radiotherapist and oncologist is concerned with giving information to a large group of people with very widely diversified interests and who require varying degrees of information, from the most advanced to the very simple. This group can be divided into:

1. The experienced medical specialist in radiotherapy and oncology who is anxious to keep up-to-date with new techniques in his attempts to push forward his own research.
2. Other members of the caring professions:
   a. Those working in the cancer field who need to acquire a particular knowledge and skill which will be assessed by examination: this includes postgraduate trainees in radiotherapy and oncology, radiographers, and post-regristration nurses.
   b. Those not so specializing; a wide group not fettered by an examination in the subject who need no more than to be conversant with malignant disease, postgraduates in other branches of medicine, undergraduates in medical school, scientists, especially those working in oncology units, ancillary workers, social workers, clergy, administrators and so on. We may well consider that these workers need more instruction than they get at present; indeed, it has been said that many of them require formal instruction and possible examination.

It is convenient to discuss the subject under three headings.

THE TRAINED SPECIALIST

The practising radiotherapist and oncologist needs to be informed of all developments in his own field and in those closely associated with it. His requirements will vary a little, depending on the work of the particular doctor, his interests and the degree of actual participation. The doctor concerned with providing the best service for his patients will need to know of recent advances or changes in techniques or new preferred methods of treatment. Thus, he will take an interest in recent reviews, current symposia and conferences and in the published results of controlled clinical trials;

these are the basic requirements needed to make him a suitable person to consult. We then have a somewhat smaller group whose chief ambition is to push forward frontiers of knowledge, to research and to provide information to be applied by the first group. The doctor here will need different information, a knowledge of the work of others in the same field and of those in closely related disciplines not only in malignant diseases but also in subjects which at first sight may have little to do with his own specialty but which may suggest new fields of research. He often has specialized in a small narrow aspect of the whole field. He will need information as soon as it is published and often at a preliminary stage. I have, of course, made an artificial division between these two groups which in practice merge one into the other. We may examine the ways in which he obtains the information.

The Spoken Word

Many meetings are arranged by the appropriate learned societies. These may be general, in which a wide range of subjects are covered with the idea of something on the programme being attractive to all members, or specific when a particular subject or problem is discussed. The aim of the general meeting is to bring together as many members as possible of the society. Such meetings will attract the first group who seek to be brought up to date and, of course, all trainees, often the second group will only be found giving the lectures. Symposia or workshops devoted to one facet of the specialized subject will attract the second group who feel that they can contribute, perhaps even learn or develop a differing or tangential point of view.

Contact through Directories

These have appeared in relatively recent years as a means of making direct contact with those responsible for research.

> There is obviously a great need for the exchange of information between laboratories working on cancer research. So many projects are in progress all over the world that it is difficult to keep abreast of current developments. It is important for researchers starting new projects to know whether similar projects are being carried out in other laboratories, and where they can learn more about techniques and ideas before starting on their own research. Directories supply the need for a type of information other than that available in journals, books, literature indices, computerised literature retrieval systems etc., World Health Organisation [2].

Similar directories have been produced by the Union Internationale Contre le Cancer and the United States of America Department of Health, Social Security and Welfare. The short summaries of work at different centres enables the worker to make a direct contact with others in his own field.

Active Participation

There can be little doubt that the current practice of large scale controlled clinical trials has led to a great exchange of information and a desire to seek more. The preparation of the protocol (a term which we have come to accept although it correctly belongs to the diplomatic service) requires a search for information, discussion and the acceptance of an agreed policy. The decision to participate in such a trial again requires a personal exploration of the available literature.

The Written Word

The method above all others is the written word contained within the literature. The volume of information is somewhat forbidding, and there are many problems in finding the information we require, of knowing that it exists, of retrieving it, and storing it for future reference. We will therefore look further into the medical library and literature retrieval systems.

THE MEDICAL LIBRARY

The rapid growth of knowledge in medical science in recent years has produced an enormous volume of medical literature. The hospital or medical school library covers the requirements of a wide range of people concerned with the care of patients; medical students needing precise readily assimilable facts, practising doctors requiring up-to-date information about new techniques, drugs, etc., postgraduate students wanting textbooks on special subjects, specialists and research workers who are seeking knowledge of new work almost as soon as it is acquired. To these medical workers must be added other interested staff working in hospitals, scientists, nurses, ancillary workers and so on. The library thus has to cater for a very wide spectrum of readers. The function of the medical library is to acquire a collection of written works, store them, catalogue them so that they can be retrieved and made available for study. We will look briefly into the ways such writings are presented:

Books

The mainstay of all written knowledge where papers are bound together to form a permanent presentation. They may be further divided into:

Textbooks

Textbooks are the basis of all training. It would take a single author several years to write a comprehensive book covering the whole subject and some parts would be outdated before publication, thus the most up-to-date books are usually written by many workers. Such multi-author books have the advantage that each chapter is written by an expert in one particular aspect of the subject. But, radiotherapy is a rapidly evolving subject and apparatus, techniques and policies of treatment are likely to get out of date very quickly.

Monographs

In our specialty it is becoming increasingly difficult to have an expert knowledge covering the whole field and many of us specialize within the broad spectrum. Thus, the appeal of monographs is that they are limited to one aspect of study and can be updated with relative ease. The subject chosen can be covered in depth and can extend its width to include contributions from associated disciplines. Again these books can be multi-author, and have an appeal to the specialist in a particular field. But they will appeal to a few only; the sale of such books will be limited and often this is reflected in the price.

Proceedings of Conferences

Proceedings should give up-to-date reviews of a particular aspect as presented verbally to a limited audience. In some cases it has been possible to produce them within one year of the meeting but unfortunately this seldom happens and it may be two or more years before they appear on the shelves – often of little importance then.

Books are listed about two to three months after publication in the National Medical Library Current Catalogue.

Reports

Reports are usually published quicker than an average bound book; they are not common in the UK, neither are they used often in medicine. In America there are the reports of the US Atomic Energy Commission, the Federal Clearing Houses and the Aeronautics Agency, issued at intervals of two to three weeks. Often they are provided as microfische, a film measuring about 6 x 4 in which represents up to 60 pages of text and requires an optical reader to enlarge each page or a printing apparatus to copy out each page.

Articles

New work is invariably communicated by means of an article in one of the many appropriate journals issued weekly, monthly or quarterly. The time taken for an article to appear in press after presentation varies tremendously, and is made up of postal time, reception and listing in editorial office, allocation to appropriate editor, reading by one or more referees, approval by editorial committee, probably alterations necessitating further correspondence with author, editing, sub-editing, allocation to an issue of the journal which may depend on the importance of the article, the length of the text and the number of other articles already accepted for publication, and then printing and distribution. It is unfortunate that modern life tends to bring about a slowing down of all of these processes and it is often several months between acceptance and publication. Some journals indicate the date of submission. Thus, prospective authors get some idea of the delay before publication in that journal and readers have an indication of the editor's interpretation of the degree of priority of that subject.

Some time can be saved if the author reads the instruction in the particular journal he is submitting his article to.

Review Articles and Current Surveys

These are frequently commissioned by the journal, the author being selected because of his particular expertise; it must, of course, be recognized that such reviews are somewhat biased by the opinion of that writer. In recent years we have seen journals devoted to such reviews, for example, *Cancer Treatment Reviews* and *Oncology Seminars.* The author may wonder how far back he should go in his review, but in radiotherapy it is relatively easy, it is not worth going back more than 5 years unless he is doing an historical review. A complete list of references will exhaust the reader and only relevant ones should be used. All references should be included in the text, a mere list of 'books I have read' does little to forward knowledge.

Other Publications

There are other useful sources of information which may be worth reading; these include:

Annotations and Leading Articles

These are usually invited by the journal from an expert on some particular subject which is topical.

Book Reviews

Book reviews are designed to help the reader to select new books; they are usually written by an expert on that subject. They should include a brief description of the aims of the book, a concise précis of its contents, the reading audience it is aimed at and the reviewer's assessment of its value to that audience. Unfortunately often they are more critical than descriptive, are concerned too much with the detection of spelling errors than with the concept of the book and occasionally are simply derogatory or misleading; it is, unfortunately, much easier to review a book than to write one. They should be signed or else the reader cannot judge the contents on his experience or knowledge of the reviewer.

Letters

These are often used as a method of obtaining early publication, or for short, pertinent comments and are well used by radiotherapists.

Trade Journals and Advertisements

Many firms distribute excellent information about new products and some give up-to-date information of a high order.

THE MOUNTAIN OF LITERATURE

It has been said that one should 'publish or be damned' and that this accounts for the large amount of literature. Perhaps we should rephrase it to 'publish *and* be damned' because this is often the only way that we can assess the work of an individual or department. Occasionally some unsuitable material escapes and is published but most journals have more material than they need, are able to choose and appoint a committee to do just this. If they fail to attract and select good articles the standing of that journal deteriorates and sales go off.

We are faced with some questions:

1. How can we manage to read all the literature, even in our own specialty, or for that matter, in one aspect of radiotherapy and oncology, and how we can keep up with developments in associated specialties which may have a bearing on our work?
2. How can we know what has been written and where?
3. We are all aware of misleading titles to articles – how can we be certain that we have not missed something?
4. How can we obtain specific information at the earliest possible time?

It is obvious that some system of indexing and abstracting is needed to appraise the reader of articles written, this can be by –

Indexes – list the title of the paper, and can be produced within a few weeks or months after the paper has been published.
Abstracts – the article is read and précis made; this, of course, takes time and it is often more than six months before the abstract of a published article appears.

Indexes and Abstracts are divided into two main groups:

1. Comprehensive – tending to deal with general medical subjects, for example, *Index Medicus,* and the *Excerpta Medica* series.
2. Specialized – dealing with one relatively small aspect of medicine, for example *Leukaemia Abstracts* and *Smoking and Health*.

Indexing Journals

Several large libraries produce their own weekly lists of articles taken from the content sheet of journals. *Current Contents* photographs content sheets and is issued two to three weeks after the publication of the journal.

A good index gives a wide coverage of the subject, and should list within a short time of publication of the article, usually the minimum time is three months, on an average it is six months but it may be a year. It should also be easily understood and usable by the average doctor or scientist and should not require a specially trained worker to understand it. As examples we may give:

Index Medicus. This is the system used by most workers, gives a good coverage of medical and scientific journals and is issued monthly but may also be obtained in a cumulative form for the whole year. The former keeps abreast of current work, but when writing a review article or seeking general references the cumulative volume saves much work.

The *Index Medicus* lists the titles of articles in the journals which are listed in the January issue each year, usually only papers of medical or para-medical interest are listed; other communications, e.g. correspondence, book reviews, news, notes are included only if they contain substantial medical information.

The subject headings for the year are designated in a separate edition of *Medical Subject Headings* (MeSH) issued in January each year. It is useful to look at this before starting a search but remember the journal is produced in America and the spelling is American English. MeSH, is divided into four parts:

1. The introduction, which explains the use of the Index and gives a list of new subheadings introduced in that year.
2. A list of new and deleted terms; these may change from year to year and represent attempts to improve the service.
3. An alphabetical list of terms and the categories to which they belong with cross references.
4. A categorized list of terms which allow various breakdowns from general groups to smaller specific groups. There is adequate cross reference between the terms.

It is recommended that all users of *Index Medicus*, experienced and inexperienced, consult the issue of MeSH each year before undertaking any project requiring a number of references.

This index lists each article under three possible cross reference headings taken from key words in the title of the article. It is thus very important that the title is correct and gives a true indication of the contents of the article. Not all journals are included, e.g. *The British Journal of Hospital Medicine* has only been listed since 1978.

Each month *Index Medicus* publishes a *Bibliography of Medical Reviews*, it is surprising how many workers have not discovered this valuable list. It gives the number of references in each review and is invaluable to all who want to keep abreast of current knowledge or who seek references.

The first issue of *Index Medicus* appeared on January 31st 1879 and listed 20 000 medical articles in the first year; one hundred years later it is expected that some 250 000 articles will be listed.

Other indexes are more limited in scope but may be concerned with a particular specialty or subspecialty.

Abstracts

The précis may be written by the author of the article or specially written by an abstracter.

Excerpta Medica covers the medical literature in separate monthly issues, each is divided into subheadings listed at the front of the issue, each issue is well indexed and there is a separate yearly index. Each abstract is short and may be sufficient to keep abreast of work but it may also suggest that the full article is worth reading further, fortunately it gives English translations of foreign articles. Particularly useful to radiotherapists who want to look-up malignant disease at other sites; for example, in the *Excerptas* on Urology, Orthopaedic Surgery, Pathology, Surgery, Neurology, etc.

There are specialized abstracts such as *Cancer Chemotherapy Abstracts, Nuclear Medicine, International Abstracts of Surgery, Leukaemic Abstracts, Carcinogenesis Abstracts, Gastro-enterology Abstracts, Biochemical and Biophysical Reviews, Chronic Bronchitis, Smoking and Health Bulletin,* and so on, which may be of particular interest to the oncologist. Some journals run an abstracting service, for example, *The Americal Journal of Roentgenology* and *Radiology, Surgery, Obstetrics and Gynaecology* and *Physics in Medicine.*

It is obviously useful to consult the indexes and abstracts journals at regular intervals. Many doctors are incompletely aware of what services are available and should make a point of consulting their librarian.

Year Books and Annuals

These contain longer abstracts of important articles. Of interest to us are the *Year Books* of Radiology, Nuclear Medicine, Cancer, Pathology, but it is also worthwhile looking at others to pursue malignant disease at the site specified. The article précis is usually very good and one is often complemented by a short commentary from the Year Book author. They make very useful 'bed-side' books, providing us with a way of keeping up with the literature. *The Medical Annual* does yearly chapters on Radiotherapy and Radiodiagnosis.

Several journals have special issues devoted wholely, or partly, to a particular study; for example, the *British Post Graduate Medical Journal* and *Practitioner.*

Science Citation Index. This index lists the authors who have made reference to a particular article. Thus, knowing the author of a certain article in which you may have interest it is possible to look up his name and find out who has used the article he wrote in a reference to their own article. By this method it is possible to work forward and find out what additional information has been added to that subject. The only disadvantage of this index is its cost and not many libraries take it.

THE USE OF A COMPUTER IN INDEXING SYSTEMS

Medical indexes are lists and it is possible to store large quantities of such information in a computer and to sort that information out rapidly and accurately in any way we wish. Such a system is provided by MEDLARS (an abbreviation for Medical Literature – Analysis and Retrieval Service).

This is based on MeSH. Each paper is read by a member of a team of indexers trained in this work and which includes a number of medical practitioners. Whilst he is reading through the article he assigns to it any of the index headings included in MeSH. Whereas *Index Medicus* is cross referenced on three index words in the title, MEDLARS uses any index word contained in the text which is included in MeSH. There is, thus, no limit to the number of headings under which an article may be indexed. In addition, it also uses several 'non-print' headings which are not included in MeSH; for example, we have metabolism, microscopy – the use of these headings may be particularly convenient at times. There is an additional list of terms called Check Tags which are always used if applicable, are specifically looked for by the indexers and are used even if more specific terms are available; concepts used in Check Tags are pregnancy, infancy, human, male, female, historical article, review. Three further groups are also added and may prove to be exceptionally useful:

Racial and Ethnic group e.g. Negro
Geographical group e.g. England
Experimental animals e.g. Guinea pig.

The information is stored on a computer and retrieval has to be carefully planned or programmed. It becomes extremely useful when we want a series of combinations; for example, if we wanted a list of publications dealing with the complications of radiotherapy in the treatment of malignant disease of the breast, it would take us a considerable time to do by hand with the *Index Medicus.* The computer can be used to select all neoplasms, then select 'breast malignant', then search through these for reference to radiotherapy and again further break down these to 'radiotherapy – complications'. There is thus unlimited possibilities of combinations of references.

It is possible to specify the language the search is to be made in; e.g. if the disease is common the search may be limited to the English language or to the more generally used languages of French, German, etc., but if the search is to be made of a very uncommon disease then all languages are used and use is then made of translation services such as that provided by the National Lending Library. A certain time period can be specified; for example, only references to articles published in the past five years.

The requested information can be arranged to be printed-out in various ways; i.e., under author, journal or title (to facilitate its finding in the Library), under language, order of year of publication, and so on. The normal print-out will give the author's name and initials, the title of the article in English, the original language, the journal article it was published in and the full list of index terms that were assigned to that article.

Medlars has been augmented with an interactive on-line computer system, MEDLINE, which is now available in many libraries.

There are advantages of using this method of search, especially when long articles or reviews are being written:

1. Little effort is needed on the part of the person requesting the search; all he needs to do is to look up MeSH, arrange his questions and send in his enquiry; he need have little, or no knowledge of computing methods or the working of MEDLARS. Many libraries now provide such a service.
2. Multiple combinations of questions can be made quite easily.
3. The index list used for compiling the MEDLARS' tape is taken from the text and it will thus contain references of articles where the required information is not immediately obvious from the title. For example, in a search for articles dealing with the association of pregnancy and malignant disease I encountered such titles as:
   a. 'Carcinoma of the uterine cervix and pregnancy'. It was obvious that this was a pertinent article.
   b. 'Management of stage I carcinoma of the Cervix'. This was not quite so obvious but needed to be looked at further; it did, in fact, include a description of pregnancy and stage I carcinoma.
   c. 'Disease distribution in South Western American Indians'. There was no indication at all that this article would be useful but it described, among other things, a number of patients with malignant disease who were pregnant. I would never have thought of looking further at it.
4. It is possible to include many more terms; for example, by Check Tags which enable the searcher to obtain information which is, or may be, specific to his enquiry.
5. The print-out of references can be limited making the information more specific; for example:
   a. by language
   b. by time period; for example, two to three years only.
   c. to a geographic site, ethnic group or age group.

THE DEPARTMENTAL LIBRARY

Whilst the hospital or medical school library is general, covering all aspects of medicine, the department will need specialized works dealing with radiotherapy and oncology and the associated sciences for day-to-day work and for the use of students. Some general journals also will be taken regularly, especially those detailing 'appointments vacant'. There are certain reference books which are necessary to any library, such as pharmacopoeias, medical and English dictionaries and also French and German dictionaries.

Journals are usually arranged in alphabetical order, but books may be classified in several ways but often on some well recognized library scheme devised for use in general libraries. Specialized libraries dealing with a fragment of the available literature, such as those in our departments, often adopt their own scheme. Nothing is worse than a system based on the author's name, because whilst many of us can remember the gist of a title few can remember the author, but whatever system is adopted some method of cross reference is essential. The specialized library must have the backing and co-operation of the main hospital or medical school library and indeed the latter may have only an incomplete selection of such special works.

Few libraries can carry a sufficiently large number of books or journals to please all their readers and so many co-operate in an inter-library loan scheme. In the UK the most comprehensive store is maintained by the National Lending Library, books and bound journals may be borrowed but often it is more expedient to request a photocopy of the particular article for permanent record, and, postage is often considerably less than on a bound copy of the journal.

All radiotherapists and oncologists must allow themselves regular, short periods of time to use the library both on a regular 'search' basis and to browse. The practice of date stamping each new journal on arrival is particularly useful, a quick look around the library will easily distinguish those journals received since the last visit.

Co-operation with the librarian will invariably reap its rewards; these workers have a particular specialized knowledge of where and how to obtain information, know of existing inter-library loan schemes, by reference to their lists of libraries they can determine which library has a particular book or journal available and for how many years it goes back. The assistance of a librarian is particularly useful when carrying out historical summaries because not many libraries are able to supply books of great age. MEDLARS' searches can usually only be carried out by a librarian.

Personal Filing of References

Radiotherapists and research workers in particular, need some method of filing the references from the literature. This can be done in several ways:

1. Reprints, articles from the journals, Xerox, or other copies may be filed in a cabinet using a personal filing system, often under the appropriate topographical systems. The advantage of this is that a copy in its entirety is available for full reference.
2. Index – a list of references placed either on index cards or in a loose-leaf folder giving the title of the article, authors, year, etc. for each subject of interest.
3. Abstracts – either, preferably, the *reader's* own abstract of the article with reference to particular points such as diagrams, tables, photographs, etc., – or an abstract made by the author or editor. Abstracts may be filed in three ways:

   a. In a book – but cross-reference is difficult;

b. On index cards, the advantage being that they can be easily moved around and grouped into an order necessary for article writing;

c. Preferably on punched cards, using peripherally punched cards. These may be arranged generally or specifically:

Generally means using the peripheral holes for the whole of radiotherapy; for example, one hole is punched for all articles dealing with carcinoma of the breast, one for carcinoma of the cervix, etc., or –

Specifically – this method is very useful for workers interested in a particular subject, one card is used for one disease; for example, on a card for carcinoma of the bronchus each hole represents a particular aspect of the disease, such as superior vena caval obstruction. The title, author, year of publication, journal, volume and page numbers are typed on the front of the card and the abstract is written or typed on the back. I have found 8 x 5 in cards the most useful because smaller cards limit the length of the abstract that can be written. Each card is numbered chronologically as it is written; this number is then used when writing a review or a long article and the card need only be referred to again when the final draft and the list of references is being typed out. This method saves the writing out of a list of authors' names on each draft with the possibilities of errors arising.

4. Computers – this is really a modified MEDLARS system on a small scale dedicated to the needs of a specific department or person.

WRITING ARTICLES

Information pertinent to a particular disease or treatment technique must be published so that other workers can benefit from the author's findings. Frequently we are concerned with reporting only that information which makes a definite advance to our knowledge or which increases the standing of a department or person. Too often we fail to report negative or unfavourable findings but this information is of considerable use because it prevents other workers starting an unprofitable line of research. All article writing demands considerable time and few service departments have the staff available or the time necessary to report, and yet this is just the information that is required by the vast majority of workers whose sole concern is the treatment and care of patients. Few articles are sent for publication without many prior drafts again demanding the time of doctor and secretaries. Whilst we accept that medicine has many specialized facets we may be accused of not utilizing the facilities of other specialists, English graduates, professional writers and illustrators. As a result many articles presented for publication have to be re-written to varying extents, the majority need shortening, often pruning, English needs to be improved, illustrations redrawn, photographs redone. It would seem sensible for medical schools, hospitals and large departments to have a unit whose responsibility would be to help prepare material for publication, this would save valuable time for more work and ensure a good standard for presentation to a journal.

OTHER MEMBERS OF THE CARING PROFESSIONS

We have two groups to consider, those in the cancer field and those who are not so specializing.

SPECIALIST TRAINING

Here we are concerned with those training specifically for a career in radiotherapy and oncology, and includes post-graduate medical students, radiographers and post-registration nurses.

There are recognized training programmes for those intending to pursue a career in radiotherapy and oncology. Syllabuses are prepared detailing the subjects that the candidate is likely to be examined on and peers in the professions undertake to assess the suitability of the candidate and to maintain the standard. This is education in the full sense and is the province of the larger radiotherapy centres. The whole subject is adequately covered and controlled by the appropriate professional bodies so that it will not be discussed further here. However, there are a few pertinent points which could be usefully considered:

1. Syllabuses must keep abreast of current advances and on the whole they do. However, this does not mean that new work is merely added to the syllabus, it is equally important to remove outdated parts and to limit the amount of information that is merely historical. Syllabuses need to be continuously reviewed in the light of clinical practice.
2. Education in malignant diseases goes further than the mere requirements of the examination and information pertinent to the care and management of the malignant patient should be added.
3. The training centre should have all the necessary facilities for the whole syllabus. Education should not be fragmented by sending candidates away to short courses covering a particular subject, such as radiobiology or statistics. We must admit that such courses may be all that is necessary for the student to pass his examinations but the centre, which has all the facilities will augment lectures with examples, discussions and the practical application of such techniques in the everyday running of the department.
4. Teaching must not only take a wide approach to the subject but must examine in detail also, thus we have four main methods:
   a. General introduction taking an overall look at the subject and relating it to adjacent subjects or specialties.

b. The formal lecture which looks at one particular aspect of the whole specialty, guiding the listener to look more closely at some aspects and suggesting reading material.
c. Individual study which follows on from the lecture, reading further, collating information, preparing personal notes, précis and references for further study or revision.
d. The tutorial or discussion where information produced by individuals looking from differing points of view is brought together to be criticized, corrected or added to.

5. There can be no excuse for grabbing a group of slides and talking around them. A lecture must be prepared specifically for that audience; often it is more desirable to build up the story on the blackboard rather than present the polished final product as a slide, otherwise students may miss the logical processes of build-up.
6. Finally, there is no place for the lecturer who brings out his notes for an annual airing; he must keep ahead of current developments.

ANCILLARY WORKERS

There are few ancillary medical workers who do not encounter patients with malignant disease. Their lack of instruction must make it very difficult for them to deal with these patients, more so when we consider the attitudes of the general public to malignant diseases. The words *cancer* and *radiotherapy* are viewed as being associated with terminal disease and it is difficult for a worker, who has not been informed, to understand what can be done for patients with malignant disease. There is an obvious need for their instruction and indeed many such workers request more information; the specialist in radiotherapy and oncology is clearly the person who can give this information. Included are social workers, physiotherapists and remedial workers, occupational therapists, surgical applicance officers, hospital chaplains, and so on. It is recommended also that administrators have at least a few lectures on the subject; to explain, the differences between radiodiagnosis and radiotherapy, the work a radiographer does, why physicists are employed in such a department, the work of radiobiologists and other scientists. They should also visit the unit to see machines. In this way we may wipe out some of the misconceptions that exist about our work and perhaps even save time by having enquiries addressed to the right person.

Scientists

Many years ago it was decided that the doctor specializing in radiotherapy should have at least an elementary knowledge of the machines he uses, the physics background to planning, an idea of the properties of radiation; in more recent years we have added a knowledge of the biological effects of irradiation, the pharmacology of anti-tumour drugs, an appreciation of immunological responses and the application of statistics and computers to this branch of medicine. In this way he is able to co-operate with the large number of scientists who are to be found in the department of radiotherapy and oncology.

The place of the scientist in the health service is now fully established, he works closely with the clinician who is ultimately responsible for patient care. The scientist has a definite career grade within the service and would benefit from more formal instruction about those aspects of medicine which apply to his training. In addition there must be adequate regular meetings and seminars within the department to allow differing workers to come together to discuss problems, new techniques, lines of research, results of treatment, controlled clinical trials and so on. The scientist can only benefit from a greater integration within the department where he is able to participate fully in discussion with his medical colleagues. He will, of course, follow the same method of obtaining information as we have previously described for the trained specialist going to meetings, both medical and scientific and consulting medical and scientific books and journals.

Nurses

Radiotherapy and oncology occupies little, if any, place in the basic nursing curriculum but is included in the diploma course. Some graduate nursing courses do include this specialty as one of those taken during elective periods. Often it is the nurses themselves who request information and visits to the centre as a result of their introduction to the specialty through a patient they have cared for either in hospital or on the district. The latter nurses take a particular interest in knowing about this therapy and requesting to see the machines involved; this is a very desirable relationship.

NON-SPECIALIST TRAINING

Undergraduate Medical Student

There is perhaps no more fruitful subject of discussion and argument than that which is stimulated by the medical curriculum. After a mere five or six years in medical school most of us feel competent to judge all aspects of the curriculum. Medicine has been described as both an art and a science but it is also an apprentice trade and we learn most from our contact with patients. Examiners are well aware of the bookish candidates with parrot-like memories who do well on theoretical questions but fail on the clinical application. To many of us practising clinicians the requirements of theoretical knowledge appears for ever to be increasing at the expense of bedside medicine. Maybe the time has come for a reassessment. The introduction of more scientists into hospitals would certainly suggest that much more of the laboratory work could be left to them, the trained experts. Medical students would then require little more than a basic understanding sufficient for them to approach and discuss problems with these scientists. Many laboratory techniques taught to undergraduates will never be used again except by the small number who specialize in that field. Patient approach, including examination, care and treatment are the special attributes of the doctor and he needs much more training in this. Cancer accounts for the second largest number of deaths, giving place only to cardiovascular diseases which are, in the main, the effects of old age and wear on the heart and arteries; a natural closure to a long life. Whatever branch of clinical medicine the student finally decides to take he will inevitably meet malignancies; indeed a considerable part of his time will be spent with these diseases. Thus he needs to be aware of the method of treatment and of what can be achieved by these. But, early diagnosis and detection means that patients come earlier for treatment, with better chances of cure, and it is the non-specialist who is responsible for first arousing suspicion of malignancy and who initiates specialized treatment. If the student is not taught about malignancy in his formative years he is unlikely to pick up knowledge or interest later.

The medical student needs to have a working knowledge of the epidemiology and aetiology of cancer, symptomology, early diagnosis and detection and an appreciation of treatment techniques. We do not wish to teach more than the rudiments of surgery, radiotherapy and chemotherapy but it is important that students recognize the appropriate treatment to be given and the possible results of that treatment. After-care is a somewhat neglected field, cancer has been diagnosed and treatment given to the best of our ability, but regrettably many consider that nothing more can be done or needs to be done. Follow-up has a definite part to play in the detection of recurrences and it is only in recent years that we have considered re-treatment or further treatment. Rehabilitation of the cancer patient has been neglected somewhat but we are beginning to take more notice and also to become involved in terminal care. The varied work carried out in the radiotherapy and oncology department offers excellent opportunities for pre-registration training.

A recent survey carried out among consultants in radiotherapy Deeley et al. [1], established that the two most important factors influencing recruitment into our specialty were lack of undergraduate training in the subject and the low academic status which it enjoys; there are a few academic units in this country. The subject involves a high academic level of training, is a true specialty overlapping and integrating with others but distinct in as far as it requires specialized training and cannot be taught by others. The time has come for this to be recognized as an academic subject represented in each medical school. Specialists in radiotherapy and oncology need to participate more in undergraduate and postgraduate training. In this way we hope to train a new generation of doctors who are fully aware of malignant disease, conversant with suspicious signs and symptoms, know of diagnostic and detection methods, can refer without delay to the appropriate therapist and appreciate the results of treatment and the need for after care. Thus, we may improve our attack on these diseases.

Postgraduate Medical Instruction

The paucity of undergraduates' training has led to requests for more postgraduate instruction. This may be of two types

1. for postgraduate training in a particular branch of medicine
2. for those who wish to keep abreast of current developments or who realize that their knowledge of the subject is inadequate.

Other medical specialties have realized the importance of including aspects of radiotherapy and oncology in the curriculum and we are actively involved in such teaching. Some centres are at present discussing the possibility of secondment to a radiotherapy and oncology department for a period of instruction.

The postgraduate centres have proved very useful for further instruction of family doctors and others requiring at least some information on the subject. This is a very desirable way of introducing the subject but invariably involves the occasional lecture only and cannot give the practical experience and contact which should be given during the undergraduate years.

Sometimes it is not easy to make our work intelligible or simplified sufficiently for those who have not the basic knowledge of physics, biology and mathematics, but suffice it to get over the application of this form of therapy and its place in the management of the patient with a malignant disease.

Lectures can be supplemented by relatively simple straightforward articles in the appropriate magazines and journals of the workers involved. Obviously such articles have to be tailored for the particular reading audience. They have to be relatively short, pertinent and if possible, tie up with the specialty concerned. They are intended as informative reading rather than a display of learning. It is important to define terms used when writing for non-specialist readers; ambiguity about the meaning of a term often leads to confusion and rejection, not only of that particular article but often of the whole subject. We are too often correctly accused of using jargon or unexplained abbreviations; when writing for workers in another specialty or discipline it is often of use to imagine the roles reversed and to consider what we know about their work, even to go further and look at some of their specialist journals.

We have dealt here with an intelligent audience who have some basic training in aspects of medicine and science, and as a consequence have frequently developed a desire to learn – sometimes for the sheer pleasure of obtaining knowledge.

REFERENCES

1. Deeley T. J., Baker J. and Brindle J. (1976) Recruitment in radiotherapy. *Med. Ed.* **10,** 313–314.
2. World Health Organisation (1977) *Directory of Laboratories working on the Biology and the Biochemistry of Tumour Cells in Asia and Europe.* Geneva, WHO.

Thomas J. Deeley

10 Cancer Information for the Public

Information about all aspects of cancer needs to be given to the general public so that they will get a better, more accurate, understanding of this disease and come to accept it as any other disease.

There are certain problems to be looked at before we can discuss methods of giving information.

We are dealing with a very wide spectrum of knowledge and intelligence; many have little or no knowledge of science, some have a limited education, some are frankly disinterested and at the other end of the scale we have the full range of academic ability.

Members of the public have their own ideas about cancer, often built up over a number of years by gossip, folk-lore and even imagination, passed on by word of mouth, seldom based on fact, only rarely augmented by personal experience or knowledge and invariably based on misconceptions.

Ignorance of the full nature and consequences of the disease often causes delay in the patient coming for definitive treatment.

We have the whole range of interest in the disease including patients, relatives, individuals who are afraid or suspicious, the frankly unconcerned and the sceptical.

In our approach we can adopt the method of the lowest common denominator on the basis that we adapt our information so that it can be understood by those of the lowest intelligence, hoping that this will not bore the others; the alternative is to attempt a more erudite attack hoping to convince at least some people. But, neither method is correct – we need to develop differing approaches depending on the audience. This now makes the problem a very complex one. We will try to cover the problems listed, to look into possible ways of remedying these and to make some recommendations about the part that can be played by the consultant in radiotherapy and oncology.

PUBLIC ATTITUDE TO CANCER

The very word 'cancer' often causes concern; fear of the disease may be stimulated by direct experience, from contact with a relative or friend, from knowledge obtained from others or from poorly conceived impressions. The established clinician, concerned as he is with the physical aspects of malignant disease and his attempts to cure or alleviate distressing symptoms, may sometimes forget the effect that the word has on his patients, their relatives, members of the caring team, his colleagues or even on himself. Each of us develops our own individual attitude, and this may be attenuated or indeed may change as a result of knowledge or experience.

It has been claimed that cancer is the scourge of modern society, more correctly we should say that it is the current scourge because man has always been subject to scourges which have produced pain, disease and suffering. We may look into some of these and see why they no longer exist or have lost the fear that they once had. We are well aware of one scourge that lasted for many years – plague. This was probably a term used to describe a number of epidemics or pestilences and went under various names, such as 'Black Death' or 'God's token'. It was found in ancient Egyptian communities: Moses removed his people from it into the wilderness; thousands died during the Middle Ages; when London was affected in 1665, 75 000 people are reputed to have died from it. We get a personal glimpse into the fear and panic it produced from Samuel Pepys' diaries (1633–1703). Those who could left London and only returned when the disease had died out. Quite early on the importance of personal contact was appreciated, the disease was found to spread from areas where ships had recently put in. But, it was not until early in the twentieth century that the importance of the rat flea as a vector was recognized. Stricter public health control and knowledge of the epidemiology and natural history of the disease has greatly reduced the incidence of this once dreaded disease. So, in the same way we can examine other diseases which were once scourges; smallpox, leprosy, cholera, syphilis, malaria, yellow fever and typhus, where the dread has been removed by control of the disease or by therapeutic measures which have produced cures.

The twentieth century has seen many changes; diabetes which once carried a hopeless prognosis is now controlled to such an extent that people are often surprised to hear that a friend or acquaintance has the disease. Tuberculosis, only a relatively few years ago, was considered a hopeless disease, thus we used such terms as 'consumption' or 'phthisis' (wasting away). Because it was often found in poor, overcrowded communities it carried a social stigma. Now, with effective anti-tubercular therapy complete recovery can be expected, sanatoria have been turned over to other uses and the disease has lost its dread. Dramatic changes have taken place with bacterial infections, pneumonia killed thousands, as did meningitis, puerperal fever, appendicitis and so on. We are reminded of the whole nation praying for a *miracle* when King Edward VII's coronation was delayed by appendicitis. Deficiencies in diet were the cause of many severe illnesses, scurvy, rickets, pellagra, beriberi etc. Pain was relieved by the discovery of anaesthetics and larger and more complex operations were possible.

Conditions which were spoken of with bated breath, feared and dreaded, have been removed by methods aimed at control, cure and prevention.

But, the removal of these diseases has brought two others into present-day prominence – cardiovascular diseases and cancer.

We see an early attitude to cancer in the account of the Greek doctor Democedes who cured Atossa, the wife of Darius 1 (522–485 BC); she at first *concealed* the growth in her breast. The literature, medical and otherwise, of the Middle Ages abounds with stories of wars, famines, plagues, all taking their tolls and sufficient scourges in themselves; the result was that few people survived to an age when cancer was common. Samuel Johnson, in his Dictionary of the English Language (1755), defined cancer as a 'virulent swelling or sore, not to be cured' – a *definite* statement. The nineteenth century saw a more objective approach although all reports stressed the inevitable result of the disease. We find such statements as 'dreadful disease', 'agonized suffering', and 'the real nature remains wholly unknown'. William Marsden (1796–1867) with amazing perspicacity saw the need for a medical specialty and a dedicated hospital. In 1851 he wrote: 'Instead of decreasing as a result of advancing science, death by cancer has increased alarmingly.' The close of the nineteenth century brought new hopes of cure by radiation. A book for the general public *Medicine for the Million* published by *The News of the World* stated 'We may lay it down, now in 1906, that nothing but early removal with the knife will give most cancer patients any chance of prolonging their lives' but, later in the same work, 'The X-ray method seems to promise us help in the future'. In 1933 Donaldson wrote, 'At the present time cancer is taboo. It is not difficult to understand why there is such a universal fear of the disease. The public believe that it must end fatally, and it appears to come like a bolt from the blue without any serious symptoms as a warning.'

So to the present day, the incidence of the disease is increasing but also the fear has continued to grow over the years. Personal experience of family or of friends has increased our appreciation of the disease; we expect the patient to suffer. Often our information of the presence of this disease is obtained only at the time of the patient's death. The patient who recovers often does not know the nature of his illness and no-one uses the word 'cancer'; only in those who die is it mentioned. Small wonder, then, that in the mind of the general public, cancer is associated with a fatal result. Now we are well aware that cancer is not one disease but a whole range of malignant diseases varying from those that have a natural history measured in days or weeks to the other extreme where known cancers have been present for many years and which do not reduce the patient's normal life expectancy. It is, then, a mixed batch of diseases ranging from those with excellent prognosis to those with little or no chance of a cure. But, as can be expected, the general public inevitably considers them as all having the worst possible prognosis, a belief which is strengthened when the word 'cancer' is used only in fatal cases.

These facts influence our attitudes to the disease. However, attitudes are complex, a mixture of something which is a basic human attribute and the effects of knowledge and experience [6]. Many factors which we encounter in our everyday lives can alter our attitudes to a situation. When we consider the attitude of the individual we must relate this to the situation. Thus, a doctor will have differing attitudes to cancer depending on whether he specializes in the disease or takes little more than passing notice. He may develop varying attitudes to certain aspects of cancer, to the epidemiological and aetiological factors which cause the disease and which could lead him to suggest methods of prevention, to diagnosis, to treatment, to rehabilitation and so on. The ancillary workers in the health service will similarly have their attitudes influenced by their association with the disease. If they see only the suffering patient in the ward or department and do not visit the follow-up clinic, they will not appreciate that such patients can be, and are, cured. The patient, relatives, friends and the general public may have little or no knowledge of the disease or what knowledge they have may be inaccurate, obtained from gossip, or badly presented information in books or the mass media. There seems little doubt that our current attitudes to cancer are greatly influenced by ignorance of the facts.

Now ignorance is an emotive word, it is relative and is associated with degree. Ignorance, derived from the Latin *ignorare*, meaning, 'not to know', implies a lack of knowledge and no more. This may have arisen from an act of commission, a deliberate refusal to learn or more usually from an omission in teaching which is little more than innocence. The student can hardly be blamed for not knowing that which he has not been taught. All of us have some degree of ignorance and none can claim otherwise. It is an attribute of Man, that he knows imperfectly.

The attitudes of the general public are deeply rooted, fear of the disease is inherent in all our minds; as we grow older hearsay from others causes a reiteration of that fear which is further accentuated by our own personal experiences. When we are young we accept the occurrence of the disease in older people and death seems logical in any case for the elderly; thus we build up in our minds an association of ideas–old age–cancer–death. As the individual himself grows older he appreciates more about the disease from his personal experience; now we have the association of age–cancer –suffering–pain–death, with perhaps the inclusion of–radiotherapy. As time progresses and one's own colleagues begin to be afflicted the age association is lost; it now becomes–contemporaries–cancer–pain–death. But, always we have the same relationship heavily weighted towards a fatal outcome. Few people have experience of a patient who has had cancer which has been cured and returned to normal life. The reason why this is so is because the word *cancer* is seldom mentioned in those who recover, few patients know the full nature of the disease, not all relatives, and many would not reveal it to others if they did know for fear of upsetting the patient, and very few friends or casual acquaintances. We have thus built up a misconception over the years, that cancer has an inevitable outcome.

The members of the public have a somewhat unusual attachment to the word 'cancer'; it is the term itself which holds the fear and use of synonymous words 'tumour', 'carcinoma', 'malignant', 'growth', may bring a sigh of relief and the sincere remark 'thank goodness that is all, at one time I thought it may be a cancer'.

Public Opinion Surveys

It is important that we know exactly what the general public knows or thinks about certain aspects of malignant disease because on this knowledge we can set about designing information techniques and programmes. There have been several surveys of public opinion in certain countries, areas, or communities and as we can imagine there are conflicting reports varying with the composition of the groups.

Paterson and Aitken-Swan [11] carried out such a survey in Manchester enquiring mainly about cancer of the breast and cervix uteri. They concluded that the majority of women were interested in knowing more about cancer and suggested that it was the clinician's responsibility to see that women were made aware of the good results of treatment. This was followed by another paper in 1958 giving details of the change in public opinion after five years of cancer education. They were pleased to report that there had been statistically significant improvement in the proportions of women aware that cancer is not always incurable, and in the number who thought that early treatment increased the chance of cure. From the same centre we have a survey of women in Lancaster reported by Briggs and Wakefield in 1966 [2]. From South Wales we have a survey carried out by the Tenovus Cancer Information Centre in 1972 by Williams, Cruickshank and Walker [19], who concluded that 'although a certain significant proportion of the population viewed the disease fairly realistically, there was a substantial proportion which was ignorant and confused in its knowledge and opinions about cancer'. The implications resulting from this survey may be summarized:

1. The mistaken belief that cancer is incurable is a major barrier in a rational approach to the disease.
2. There was considerable doubt in the public's mind about the early signs and symptoms of the disease.
3. Communications about cancer need to be adjusted to the groups forming the audience and talks addressed to the lower common denominator will need to be augmented.
4. It is important to co-operate with leaders of the local communities, especially doctors, nurses and teachers and the need for basic instruction to those in training is emphasized.
5. Whilst instruction can be given relatively easily to women this is not so with men and programmes are suggested for use in industry.
6. The public is not a passing receiver of communication, it evolves its own patterns of opinion and knowledge.

In the same area Bluck [1] carried out a survey which included general practitioners and members of the public which showed that attitudes were dependent upon social class and concluded that the public were becoming increasingly knowledgeable and questioning about all health matters. This suggested that cancer programmes should be part of a more general health programme.

Similar surveys have been reported from Merseyside [7], from the USA [8, 9], Canadian opinion is presented by Phillips [13, 14], and Phillips and Taylor [15] from Western Australia by the Cancer Council [3], the Institute of Public Opinion Research, Czechoslovakia [10] and by Seeber of Argentine in the same year [17]. We thus have considerable information from such sources.

The importance of different communities, educational standards, social classes and age groups of the individuals must be stressed. Of particular interest to us is a survey of doctors' opinions reported by Bluck [1], of medical students by Sherman and Williams [18] and of nurses by Davison [4].

We must not lose sight of the fact that there may be considerable variation in the collection and analysis of the views expressed by the public. What we eventually end up with is an impression of the attitudes of a group of people in a certain place, at a certain point in time, who were willing to be questioned by a group of people with varying ability to carry out such work, who may be biased, may unwittingly force or stress a reply to a question which may not be entirely clear to the person they are interviewing, who may treat the whole situation seriously, maturely or otherwise; exaggeration, bravardo and unco-operation are likely to arise. There is thus a very large subjective influence and our interpretation of the results must take this into account. In carrying out such surveys we need to appreciate the reticence of the public to discuss this disease and remember the secrecy with which for many years it has been enshrined. In addition, in some people's minds this disease has some connection of shame, perhaps God's retribution for something done wrong in the past and such thinking may cause considerable inhibition in answering.

Delay

We must now look at a very disturbing aspect of the public's approach: delay in presenting for definitive treatment. To some extent we can understand part of this delay because procrastination is a basic human failing. In most of our dealings it is logical to suppose that expedience has obvious merits in achieving a conclusion, satisfactory or otherwise, and that the majority of people wish to know the result of their fate. Perversely, often this is not so. We may ask what causes these delays in dealing with everyday affairs because somewhat the same philosophy may govern the patient's response to the signs and symptoms of cancer. Reasons given in excuse include:

Too busy: there is little doubt that we live in a busy age, there is always something more important to do, conflicting interests compete for attention, the need for urgency in so many things commits us to delay those that appear less pressing.

Inconvenience: time off to be ill may not be desirable especially to those who are indispensable or seek promotion.

Conflicting interests: we all prefer to do those things that we enjoy most.

Unseemly haste: our first impulse to do may be followed by the suggestion that haste is unseemly; that delay will reveal a true state and that which we precipitously applied ourselves to may not need such application.

Self-delusion: ostrich-like we may delude ourselves that what at first appeared to have unpleasant connotations may not occur if we ignore it.

Fear: an elementary response which prefers *status quo* and shrinks from an unknown new experience.

Ignorance: many simply do not appreciate the need for urgency.

We seemingly have adequate excuses for delay, seldom is it premeditated and few of us would accept responsibility for our tardiness. All the causes of delay we have given can be applied to the patient with cancer; I will not elaborate further, but readers may like to consider that these causes for delay can apply also to the general practitioner who first sees the patient, as they do to the hospital consultant.

We must consider now the presenting symptoms. Pain is always a symptom which causes concern and acute pain sends the patient immediately to the doctor, contrary to popular public belief pain is not associated with early cancer and it may be that because symptoms are painless the patient is reassured that it can not be serious. Bleeding is unnatural and leads to uneasiness, suspicion and concern. If it increases in amount the patient invariably seeks advice, often it is intermittent and optimism about its impending cessation will often lead to delay. Superior vena caval obstruction is always worrying, the patient goes to the doctor and is referred for treatment with the minimum of delay. Other symptoms may cause concern, a mass is examined daily for increase in size, a sore to see if healing is taking place, changes in body functions are initially associated with changes in habits, environment, diet and so on until they are proved to be unrelated. So often we are dealing with symptoms which are not progressive, any fluctuation being taken as a sign that is not as important or as ominous as was first thought. Some patients may suspect the diagnosis but imagine that nothing can be done. Wives in particular defer because they do not want to cause worry or even inconvenience to their spouse and family.

Whatever the cause of the delay often we are presented with a patient who has had symptoms for some considerable time and could have come earlier for medical advice.

Symptomatology

There are very few symptoms or clinical signs which can be attributed unequivocably to malignant disease, differing symptoms suggest varying degrees of probability of malignancy. Superior vena caval obstruction is invariably due to malignancy and only occasionally not, some para-malignant syndromes of the skin are almost pathognomonic, and so we can go on. We are concerned here with the symptoms or signs observed by the public; these are too familiar to need elaboration here, but include a mass, a sore that does not heal, unusual bleeding, changes in regular habits, difficulty in swallowing and so on. People are often more concerned with their cars or television sets, for which they will seek expert advice if everything is not perfect, than they are for their general health. We are offered seemingly adequate excuses for failure of health, the time of life, old age, a 'natural thing', diet, habits, and so on, often illustrated by reference to someone they know who has, in their opinion, had similar symptoms. Perhaps the medical profession are to blame by not encouraging discussion, for discouraging questions and for failing to inform.

Early Diagnosis

The difference between a cancer and a benign tumour is the propensity of the former to metastasize. Often the difference between a curable and a hopeless malignancy is whether or not it is localized and can be removed completely or covered by a field of radiation. So spread is all important. Now it is specious to suppose that a tumour starts small and grows uniformly and further to suggest that the larger it is, the greater is its surface area and the greater the chance of lymphatic dissemination or invasion of a blood vessel. It is logical therefore to suggest that the longer a lesion is present, the greater are the chances of dissemination and this, on the whole, is borne out clinically. Therefore, we need to get the patient to come for advice as early as possible and possible ways of doing this are:

1. The development of some test to diagnose cancer in a pre-symptomatic stage – some work is in progress, and we may optimistically hope that this may be possible in the near future. At the moment it is not.
2. To suggest ways of self-examination – here we have the excellent example of self-examination of the breast. Observation and palpation are what the doctor does and the patient can do them herself, routinely and regularly after suitable instruction; but when she finds anything suspicious she should be well aware that something can be done. We must be careful that she does not presume the worst and give up. Thus, instruction in self-examination must stress that early diagnosis is associated with greater chance of cure.

3. Cytology – again this is too well known to demand more than a passing reference. There is no doubt that a cancer of the cervix can be detected at a stage when it is confined to the epidermis and has no opportunity of involving lymphatic or blood vessels; at this stage it can be removed completely. We need to be aware of changing sex habits, new contraceptives have removed the fear of pregnancy, and have encouraged intercourse at an earlier age when any resistance that the mucosa may subsequently develop is not present, they favour promiscuity and there is no longer the barrier present between male and female as in other methods so that exciting causes may be passed from male to female. Bearing this in mind we should suggest smears should start being taken at an earlier age than the 35 years recommended. The enormity of the task of taking regular sputums means that these tests can only be carried out in those at high risk, male, smokers, over forty years with chronic cough. Cytology at other sites is usually used to confirm clinical diagnosis rather than for detection.
4. Well-patient clinics – these would appear to be very desirable, giving an opportunity for some health education, for the measurement of blood pressure, examination of the urine, clinical examination of the breast supplemented by mammography, or thermography, for chest X-ray and for a cervical smear. Such clinics would naturally be expensive but desirable and this would be offset if they detected a proportion of early lesions. They will appeal most to those of a higher intelligence and for the higher social levels who can see the necessity for such examination.

We have discussed methods of early diagnosis; obviously the earlier this comes in the natural history of the disease the better the prognosis but it would be preferable to prevent the process ever starting.

Prevention

When we come to consider prevention we are aware of the many faces of malignancy exemplified by variations in presentation, progress, response to treatment, prognosis and of course, causes. Cancer is not one disease caused by one agent, more correctly it is a generic term implying a group of diseases which have one thing in common, growth and dissemination, and which may result from many exciting causes. Accept this and we are a long way to instructing the general public. Epidemiological surveys and aetiological investigations have given us a considerable amount of information about the causes of cancer and from this we can promote preventative measures.

Briefly the causes may be considered under the following headings:

a. genetic factors;

b. familial, this may be no more than an increased susceptibility to respond to an exciting cause or alternatively a decreased host resistance;
c. chronic irritation;
d. radiation;
e. occupation – industrial chemicals and irritants;
f. diet, including deficiencies and food contaminants;
g. tobacco;
h. drugs, including immunosuppressive agents and hormones;
i. biological agents, including viruses and bacteria; and
j. social habits, including sexual intercourse;

To this list may be added the various interactions of exciting causes such as:

k. alcohol and smoking, working together in cancer of the mouth;
l. smoking and asbestos fibres in cancer of the lung; and
m. host susceptibility and the available carcinogens.

The complexity of the situation has been shown for cancer of the cervix [5]; this is a sexually transmitted disease but the factors which have been incriminated are many: marriage, poverty, intercourse, circumcision, hygiene, infection, contraception, religion, ethnic type, socio-economic status, the most important single factor being age of first intercourse. Now none of these factors are found as sole causes and we can group some of them together where more than one factor may be present, such as:

Adolescent intercourse, which involves early sexual knowledge, promiscuity, early marriage, increased parity, perhaps poor sexual hygiene.

Promiscuity, with the association of broken marriage and remarriage, an increased possibility of meeting a consort with a carcinogen, a greater chance of contracting a venereal disease, and the practice of prostitution.

Economic factors, may result in neglect and ignorance which lead to insecurity and possible early sexual pressures, unstable marriages, inability to buy contraceptives and poor hygiene.

The complexities of such interactions and the combination of aetiological causes shown here can be present in other lesions of the body.

Worldwide variations in the occurrence of certain malignancies may help us to determine some of the causative factors and could help to draw attention to those factors which are known to produce certain malignancies. Such variations include the postcricoid carcinoma seen in Scandinavian women, stomach cancer in rice eaters, naso-pharyngeal tumours in Chinese, the high incidence of breast cancer in the USA and low in Japan, oesophageal and liver cancers in Bantu and so on.

Much work needs to be done on aetiology but we already have much information.

Treatment

The average member of the public has little knowledge of treatment techniques. Surgical removal is accepted, it seems logical, diseased branches of trees are lopped, infected vegetables are removed and so on. The public have taken an interest in surgical procedures and are kept up-to-date by the press and other media. Radiotherapy is very much an unknown field, few have even heard of it, many have a totally wrong idea, the majority confuse radiotherapy, radiodiagnosis, radiography and radiobiology, few, even among doctors, recognize it as a separate medical specialty. A few, who have had personal experience of its use for relatives and friends, view it with foreboding, a kind of 'last ditch' between life and death. Chemotherapy, although not understood, is more acceptable: it is the use of drugs and implies no more than the bottle of medicine of old, brought up-to-date as tablets, capsules, injections – therefore nothing new.

The very fact that treatment has been instituted raises the hopes of cure, the public will accept inconvenience, a certain amount of suffering, convalescence, some complications, provided that cure is in sight.

We may well be reaping the results of the past injudicious use of radiation given in a vague hope to terminal patients, in expectation of miracles, to please a surgeon who requested it, or referred the patient because there was nothing else to be done and he wished to dispose of the patient to be able to refill the bed. Regrettably in the past radical treatment was sometimes given to terminal patients and this did nothing to improve the standing of the specialty. Fortunately we are selecting patients for radical treatment more discriminately now; radioactive isotope investigations enable us to detect occult metastases and we do not submit these patients to local therapy.

After-care

The importance of after-care has not received the publicity that it demands. Follow-up clinics have a definite purpose:

1. For continuing patient care, further treatment may be possible for a recurrence, or excision may still be possible, or palliation may be given in the hopeless case and can often be repeated should symptoms recur.
2. For reassurance of the patient; he builds up an association with the oncology team. He attends regularly to be reassured that his disease is under control, he knows that new symptoms will be investigated, if they represent regrowth they can be dealt

with, that the possibility of recurrence is considered first and excluded before he is referred to another consultant for treatment of another disease.
3. To assess the results of treatment.

An important aspect of after-care is rehabilitation. It is not sufficient merely to achieve immediate control so that the patient goes home or to obtain a statistic – a 1-, 2-, 5-year survivor; we also have a responsibility to return him to normal life. We have insufficient knowledge of what happens to the patient when he returns home. Apart from one brief sentence the problem of the cancer patient was completely ignored in the Report of a Sub-Committee of the Standing Medical Advisory Committee in 1972 [16], probably because the concept of needing to rehabilitate a cancer patient is somewhat novel. It may also be due to the profound pessimism with which most people, doctors included, view the disease, and that the responsibility of rehabilitation of such patients has never been clearly apportioned between surgeon, radiotherapist, rehabilitation officer, rheumatologist and general practitioner.

To protect the person who has had cancer the relatives shield him from worry, do not involve him in family affairs, ask for no contribution to the running of the household, persuade him not to try to go back to work, do not 'chivvy' or persuade as they would with a less serious, more hopeful disease. In time he feels almost neglected, useless. Now the majority of men wish to retain their dignity of working and providing for the family and indeed many of our patients return to an active life, often the same occupation or sometimes a lighter, less exacting occupation. But, they and their families need to know what they can do and how much they should be forced.

After-care also includes provision of prostheses when necessary, and corrective operations, such as skin grafts. Mastectomy patients can be helped considerably by discussion of their operation and provision of a suitable artificial breast, which can be worn with a normal dress brassière and normal clothes, including swimwear. This demands patience and determination on the part of the patient to find out the best prosthesis for her own use. Cottonwool and stuffed silk scarves fail because they have no weight and do not move, they are inanimate; balloons, whilst giving shape, have insufficient weight; fluid-filled are better, having weight, moving with the patient, but may have a wave motion if the fluid is not viscous enough. Small plastic spheres are very acceptable, they have weight, hold on to the chest wall and the whole moves with patient movement very much in the way that the normal breast does. Wigs go far to increase confidence when hair is lost. Colostomy patients need to be prepared well before the operation, although it seems the end of the world at the time it is surprising how quickly they adapt; often their chief concern is that they may smell. They invariably benefit from an early introduction to a patient who already has had the operation. Much can be done to restore the patient's confidence and this is part of 'after-care'.

Support

After leaving hospital the patient and his relatives may need social support. This may include home help, nursing, night watching, bedpans, wheelchairs, laundry, financial support, visits, reading material, and so on; whilst much of this is available on request, not all relatives know how they can get help or what help is available. Moral support may be given by joining a society or club of patients similarly afflicted.

Results of Treatment

The vast majority of the public are totally unaware of what can be done and what survival rates can be achieved. Once informed of the nature of the disease they assume and accept the worst possible prognosis. If cancer is mentioned only when the patient dies it is to be expected that the public think all patients die immediately and there is no cure: 'Everyone I have known with cancer dies quickly', the operative phrase here is 'I have known' – the general public just are not aware that a patient who lives may have had a cancer and have been cured. There is a natural reticence to publish survival rates, even a 90 per cent chance of a cure is not certain, 50 per cent sounds much worse, and so on. It must be remembered that we do not publish survival rates for other diseases such as hepatitis, coronary thrombosis, cirrhosis and so on.

Somehow we have to get it across that cures can occur without mentioning the 'odds' more specifically. Prognostication is always difficult but it is surprising how many patients referred have relatives who have got the impression from a previous clinician that the survival will be so many months, or weeks, definite estimates usually, not 'about', with no explanation of the unreliability of such estimates. The public expect a date to be given, and presumably the future of the patient revolves about that date; if he survives longer the diagnosis is more likely to be considered incorrect than that the treatment was successful.

We must remember that survival rates are based on a mass response and we are not justified in applying them to the individual. Normal life expectancy calculations really are more meaningful; we can say that at a certain point of time after his treatment the patient has an expectation of life equivalent to the normal population of the same age and sex who have not had that malignancy.

Pain and Suffering

The public expect pain and suffering in the cancer patient and are surprised if this is not so, even to the extent of questioning the diagnosis. Pain does occur but with current practices it can be controlled in the vast majority of patients. We sometimes forget the value of radiotherapy, bone pain can often be relieved with one or two treatments without all the sequelae of strong analgesics. Distress may result from bleeding, ulceration, infection, an unsightly mass, nausea, vomiting, indigestion and so on, all of which can be alleviated.

Terminal Care

A new experience always causes concern. What will happen? Will I be able to cope when my time comes? Will my relatives be able to manage? Where can I get help? What about the children? Will it be distressing for them to see me approaching death? All questions which need help; in fact we do not fully know all the problems, real or imagined of the terminal patient and considerable work remains to be done to sort them out. Terminal homes, a name dreaded by many, even doctors, even though we fully realize that we will die some day, have a very definite place. The atmosphere in such a home has to be seen to be believed and they are certainly better places to die in than the overcrowded home or the busy acute ward or some geriatric ward. Many of our patients are unprepared for death and we need to advise much earlier on in the course of the disease.

Conclusion

We have looked through a few of the problems associated with public information and have concluded that current attitudes to malignant diseases are based mainly on a lack of information; this produces uncertainty, suspicion, and fear. We have seen also that the public needs to be informed of what can be done for the established disease, to be encouraged to attend hospital for early diagnosis and detection and that they should be fully aware of those factors which may cause a cancer. There is a great need for simple information and we must now look to ways of providing this.

INFORMATION METHODS

Information may be given in several ways, which may complement each other:

Personal

The doctor is in the unique position of having a direct personal approach of one-to-one and so is able to give information directly to a particular patient on a specific topic. However, this limits the audience he meets, to patients or their relatives and there are obvious limits to how much information may be spread in this way. He will, of course, be joined in this approach by other members of the caring team, nurses, radiographers and so on, but they will need initial instruction from the specialist.

Cancer Information Centres

A few centres in the country exist for the sole purpose of disseminating information to the public about malignant diseases. I have the honour to work with the Tenovus Cancer Information Centre in Cardiff which covers a large area in South Wales. An executive committee has lay members with a particular interest in malignant diseases, health education officers, scientists, family doctors and hospital consultants, some of whom are radiotherapists. The centre has its own education officers who are primarily responsible for meeting the public, distributing information, answering queries, giving lectures and film shows and calling on a group of doctors or scientists to give expert advice if required. This centre has carried out investigations of public opinion about cancer, produces its own literature and posters, distributes other literature and deals with a large number of enquiries each year. Meetings are organized for interested organizations at which a film may be shown or a talk given followed by questions from the audience. A well-stocked film library is available for loan. Not least of the work done is that of answering telephone queries, sending out the appropriate literature to help the enquirer or putting him in contact with someone who will help him, his own family doctor, his doctor at hospital or a helping organization of people with the same complaint. The ambiguity of a telephone often helps patients to ask questions which they are reluctant to ask from those who are treating them but reassurance that the question is not silly may be all that they require and after talking to the Information Centre they are sufficiently confident to go to their own doctor and ask. The service always recommends that the patient asks the doctor who is treating him.

Talks to the public can be quite illuminating, although we may sometimes feel that we are filling a gap in a programme, the interest of the public is rewarding but more important, perhaps, are the somewhat diffident questions asked by an individual when she gets you on to one side. Frequently such questions are pertinent to that individual and may be a plea for help.

Some industries are co-operative and allow time for talks during lunch breaks and schools may be particularly interested even to the extent of setting projects for senior students.

The great advantage of such centres is that they are community orientated and know the requirements of the local people, their attitudes to cancer and local idiosyncrasies.

Publications

Articles in magazines and journals have tremendous potential, especially if they are factual, written in simple, easily understood language and unemotive. Many doctors do not have the right approach to the public and articles may well be better written by professional writers, who are experienced in the public's needs and tastes, working in close co-operation with a doctor. Information about the hospital's radiotherapy service in a local paper can do much to break down the fear of radiotherapy and cancer. There is a natural reluctance by doctors to talk or write about cancer but this only perpetuates the problem and pertinent articles and interesting details may do much to help create a more favourable atmosphere.

Radio and Television

These have a definite place in any information programme, we have virtually a captive audience, many of whom will watch right through. But, here we do have to be particularly careful, we must cater for the majority, remembering that the large proportion of these are watching for entertainment only. More complicated programmes full of technical phrases, the use of specialized medical or scientific jargon and a doctor who is unable to come down to the audience level, probably do more harm than anything else. The audience have their fears about cancer increased and often learn nothing. What is needed are short snappy informative features, lasting 10–20 minutes only, where simple facts can be put across. We have much to learn about presentation from the producers of television programmes. Such programmes do, however, need very close co-operation between doctor and presenter.

We have something to learn from advertising programmes, a simple message can be put over very easily either with 'stills' or with animated diagrams. In this way we could counter tobacco advertising with similar adverts of the dangers, inform the public of potentially dangerous symptoms or signs, encourage them to have cervical smears, and so on. Radio will meet the requirements of a different audience, local radio programmes may do much to bring information to the public in a local community.

The information we give is aimed to be understood by the least intelligent, but it must be augmented for others by a few more erudite programmes and supplemented by a list of books or articles for further reading.

Health Education Programmes

Most Area Health Authorities have viable health education programmes in their area where information usually from the Health Education Council is available. Some carry out definite programmes of public instruction and would welcome the co-operation of a cancer information service or the help of an interested consultant oncologist.

Posters

Posters in appropriate places may be particularly useful, anti-smoking at the place of work or in schools, cervical smears at areas frequented by ladies, in family doctors' waiting rooms, and so on. A somewhat unexplored field, apart from smoking, it could possibly be extended. Posters may be used to publicize the information service.

We must remember that what we say to lay audiences will be interpreted by the individual and by the audience in a way that fits in with the individual's and the group's own thinking. I am reminded of a quotation from a story about that likeable rascal William and his Gang who were being instructed by Cousin Percy who was 'wonderful with boys and always got on well with them' –

> He took them through the wood, and, with the offensive jocularity of one who thinks he is imparting instruction so subtly that the recipient has no idea that he is being instructed – a manner that the Outlaws detested beyond all others – he taught them how to tell the various trees from their shape and twigs though there were no leaves on them. The Outlaws had not the slightest desire to be able to tell the various trees from their shape and twigs though there were no leaves on them. Trees were not divided into oaks and beeches and elms in the Outlaws' eyes. They were divided into trees that could be climbed and trees that could not be climbed; into trees that would do for tents, or trees that would do for ships, or trees that were simply trees and nothing else.
>
> 'The Outlaws and Cousin Percy', in *William's Crowded Hours.*
> Richmal Crompton, 1931.

The information imparted to the public has to be carefully geared to the audience and, if possible, is based on a knowledge of the people making up that audience. The lecturer thus needs to do a little research and enquiry about who will be there before he embarks on the preparation of his talk. The author needs to know who will buy the magazine or journal and to pitch the level accordingly.

Schoolchildren

We have talked mostly of adults who already have preconceived ideas about cancer, built up on erroneous information. It is hard to remove or change these attitudes but children's minds are unfettered in this way. It is just at this time, the formative years, that the child is ready to accept a whole mass of facts, digest them and evaluate them. There is little doubt that to change the public's attitude to cancer, to bring people to earlier diagnosis, and to prevent some cancers we must start with the school child, preferably at the secondary school level.

In Cardiff, the Tenovus Cancer Information Centre, together with the Local Education Authority and the Area Health Authority, have appointed a Schools Health Education Teacher whose responsibility will be to conduct a cancer education project in local schools. Her work will include:

1. An assessment of the level of knowledge and attitudes to cancer among secondary school children.
2. An assessment of the teaching techniques available.
3. To create a school teaching pack for teachers.
4. To establish a method of conducting the teaching of cancer.
5. To assess the value of her work and disseminate the results to interested bodies in education, health and cancer information.

We have been encouraged by the response of the three organizations concerned and of the schools visited.

The Role of the Radiotherapist and Oncologist

No therapist can be satisfied with the results he gets from treating his cancer patients, the majority of our failures are due to dissemination of the disease and so we must turn back to try and get patients to come for diagnosis and treatment at an earlier stage in the natural history of the disease. If possible we should get them before symptoms have developed. But, we can go back even further – we know some of the causes of cancer and removal of these may prevent cancer. There is an obvious need for public information to achieve this.

We are all aware of the public attitudes to cancer based on incomplete knowledge; relevant information given to the public will help to allay their fears, to have cancer accepted as any other disease and not as a scourge, and factual information given in the formative years at school may well produce a new generation who have a more rational approach.

The radiotherapist is in the somewhat unique position of having an interest in all facets of cancer, he is a true oncologist, and thus can play an important role in passing on information. He has a responsibility, indeed a duty, to participate actively in all the aspects of cancer information we have mentioned, keeping up-to-date himself, training future specialists in the same field, assisting in the education of young doctors and scientists and ancillary workers and in giving more simple information to the public.

REFERENCES

1. Bluck M. E. (1975) *Public and Professional Opinion on Preventive Medicine.* Report on a study of knowledge and attitudes among general practitioners and members of the public in areas of South East Wales with special reference to cancer prevention. Cardiff, Tenovus Cancer Information Centre.
2. Briggs J. E. and Wakefield J. (1967) *Public Opinion on Cancer.* A survey of knowledge and attitudes among women in Lancaster, 1966. Manchester, Christie Hospital and Holt Radium Institute.
3. Cancer Council of Western Australia (1966) *A Social Survey of Community Attitudes to Cancer.*
4. Davison R. L. (1965) Opinion of nurses on cancer, its treatment and curability. *Br. J. Prev. and Soc. Med.* **19**, 24–29.
5. Deeley T. J. (1976) Cancer of the cervix uteri – an epidemiological survey. *Clin. Radiol.* **27**, 43–51.
6. Deeley T. J. (1979) *Attitudes to Cancer.* London, SPCK.
7. Hobbs P. (1968) *Public Opinion on Cancer.* A survey of knowledge and attitudes among women in Merseyside. Liverpool, Merseyside Cancer Education Council.
8. Horn D. (1956) *Public Opinion on Cancer and the American Cancer Society.* A report of a National Sample Survey. New York, American Cancer Society Inc.
9. Horn D. and Waincrow S. (1964) What changes are occurring in public opinion towards cancer? A National Public Opinion Survey. *Am. J. Public Health.* **54**, 431–440.
10. Institute for Public Opinion Research (1964) *Question of Health and Illness – Preliminary Results of a Nationwide Survey on Public Knowledge of Cancer.* English Summary. Prague, Czechoslovakian Academy of Science.

11. Paterson R. and Aitken-Swan J. (1954) Public opinion on cancer: a survey among women in the Manchester area. *Lancet* 2, 857–861.
12. Paterson R. and Aitken-Swan J. (1958) Public opinion on cancer: changes following five years of cancer education. *Lancet* 2, 791–793.
13. Phillips A. J. (1955) Public opinion on cancer in Canada. *Can. Med. J.* 73, 639–647.
14. Phillips A. J. (1968) *Knowledge of Cancer among Canadian men.* Public opinion about Current Cancer Programmes and Surveys. Geneva, International Union Against Cancer.
15. Phillips A. J. and Taylor R. M. (1961) Public opinion on cancer in Canada, a second survey. *Can. Med. J.* 84, 142–147.
16. Report of a Sub-Committee of the Standing Medical Advisory Committee (1982). *Rehabilitation.* London, HMSO.
17. Seeber A. B. de S. (1964) *Public Opinion on Cancer in Argentine.* Bulletin 2. Geneva, International Union Against Cancer.
18. Sherman C. D. and Williams O. M. (1970) A Survey of the Attitudes of Second, Third and Fourth Year Medical Students towards the 'Curability' of Breast Cancer. *CA* 20, 365.
19. Williams E. M., Cruikshank A. and Walker W. M. (1972) *Public Opinion on Cancer in South East Wales.* Cardiff, Tenovus Cancer Information Centre.

Index